THE TOP
100 DRUGS

CLINICAL PHARMACOLOGY
AND PRACTICAL PRESCRIBING

Dedication and acknowledgement

Dedication

This book is dedicated to our families, without whose support and patience we would not have been able to write it.

Acknowledgement

Many students at St George's, University of London contributed to the development of this book. We wish to express our gratitude to them all, but particularly to those who participated in the projects that generated the original 'Top 100 Drugs' list, and to the members of a focus group convened to ensure the book would meet their needs. We also thank Dr Selma Audi and, from the University of Birmingham, Dr Sarah Pontefract and Professor Jamie Coleman for their contributions to the analysis that underpinned the second edition. This third edition is again informed by an updated analysis of prescribing frequencies. For their assistance in providing inpatient electronic prescribing data, we would like to thank the Clinical Informatics team at St George's University Hospitals NHS Foundation Trust, in particular Samir Rumjaun and Dr Matthew Laundy.

THIRD EDITION

THE TOP 100 DRUGS

CLINICAL PHARMACOLOGY AND PRACTICAL PRESCRIBING

Andrew Hitchings BSc(Hons) MBBS PhD FRCP FHEA FFICM FBPhS
Reader in Clinical Pharmacology, St George's, University of London;
Honorary Consultant in Neurointensive Care, St George's University Hospitals NHS
Foundation Trust, London, UK

Dagan Lonsdale BSc(Hons) MBBS PhD MRCP FHEA FFICM
Senior Lecturer in Clinical Pharmacology, St George's, University of London;
Honorary Consultant Intensivist, St George's University Hospitals NHS Foundation
Trust, London, UK

Daniel Burrage BSc(Hons) MBBS MSc (Med Ed) PhD MRCP FHEA
Honorary Senior Lecturer, St George's, University of London;
Consultant in Clinical Pharmacology and Acute Medicine, St George's University
Hospitals NHS Foundation Trust, London, UK

Emma Baker MBChB PhD FRCP FBPhS
Professor of Clinical Pharmacology, St George's, University of London;
Honorary Consultant Physician, St George's University Hospitals NHS Foundation
Trust, London, UK

ELSEVIER

First edition 2015
Second edition 2019

The right of Andrew Hitchings, Dagan Lonsdale, Daniel Burrage and Emma Baker to be identified as authors of this work has been asserted by them in accordance with the Copyright, Designs and Patents Act 1988.

Notices

Practitioners and researchers must always rely on their own experience and knowledge in evaluating and using any information, methods, compounds or experiments described herein. Because of rapid advances in the medical sciences, in particular, independent verification of diagnoses and drug dosages should be made. To the fullest extent of the law, no responsibility is assumed by Elsevier, authors, editors or contributors for any injury and/or damage to persons or property as a matter of products liability, negligence or otherwise, or from any use or operation of any methods, products, instructions, or ideas contained in the material herein.

ISBN: 978-0-323-83445-2

Content Strategist: Alexandra Mortimer
Content Project Manager: Taranpreet Kaur
Design: Miles Hitchen
Marketing Manager: Deborah Watkins

Printed in Scotland

Last digit is the print number: 9 8 7 6 5 4 3 2 1

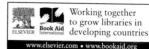

Working together
to grow libraries in
developing countries

www.elsevier.com • www.bookaid.org

Contents

List of abbreviations

5-ASA	5-aminosalicylic acid
5-HT	5-hydroxytryptamine (serotonin)
ACE	Angiotensin-converting enzyme
ACS	Acute coronary syndrome
ACTH	Adrenocorticotropic hormone
ADH	Antidiuretic hormone
ADP	Adenosine diphosphate
AE	Adverse effect
AF	Atrial fibrillation
ALS	Advanced Life Support
ALT	Alanine aminotransferase/transaminase
AMP	Adenosine monophosphate
AMPA	α-amino-3-hydroxy-5-methyl-4-isoxazoleproprionic acid
APTR	Activated partial thromboplastin time ratio
APTT	Activated partial thromboplastin time
ARB	Angiotensin receptor blocker
AT_1	Angiotensin type 1 (receptor)
ATP	Adenosine triphosphate
ATPase	Adenosine triphosphatase
AV	Atrioventricular
BCG	Bacillus Calmette–Guérin
BMI	Body mass index
BNF	British National Formulary
BP	Blood pressure
Ca^{2+}	Calcium ion
cGMP	Cyclic guanosine monophosphate
CGRP	Calcitonin gene-related peptide
CHC	Combined hormonal contraception
CKD	Chronic kidney disease
Cl^-	Chloride ion
CNS	Central nervous system
CO	Carbon monoxide
CO_2	Carbon dioxide
COC	Combined oral contraceptive
COPD	Chronic obstructive pulmonary disease
COX	Cyclooxygenase
CPR	Cardiopulmonary resuscitation
CQC	Care Quality Commission
CRH	Corticotropin-releasing hormone
CRP	C-reactive protein
CT	Computerised tomography
CTZ	Chemoreceptor trigger zone
CV	Cardiovascular
CVS	Cardiovascular system
CYP	Cytochrome P450
CysLT1	Cysteinyl leukotriene receptor 1
DEXA	Dual-energy X-ray absorptiometry
DMARD	Disease-modifying antirheumatic drug
DNA	Deoxyribonucleic acid
DOAC	Direct oral anticoagulant
DPP-4	Dipeptidylpeptidase-4
DVT	Deep vein thrombosis
ECF	Extracellular fluid
ECG	Electrocardiogram
eGFR	Estimated glomerular filtration rate
ENaC	Epithelial sodium channels
ER	Estrogen (oestrogen) receptor
FBC	Full blood count
FDC	Fixed-dose combination
FH4	Tetrahydrofolate
FSH	Follicle-stimulating hormone
FSRH	Faculty of Sexual and Reproductive Healthcare
G	Gauge
g	Gram

G6PD	Glucose-6-phosphate dehydrogenase	L	Litre
GABA	γ-aminobutyric acid	LABA	Long-acting β_2-agonist
GCS	Glasgow Coma Scale	LAMA	Long-acting antimuscarinic
G-CSF	Granulocyte colony-stimulating factor	LDL	Low-density lipoprotein
		L-dopa	Levodopa
GFR	Glomerular filtration rate	LH	Luteinising hormone
GI	Gastrointestinal	LMWH	Low molecular weight heparin
GIP	Glucose-dependent insulinotropic peptide	LRTI	Lower respiratory tract infection
GLP-1	Glucagon-like peptide-1	m	Metre
GMP	Guanosine monophosphate	mAb	Monoclonal antibody
GORD	Gastro-oesophageal reflux disease	MDI	Metered dose inhaler
		mg	Milligram
GP	General practitioner	MHRA	Medicines and Healthcare Products Regulatory Agency
GTN	Glyceryl trinitrate		
GU	Genitourinary	min	Minute
H^+	Hydrogen ion	mL	Millilitre
HAS	Human albumin solution	mmHg	Millimetres of mercury
HbA_{1c}	Haemoglobin A_{1c} (glycated haemoglobin)	mmol	Millimole
		MR	Modified release
HER2	Human epidermal growth factor receptor 2	MRSA	Meticillin-resistant *Staphylococcus aureus*
HIT	Heparin-induced thrombocytopenia	MSK	Musculoskeletal
		Na^+	Sodium ion
HIV	Human immunodeficiency virus	NAPQI	N-acetyl-p-benzoquinone imine
HMG CoA	3-hydroxy-3-methyl-glutaryl coenzyme A	NHS	National Health Service
		NICE	National Institute for Health and Care Excellence
hr	Hour		
hrly	Hourly	NMS	Neuroleptic malignant syndrome
HRT	Hormone replacement therapy		
		NO	Nitric oxide
HUS	Haemolytic–uraemic syndrome	NPH	Neutral protamine Hagedorn
		NRT	Nicotine replacement therapy
IBS	Irritable bowel syndrome		
ICS	Inhaled corticosteroid	NSAID	Non-steroidal antiinflammatory drug
Ig	Immunoglobulin		
IL	Interleukin	OPAT	Outpatient parenteral antimicrobial therapy
IM	Intramuscular		
INR	International normalised ratio	p	Pence
		PaO_2	Partial pressure of oxygen in arterial blood
ISMN	Isosorbide mononitrate		
IV	Intravenous	P_AO_2	Partial pressure of oxygen in alveolar gas
K^+	Potassium ion		
kg	Kilogram		

PCR	Polymerase chain reaction	SSRI	Selective serotonin reuptake inhibitor
PD	Pharmacodynamic		
PDE	Phosphodiesterase	SV2A	Synaptic vesicle protein 2A
PE	Pulmonary embolism	SVT	Supraventricular tachycardia
PGE$_2$	Prostaglandin E$_2$		
PK	Pharmacokinetic	T$_3$	Triiodothyronine
PO$_2$	Partial pressure of oxygen	T$_4$	Thyroxine
POP	Progesterone-only pill	TIA	Transient ischaemic attack
PPI	Proton pump inhibitor		
RNA	Ribonucleic acid	TNF	Tumour necrosis factor
SA	Sinoatrial	TPMT	Thiopurine methyltransferase
SC	Subcutaneous		
sec	Second	TSH	Thyroid-stimulating hormone
SERM	Selective estrogen (oestrogen) receptor modulator		
		UC	Ulcerative colitis
		UFH	Unfractionated heparin
SGLT-2	Sodium–glucose co-transporter 2	UK	United Kingdom
		UTI	Urinary tract infection
SIADH	Syndrome of inappropriate antidiuretic hormone	VF	Ventricular fibrillation
		VRE	Vancomycin-resistant enterococcus
SL	Sublingual		
SNRI	Serotonin and noradrenaline reuptake inhibitor	VT	Ventricular tachycardia
		VTE	Venous thromboembolism
SpO$_2$	Saturation of oxygen by pulse oximetry	WCC	White cell count
		WHO	World Health Organization

ix

Introduction

Why should you use this book?

Learning pharmacology is hard. Over 2000 drugs are available in the UK, and the amount of information you could obtain for each one is almost limitless. Conventional pharmacology textbooks and online resources cover the science of these drugs in detail—often more than you need—but generally neglect the crucial practical aspects of prescribing. Conversely, protocols and formularies used by more experienced prescribers may seem impenetrable and provide insufficient detail on the clinical pharmacology that underpins the use and understanding of drugs.

Against this backdrop, you need a place to start. You need to focus most of your attention on the most important information about the most important drugs. You need a bridge between a student's textbook and a prescriber's formulary, in which scientific and practical aspects receive equal attention. Fundamentally, you need to know what you need to know about the drugs you are going to prescribe in practice. That is what this book seeks to provide.

What are 'the top 100 drugs'?

For this third edition, we have fully updated our analysis[1] to identify which drugs are prescribed most often in hospital and community settings. We analysed data from over 1 billion community prescriptions,[2] and nearly 900,000 inpatient prescriptions, over a 1-year period that straddled 'pre-pandemic' and 'pandemic' periods. In a change to our previous methodology, we identified the top 100 drugs entirely from their prescribing frequencies. These drugs account for over 95% of all prescriptions in both settings of care. The small number of 'emergency drugs' that do not make it into the top 100, but which are still important to know about, are now covered in a dedicated section, as are intravenous (IV) fluids. Demonstrating the continued stability of the list despite the shock to the healthcare system from the COVID-19 pandemic, 88 drugs from the previous analysis retain their places. New entrants include drugs that have increased in use progressively over several years (e.g. sodium–glucose co-transporter 2 inhibitors) or more abruptly due to the pandemic (e.g. antiviral drugs, monoclonal antibodies).

How to use this book

Organisation of the book

The top 100 drugs are arranged in alphabetical order. We have generally identified them by the name of the class to which they belong: thus 'bisoprolol' is found under 'β-blockers'. As necessary, we have applied our judgement on how to group drugs for practical and learning purposes, even if this does not correspond to a conventional pharmacological class. We have listed common examples in order of the frequency with which they are used, with less common but still important drugs added where appropriate. Where a drug is effectively in a class of its own, we have identified it simply by its name: thus we use 'metformin' rather than 'biguanides'. In addition to the top 100 drugs, we have provided details of important emergency drugs and commonly used IV fluid preparations in their own sections.

To help you test and reinforce your knowledge, we have included self-assessment questions. The answers to these direct you to the relevant drug entries as appropriate. They also provide an opportunity to bring together information from several drugs and show how it may be integrated in practice.

Using the book

We anticipate this book being used in two main ways. One is as a 'quick reference source' for when you encounter a drug on the ward or in clinic and want to read up on it quickly. The alphabetical arrangement aims to facilitate this. The other way you might use it is when learning about an area of clinical practice or a particular disease and want core information about the relevant drugs. To support this way of working, we have provided two additional tables of contents: one listing the drugs relevant to each specialty area, and the other listing drugs used in specific indications.

In your early years of study, you will probably concentrate on learning clinical pharmacology. As you progress, you will increasingly need to supplement this with knowledge and skills in practical prescribing. Reflecting this, we have arranged the information under these two main headings in a consistent way throughout the book. We have further divided the information with standard subheadings, the purpose of which is outlined in Table 1.1. We use bold text and icons to draw out key points, as indicated in Box 1.1. When cross-referencing other drugs that are discussed elsewhere in the book, we indicate this using **coloured text**.

Using the information

We provide information that we hope will inform your understanding of drugs and their practical use, but this is not a prescribing formulary. This is particularly important in relation to cautions and contraindications (which we refer to collectively as 'Warnings'). To reproduce all the points that might need to be considered in practice would be overwhelming and defeat the point of the book. Likewise, for drug doses, we will often provide a 'typical starting dose' (for adults unless otherwise specified) because we think it's useful for you to have an idea of the kind of doses you will see used in practice. However, it is not our intention that when writing real prescriptions you will look up doses in this book. The key point is this: this book is for *learning*. When you are *making decisions* in practice, you will need also to consult formularies (in the UK, the *British National Formulary* (BNF)), protocols, policies, and guidance, as appropriate to the clinical context. You can practise this now—the knowledge you will acquire from this book will make the prescribing reference sources more useful and accessible.

Where next?

This book provides, in our judgement, the most important information that you need to know about drugs to pass your examinations and become a safe and effective prescriber. However, in providing you with this 'starting point', it is not our intention to stifle your inquisitiveness. We would actively encourage you to learn more, both about the drugs in this book and others that are less commonly used. We just know, from years of experience teaching prescribers and students, that when confronted with such an overwhelming number of drugs, and all the things you could possibly know about them, it is sometimes difficult to see the wood for the trees.

TABLE 1.1 Anatomy of the 'drug' pages

Drug class (or drug name, if it is in a class of its own)

CLINICAL PHARMACOLOGY

Common indications	A list of the **situations in which the drug is commonly used**, along with a brief discussion of its **place in therapy;** in other words, where it fits in alongside other treatment options.
Spectrum of activity (antibiotics only)	For antibiotics only, a brief description of the spectrum of their antibacterial activity.
Mechanisms of action	A brief discussion of how the drug works in the indications specified.
Important adverse effects	The most common and important adverse effects of the drug, with a discussion of their mechanism where this aids understanding.
Warnings	The situations in which the drug should be avoided (i.e. is **contraindicated**) or where extra **caution** should be used.
Important interactions	The most important interactions with other drugs.

Common examples

PRACTICAL PRESCRIBING

Prescription	A discussion of how the drug is usually prescribed, including, as appropriate, typical starting dosage and route of administration. All dosages are for adults unless otherwise specified.
Administration	A discussion of any important considerations about how the drug should be administered, beyond those already covered by the prescription.
Communication	A brief discussion of the important information that should be conveyed to the person, written in non-technical language.
Monitoring and stopping	Details about how the efficacy safety of the drug should be monitored, and the considerations around when it should be stopped.
Cost	A brief mention of cost, particularly to highlight where savings can be made without affecting treatment efficacy.

Clinical tip—an interesting or useful fact or tip about the drug, generally derived from clinical experience.

Box 1.1 Text features used throughout the book

Bold text is used to highlight key points for quick identification.

Coloured text is used to identify drugs that are covered elsewhere in the **Top 100 drugs, Emergency drugs** or **Intravenous fluids** sections.

A ▲ **red triangle** is used to identify important circumstances such as co-morbidities (cautions) or concurrent medications (interactions) in which use of the drug is risky. Although the drug may occasionally be used in these situations, this would be appropriate only after careful risk–benefit assessment and some extra safety measures, such as lower dosage and more intensive monitoring. As a novice prescriber, you would generally be expected to seek senior or specialist guidance in these situations.

A ✖ **red cross** is used to identify circumstances (contraindications or interactions) in which use of the drug is generally regarded to be dangerous and inappropriate.

References

1. Audi S et al. The 'top 100' drugs and classes in England: an updated 'starter formulary' for trainee prescribers. British Journal of Clinical Pharmacology 2018;84(11):2562-2571.
2. NHS Business Services Authority. Prescription Cost Analysis (PCA) data (2021). Available online: https://www.nhsbsa.nhs.uk/prescription-data/dispensing-data/prescription-cost-analysis-pca-data.

Drugs listed by specialty area

Specialty	Drugs
Cardiovascular medicine	Adenosine
	Adrenaline (epinephrine)
	Aldosterone antagonists
	α-blockers
	Amiodarone
	Angiotensin receptor blockers
	Angiotensin-converting enzyme (ACE) inhibitors
	Antimuscarinics, cardiovascular, and gastrointestinal uses
	Antiplatelet drugs, ADP-receptor antagonists
	Antiplatelet drugs, aspirin
	β-blockers
	Calcium channel blockers
	Colloids (plasma substitutes)
	Compound sodium lactate
	Digoxin
	Direct oral anticoagulants
	Diuretics, loop
	Diuretics, thiazide, and thiazide-like
	Fibrinolytic drugs
	Heparins and fondaparinux
	Nitrates
	Opioids
	Prostaglandins and analogues
	Sodium chloride
	Sodium–glucose co-transporter 2 inhibitors
	Statins
	Warfarin
Critical care, peri-operative medicine, and pain	Adenosine
	Adrenaline (epinephrine)
	Anaesthetics, general
	Anaesthetics, local
	Antidepressants, tricyclics, and related drugs
	Antiemetics, dopamine D_2-receptor antagonists
	Antiemetics, histamine H_1-receptor antagonists
	Antiemetics, serotonin 5-HT_3-receptor antagonists
	Benzodiazepines
	Carbamazepine
	Colloids (plasma substitutes)
	Compound sodium lactate
	Fibrinolytic drugs
	Gabapentinoids
	Glucose (dextrose)

Naloxone
Non-steroidal antiinflammatory drugs and COX-2 inhibitors
Opioids
Oxygen
Paracetamol
Potassium, intravenous
Red cells
Serotonin 5-HT$_1$-receptor agonists (triptans)
Sodium chloride
Valproate (valproic acid)

Dermatology, ophthalmology, and otolaryngology

Antihistamines (H$_1$-receptor antagonists)
Clindamycin
Corticosteroids, topical
Emollients
Methotrexate
Ocular lubricants (artificial tears)
Prostaglandin analogue and carbonic anhydrase inhibitor eye drops
Tetracyclines and glycylcyclines
Tranexamic acid

Endocrinology and metabolic medicine

Aldosterone antagonists
Angiotensin receptor blockers
Angiotensin-converting enzyme (ACE) inhibitors
Antidepressants, tetracyclic, and serotonin-noradrenaline reuptake inhibitors
β-blockers
Calcium and vitamin D
Corticosteroids, systemic
Dipeptidylpeptidase-4 inhibitors
Glucose (dextrose)
Insulin
Iron
Metformin
Potassium, oral
Sodium–glucose co-transporter 2 inhibitors
Statins
Sulfonylureas
Thyroid hormones
Vitamins

Gastroenterology and hepatology

Aldosterone antagonists
Alginates and antacids

Aminosalicylates
Antidepressants, tricyclics, and related drugs
Antiemetics, dopamine D_2-receptor antagonists
Antiemetics, histamine H_1-receptor antagonists
Antiemetics, serotonin 5-HT_3-receptor antagonists
Antimuscarinics, cardiovascular, and gastrointestinal uses
Antiviral drugs, other
Colloids (plasma substitutes)
Corticosteroids, systemic
Glycopeptide antibiotics
H_2-receptor antagonists
Laxatives, oral
Laxatives, rectal
Methotrexate
Proton pump inhibitors
Vitamins

Haematology and immunology

Antihistamines (H_1-receptor antagonists)
Antiplatelet drugs, ADP-receptor antagonists
Antiplatelet drugs, aspirin
Antiviral drugs, other
Corticosteroids, systemic
Direct oral anticoagulants
Fibrinolytic drugs
Heparins and fondaparinux
Iron
Leukotriene receptor antagonists
Monoclonal antibodies
Red cells
Vaccines and immunoglobulins
Vitamins
Warfarin

Infectious diseases

Aminoglycosides
Antifungal drugs
Antiviral drugs, aciclovir
Antiviral drugs, other
Cephalosporins and carbapenems
Chloramphenicol
Clindamycin
Corticosteroids, systemic
Glycopeptide antibiotics
Macrolides
Metronidazole
Monoclonal antibodies

Nitrofurantoin
Penicillins, antipseudomonal
Penicillins, broad-spectrum
Penicillins, narrow-spectrum
Quinine
Quinolones
Tetracyclines and glycylcyclines
Trimethoprim
Vaccines and immunoglobulins

Neurology and psychiatry

Acetylcholinesterase inhibitors
Antidepressants, selective serotonin reuptake inhibitors
Antidepressants, tetracyclic and serotonin-noradrenaline reuptake inhibitors
Antidepressants, tricyclics, and related drugs
Antiemetics, histamine H_1-receptor antagonists
Antiplatelet drugs, ADP-receptor antagonists
Antiplatelet drugs, aspirin
Antipsychotics, first-generation (typical)
Antipsychotics, second-generation (atypical)
Benzodiazepines
β-blockers
Carbamazepine
Dopaminergic drugs for Parkinson's disease
Fibrinolytic drugs
Gabapentinoids
Lamotrigine
Levetiracetam and brivaracetam
Monoclonal antibodies
Naloxone
Quinine
Serotonin $5-HT_1$-receptor agonists (triptans)
Vaccines and immunoglobulins
Valproate (valproic acid)
Vitamins
Z-drugs

Obstetrics and gynaecology

Oestrogens and progestogens
Prostaglandins and analogues
Tranexamic acid
Uterotonics
Vitamins

Oncology and palliative care

Allopurinol
Antiemetics, dopamine D_2-receptor antagonists

Antiemetics, histamine H_1-receptor antagonists
Antiemetics, serotonin 5-HT_3-receptor antagonists
Antimuscarinics, cardiovascular, and gastrointestinal uses
Antipsychotics, first-generation (typical)
Benzodiazepines
Bisphosphonates
Corticosteroids, systemic
Hormone antagonists and agonists used in breast and prostate cancer
Methotrexate
Monoclonal antibodies
Opioids
Paracetamol

Renal medicine and urology

5α reductase inhibitors
α-blockers
Angiotensin receptor blockers
Angiotensin-converting enzyme (ACE) inhibitors
Antimuscarinics, genitourinary uses
Calcium and vitamin D
Compound sodium lactate
Diuretics, loop
Diuretics, thiazide, and thiazide-like
Glucose (dextrose)
Phosphodiesterase (type 5) inhibitors
Potassium, intravenous
Prostaglandins and analogues
Sodium chloride
Sodium–glucose co-transporter 2 inhibitors

Respiratory medicine

Acetylcysteine and carbocisteine
Adrenaline (epinephrine)
Antimuscarinics, bronchodilators
β_2-agonists
Corticosteroids, inhaled
Corticosteroids, nasal
Corticosteroids, systemic
Heparins and fondaparinux
Leukotriene receptor antagonists
Monoclonal antibodies
Oxygen

Rheumatology

Allopurinol
Aminosalicylates
Bisphosphonates

Calcium and vitamin D
Corticosteroids, systemic
Methotrexate
Non-steroidal antiinflammatory drugs and COX-2 inhibitors
Opioids
Paracetamol

Toxicology

Acetylcysteine and carbocisteine
Benzodiazepines
Naloxone
Oxygen
Vitamins

Drugs listed by indication

Indication	Drugs
Acne vulgaris	Clindamycin
	Oestrogens and progestogens
	Tetracyclines and glycylcyclines
	Trimethoprim
Acute coronary syndrome	Antiplatelet drugs, ADP-receptor antagonists
	Antiplatelet drugs, aspirin
	β-blockers
	Fibrinolytic drugs
	Heparins and fondaparinux
	Nitrates
	Statins
Adrenal insufficiency	Corticosteroids, systemic
Alcohol withdrawal reactions	Benzodiazepines
	Vitamins (thiamine)
Allergic rhinitis	Antihistamines (H_1-receptor antagonists)
	Corticosteroids, nasal
	Leukotriene receptor antagonists
Alzheimer's disease	Acetylcholinesterase inhibitors
Anaemia	Iron
	Red cells
	Vitamins
Anaesthesia	Adrenaline (epinephrine)
	Anaesthetics, general
	Anaesthetics, local
	Benzodiazepines
Anaphylaxis	Adrenaline (epinephrine)
	Antihistamines (H_1-receptor antagonists)
	Corticosteroids, systemic
Androgenetic alopecia	5α reductase inhibitors
Anxiety	Antidepressants, tetracyclic, and serotonin-noradrenaline reuptake inhibitors
	Benzodiazepines
	Gabapentinoids

Arrhythmias

Adenosine
Amiodarone
Antimuscarinics, cardiovascular, and gastrointestinal uses
β-blockers
Calcium channel blockers
Digoxin

Ascites

Aldosterone antagonists
Diuretics, loop

Asthma

Antimuscarinics, bronchodilators
β_2-agonists
Corticosteroids, inhaled
Corticosteroids, systemic
Leukotriene receptor antagonists
Monoclonal antibodies

Atrial fibrillation

Amiodarone
β-blockers
Digoxin
Direct oral anticoagulants
Warfarin

Atrial flutter

Amiodarone

Bacterial conjunctivitis

Chloramphenicol

Bacterial vaginosis

Clindamycin
Metronidazole

Benign prostatic enlargement

5α reductase inhibitors
α-blockers

Bipolar disorder

Antipsychotics, first-generation (typical)
Antipsychotics, second-generation (atypical)
Lamotrigine
Valproate (valproic acid)

Bone and joint infection

Clindamycin
Glycopeptide antibiotics
Penicillins, broad-spectrum
Penicillins, narrow-spectrum

Bowel preparation	Laxatives, oral Laxatives, rectal
Bradycardia	Antimuscarinics, cardiovascular, and gastrointestinal uses
Cancer	Bisphosphonates Corticosteroids, systemic Hormone antagonists and agonists used in breast and prostate cancer Methotrexate Monoclonal antibodies
Carbon monoxide poisoning	Oxygen
Cardiac arrest	Adrenaline (epinephrine) Amiodarone
Chronic kidney disease	Angiotensin receptor blockers Angiotensin-converting enzyme (ACE) inhibitors Calcium and vitamin D Sodium–glucose co-transporter 2 inhibitors
Chronic obstructive pulmonary disease	Antimuscarinics, bronchodilators β_2-agonists Corticosteroids, inhaled Macrolides Vaccines
Cirrhotic liver disease	Colloids (plasma substitutes) Aldosterone antagonists Laxatives, oral Laxatives, rectal
***Clostridioides difficile* colitis**	Glycopeptide antibiotics Metronidazole
Conjunctivitis	Chloramphenicol
Constipation	Laxatives, oral Laxatives, rectal
Contraception	Oestrogens and progestogens

COVID-19

Antiviral drugs, other
Corticosteroids, systemic
Monoclonal antibodies
Vaccines and immunoglobulins

Croup

Adrenaline (epinephrine)
Corticosteroids, systemic

Deep vein thrombosis

Direct oral anticoagulants
Heparins and fondaparinux
Warfarin

Dementia

Acetylcholinesterase inhibitors

Dementia in Parkinson's disease

Acetylcholinesterase inhibitors

Dental infection

Metronidazole

Depression

Antidepressants, selective serotonin reuptake inhibitors
Antidepressants, tetracyclic, and serotonin-noradrenaline reuptake inhibitors
Antidepressants, tricyclics and related drugs

Diabetic ketoacidosis

Insulin

Diabetic nephropathy

Angiotensin receptor blockers
Angiotensin-converting enzyme (ACE) inhibitors
Sodium–glucose co-transporter 2 inhibitors

Diabetic neuropathy

Antidepressants, tetracyclic, and serotonin-noradrenaline reuptake inhibitors
Gabapentinoids

Dry eyes

Acetylcysteine
Ocular lubricants (artificial tears)

Dry skin

Emollients

Dyslipidaemia

Monoclonal antibodies
Statins

Dyspepsia	Alginates and antacids
	H_2-receptor antagonists
	Proton pump inhibitors
Eczema	Corticosteroids, topical
	Emollients
	Monoclonal antibodies
Endocarditis	Aminoglycosides
	Glycopeptide antibiotics
	Penicillins, narrow-spectrum
Epiglottitis	Cephalosporins and carbapenems
	Chloramphenicol
Epilepsy	Benzodiazepines
	Carbamazepine
	Gabapentinoids
	Lamotrigine
	Levetiracetam and brivaracetam
	Valproate (valproic acid)
Epistaxis	Tranexamic acid
Erectile dysfunction	Phosphodiesterase (type 5) inhibitors
	Prostaglandins and analogues
Faecal impaction	Laxatives, rectal
Fever	Antiplatelet drugs, aspirin
	Non-steroidal antiinflammatory drugs and COX-2 inhibitors
	Paracetamol
Fungal infections	Antifungal drugs
Gastro-oesophageal reflux disease	Alginates and antacids
	H_2-receptor antagonists
	Proton pump inhibitors
Gastroenteritis (severe)	Quinolones
Glaucoma	Prostaglandin analogue and carbonic anhydrase inhibitor eye drops

Gout	Allopurinol
	Non-steroidal antiinflammatory drugs and COX-2 inhibitors
Guillain–Barré syndrome	Vaccines and immunoglobulins
Haemorrhage	Adrenaline (epinephrine)
	Red cells
	Tranexamic acid
Haemophilia A	Monoclonal antibodies
Heart failure	Aldosterone antagonists
	Angiotensin receptor blockers
	Angiotensin-converting enzyme (ACE) inhibitors
	β-blockers
	Digoxin
	Diuretics, loop
	Sodium–glucose co-transporter 2 inhibitors
***Helicobacter pylori* infection**	Macrolides
	Metronidazole
	Penicillins, broad-spectrum
	Proton pump inhibitors
Hepatic encephalopathy	Laxatives, oral
	Laxatives, rectal
Hepatitis virus B or C infection	Antiviral drugs, other
	Vaccines
Herpesvirus infection	Antiviral drugs, aciclovir
HIV infection	Antiviral drugs, other
	Trimethoprim (co-trimoxazole)
Hormone replacement therapy	Oestrogens and progestogens
Hypercalcaemia	Bisphosphonates
	Diuretics, loop
	Sodium chloride

Hyperosmolar hyperglycaemic state	Insulin Potassium chloride Sodium chloride
Hyperkalaemia	β₂ agonists Glucose (dextrose) Calcium and vitamin D Insulin
Hypertension	α-blockers Angiotensin receptor blockers Angiotensin-converting enzyme (ACE) inhibitors β-blockers Calcium channel blockers Diuretics, thiazide, and thiazide-like Nitrates
Hyperuricaemia	Allopurinol
Hypocalcaemia	Calcium and vitamin D
Hypoglycaemia	Glucose (dextrose)
Hypokalaemia	Potassium, intravenous Potassium, oral
Hypopituitarism	Corticosteroids, systemic Thyroid hormones
Hypothyroidism	Thyroid hormones
Hypoxaemia	Oxygen
Immunisation	Vaccines and immunoglobulins
Induction of labour	Prostaglandins and analogues Uterotonics
Infective exacerbation of COPD	Corticosteroids, systemic Macrolides Penicillins, broad-spectrum Quinolones Tetracyclines and glycylcyclines

Inflammatory arthritis

Aminosalicylates
Corticosteroids, systemic
Methotrexate
Monoclonal antibodies
Non-steroidal antiinflammatory drugs and
COX-2 inhibitors

Inflammatory bowel disease

Aminosalicylates
Corticosteroids, systemic
Methotrexate
Monoclonal antibodies

Influenza

Antiviral drugs, other
Vaccines

Insomnia

Benzodiazepines
Z-drugs

Intraabdominal infection

Aminoglycosides
Clindamycin
Metronidazole
Penicillins, antipseudomonal
Penicillins, broad-spectrum
Tetracyclines and glycylcyclines

Irritable bowel syndrome

Antimuscarinics, cardiovascular, and gastrointestinal uses
Antidepressants, tricyclics and related drugs

Ischaemic heart disease

Angiotensin receptor blockers
Angiotensin-converting enzyme (ACE) inhibitors
Antiplatelet drugs, ADP-receptor antagonists
Antiplatelet drugs, aspirin
β-blockers
Calcium channel blockers
Heparins and fondaparinux
Nitrates
Statins

Leg cramps

Quinine

Lower urinary tract symptoms

5α reductase inhibitors
α-blockers

Lyme disease	Tetracyclines and glycylcyclines
Malaria	Clindamycin Quinine Tetracyclines and glycylcyclines
Mechanical heart valves	Warfarin
Medical termination of pregnancy	Prostaglandins and analogues
Megaloblastic anaemia	Vitamins
Meningitis	Cephalosporins and carbapenems Corticosteroids, systemic Penicillins, narrow-spectrum
Menopause	Oestrogens and progestogens
Menorrhagia	Iron Tranexamic acid
Migraine	Antidepressants, tricyclics and related drugs β-blockers Monoclonal antibodies Serotonin 5-HT$_1$-receptor agonists (triptans) Valproate (valproic acid)
Motion sickness	Antiemetics, histamine HT$_1$-receptor antagonists
Mucolytics	Acetylcysteine and carbocisteine
Myeloma	Bisphosphonates Corticosteroids, systemic
Nasal polyps	Corticosteroids, nasal Monoclonal antibodies
Nausea and vomiting	Antiemetics, dopamine D$_2$-receptor antagonists Antiemetics, histamine H$_1$-receptor antagonists Antiemetics, serotonin 5-HT$_3$-receptor antagonists Antihistamines (H$_1$-receptor antagonists) Antipsychotics, first-generation (typical)

Neuropathic pain	Antidepressants, tetracyclic, and serotonin-noradrenaline reuptake inhibitors
	Antidepressants, tricyclics and related drugs
	Carbamazepine
	Gabapentinoids
Obsessive compulsive disorder	Antidepressants, selective serotonin reuptake inhibitors
Ocular hypertension	Prostaglandin analogue and carbonic anhydrase inhibitor eye drops
Oedema, peripheral or pulmonary	Aldosterone antagonists
	Diuretics, loop
	Nitrates
	Opioids
	Oxygen
Opioid toxicity	Naloxone
Osteoarthritis	Non-steroidal antiinflammatory drugs and COX-2 inhibitors
	Opioids
	Paracetamol
Osteoporosis	Bisphosphonates
	Calcium and vitamin D
	Monoclonal antibodies
Otitis externa	Aminoglycosides
	Chloramphenicol
	Macrolides
	Penicillins, narrow-spectrum
Otitis media	Macrolides
	Penicillins, broad-spectrum
Overactive bladder	Antimuscarinics, genitourinary uses
Paget's disease	Bisphosphonates

Pain	Anaesthetics, local
	Anaesthetics, general
	Antiplatelet drugs, aspirin
	Non-steroidal antiinflammatory drugs and COX-2 inhibitors
	Opioids
	Paracetamol
Panic disorder	Antidepressants, selective serotonin reuptake inhibitors
Paracentesis	Colloids (plasma substitutes)
Paracetamol poisoning	Acetylcysteine and carbocisteine
Parkinson's disease	Acetylcholinesterase inhibitors
	Dopaminergic drugs for Parkinson's disease
Pelvic inflammatory disease	Cephalosporins and carbapenems
	Metronidazole
	Quinolones
	Tetracyclines and glycylcyclines
People unable to meet their water and electrolyte requirements	Compound sodium lactate
	Glucose (dextrose)
	Potassium, intravenous
	Sodium chloride
Peptic ulcer disease	H_2-receptor antagonists
	Metronidazole
	Macrolides
	Penicillins, broad-spectrum
	Proton pump inhibitors
Peri-operative glycaemic control	Insulin
Peripheral vascular disease	Antiplatelet drugs, ADP-receptor antagonists
	Antiplatelet drugs, aspirin
	Prostaglandins and analogues
	Statins

Pneumocystis pneumonia	Trimethoprim (co-trimoxazole)
Pneumonia	Cephalosporins and carbapenems
	Macrolides
	Metronidazole
	Penicillins, antipseudomonal
	Penicillins, broad-spectrum
	Penicillins, narrow-spectrum
	Quinolones
	Tetracyclines and glycylcyclines
Pneumothorax	Oxygen
Post-exposure prophylaxis	Antiviral drugs, other
Post-partum haemorrhage	Red cells
	Tranexamic acid
	Uterotonics
Potassium depletion	Potassium, intravenous
	Potassium, oral
Pre-exposure prophylaxis	Antiviral drugs, other
Prevention of neural tube defects	Vitamins
Prevention of Rh0(d) sensitisation	Vaccines and immunoglobulins
Primary hyperaldosteronism	Aldosterone antagonists
Primary prevention of major adverse cardiovascular events	Statins
Prostate cancer	Hormone antagonists and agonists used in breast and prostate cancer

Prostatitis	Aminoglycosides
	Cephalosporins and carbapenems
	Quinolones
	Trimethoprim
Protozoal infections	Metronidazole
Pruritus	Antihistamines (H_1-receptor antagonists)
	emollients
Psoriasis	Corticosteroids, topical
	Emollients
	Methotrexate
	Monoclonal antibodies
Psoriatic arthritis	Corticosteroids, systemic
	Methotrexate
	Monoclonal antibodies
Pulmonary embolism	Fibrinolytic drugs
	Direct oral anticoagulants
	Heparins and fondaparinux
	Warfarin
Pulmonary hypertension	Phosphodiesterase (type 5) inhibitors
	Prostaglandins and analogues
Pyelonephritis	Aminoglycosides
	Cephalosporins and carbapenems
	Penicillins, broad-spectrum
Rapid tranquilisation	Antipsychotics, first-generation (typical)
	Benzodiazepines
Reconstitution and dilution of drugs	Glucose (dextrose)
	Sodium chloride
Reduced gut motility	Antiemetics, dopamine D_2-receptor antagonists
Renal stones	Allopurinol

Respiratory secretions	Acetylcysteine and carbocisteine
	Antimuscarinics, cardiovascular, and gastrointestinal uses
	Antimuscarinics, bronchodilators
Respiratory tract infection	Cephalosporins and carbapenems
	Macrolides
	Monoclonal antibodies
	Penicillins, antipseudomonal
	Penicillins, broad-spectrum
	Quinolones
	Tetracyclines and glycylcyclines
Reversal of warfarin anticoagulation	Vitamins
Rheumatoid arthritis	Aminosalicylates
	Corticosteroids, systemic
	Methotrexate
	Monoclonal antibodies
	Non-steroidal antiinflammatory drugs and COX-2 inhibitors
Schizophrenia	Antipsychotics, first-generation (typical)
	Antipsychotics, second-generation (atypical)
Seasonal allergic rhinitis	Antihistamines (H_1-receptor antagonists)
	Corticosteroids, nasal
	Leukotriene receptor antagonists
Secondary parkinsonism	Dopaminergic drugs for Parkinson's disease
Secondary prevention of major adverse cardiovascular events	Angiotensin receptor blockers
	Angiotensin-converting enzyme (ACE) inhibitors
	Antiplatelet drugs, ADP-receptor antagonists
	Antiplatelet drugs, aspirin
	Statins
Sedation	Anaesthetics, general
	Benzodiazepines

Sepsis	Aminoglycosides
	Cephalosporins and carbapenems
	Metronidazole
	Penicillins, antipseudomonal
	Penicillins, broad-spectrum
	Penicillins, narrow-spectrum
Shock	Colloids (plasma substitutes)
	Compound sodium lactate
	Sodium chloride
Sickle cell disease	Monoclonal antibodies
Sinusitis	Macrolides
	Penicillins, broad-spectrum
	Penicillins, narrow-spectrum
	Tetracyclines and glycylcyclines
Sjögren's syndrome	Ocular lubricants (artificial tears)
Skin and soft tissue infection	Antifungal drugs
	Clindamycin
	Glycopeptide antibiotics
	Macrolides
	Metronidazole
	Penicillins, antipseudomonal
	Penicillins, broad-spectrum
	Penicillins, narrow-spectrum
	Tetracyclines and glycylcyclines
Status epilepticus	Benzodiazepines
	Levetiracetam and brivaracetam
	Valproate (valproic acid)
Stroke/cerebrovascular disease	Fibrinolytic drugs
	Angiotensin receptor blockers
	Angiotensin-converting enzyme (ACE) inhibitors
	Antiplatelet drugs, ADP-receptor antagonists
	Antiplatelet drugs, aspirin
	Statins
Subacute combined degeneration of the cord	Vitamins

Supraventricular tachycardia

Adenosine
Amiodarone
β-blockers
Calcium channel blockers

Tonsillitis

Penicillins, narrow-spectrum

Trauma

Opioids
Non-steroidal antiinflammatory drugs and COX-2 inhibitors
Paracetamol
Tranexamic acid
Red cells

Trigeminal neuralgia

Carbamazepine

Tumour lysis syndrome

Allopurinol

Type 1 diabetes

Insulin

Type 2 diabetes

Dipeptidylpeptidase-4 inhibitors
Insulin
Metformin
Sodium–glucose co-transporter 2 inhibitors
Sulfonylureas

Typhoid

Tetracyclines and glycylcyclines

Ulcerative colitis

Aminosalicylates
Corticosteroids, systemic
Monoclonal antibodies

Urinary tract infection

Aminoglycosides
Cephalosporins and carbapenems
Nitrofurantoin
Penicillins, antipseudomonal
Penicillins, broad-spectrum
Quinolones
Trimethoprim

Urticaria

Antihistamines (H_1-receptor antagonists)

Venous thromboembolism	Direct oral anticoagulants Heparins and fondaparinux Warfarin
Ventricular fibrillation	Amiodarone
Ventricular tachycardia	Amiodarone Anaesthetics, local
Vertigo	Antiemetics, histamine H_1-receptor antagonists
Viral infection	Antiviral drugs, aciclovir Antiviral drugs, other
Vitamin D deficiency	Calcium and vitamin D
Vitamin deficiency	Vitamins
Wernicke's encephalopathy and Korsakoff's psychosis	Vitamins

The top 100 drugs

5α-reductase inhibitors

CLINICAL PHARMACOLOGY

Common indications	❶ In men with **lower urinary tract symptoms** due to **benign prostatic enlargement,** 5α-reductase inhibitors are offered if the prostate is bulky (estimated mass >30 g or prostate-specific antigen (PSA) level >1.4 ng/mL). They improve symptoms, which include difficulty passing urine, urinary retention, and poor urinary flow, and reduce the need for prostate-related surgery. **α-blockers** are also used for this indication and have a more rapid onset of effect. ❷ Finasteride is also an option for treatment of **androgenetic alopecia** (male-pattern baldness) in men.
Mechanisms of action	5α-reductase inhibitors reduce the size of the prostate gland. They do this by **inhibiting** the intracellular enzyme **5α-reductase,** which converts testosterone to its more active metabolite dihydrotestosterone. As dihydrotestosterone stimulates prostatic growth, inhibition of its production by 5α-reductase inhibitors reduces prostatic enlargement and improves urinary flow. However, it can take several months for this effect to become evident clinically. For this reason, an **α-blocker**, which is likely to have a more rapid effect, is usually offered to men with moderate or severe symptoms in the first instance. 5α-reductase inhibitors are most useful when the prostate is particularly bulky, either on clinical examination or inferred from the PSA level. An additional effect of androgen inhibition is hair growth, which can be exploited to advantage in treatment of androgenetic alopecia.
Important adverse effects	The most common adverse effects of 5α-reductase inhibitors relate to their antiandrogen action. These include **impotence** and **reduced libido,** which are usually transient, and breast tenderness and enlargement (**gynaecomastia**), which can affect adherence to treatment. **Hair growth** may occur, and this could be an unwanted effect, a desirable side effect or the therapeutic objective, depending on the clinical context. This effect will reverse slowly (over several months) if treatment is stopped. Rarely but importantly, **breast cancer** and **suicidal thoughts** have been reported in men taking finasteride.
Warnings	Exposure of a male fetus to 5α-reductase inhibitors may cause abnormal development of the external genitalia. It is therefore important that ✖ **women of childbearing potential** do not take these drugs and are not exposed to them, e.g. by handling broken or damaged tablets or through semen during unprotected sex with a man taking these drugs.
Important interactions	Finasteride has no clinically important drug interactions. Dutasteride is metabolised by cytochrome P450 enzymes, but the interactions predicted from this are not severe.

PRACTICAL PRESCRIBING

Prescription	For treatment of **benign prostatic enlargement,** dutasteride is given at a dose of 500 micrograms orally daily, or finasteride at 5 mg orally daily. For **androgenetic alopecia,** finasteride is used at a dose of 1 mg orally daily. Dutasteride is not licensed for this indication.
Administration	Tablets must be prepared, stored, and administered carefully. They should be swallowed whole, with or without food. Women who are, or could be, pregnant, must not touch crushed or broken tablets.
Communication	For the more common indication of **benign prostatic enlargement,** explain that the reason for difficulty passing urine is because the prostate has grown and is squashing the tube coming out of the bladder. Explain that the aim of treatment is to **reduce the bulk of the prostate gland,** which will relieve compression on the tube and make it **easier to pass urine.** However, it may take **up to 6 months** for symptoms to improve, and if treatment is stopped, the benefit will subside over a few months. The same applies if used for **androgenetic alopecia.** Warn of the **main side effects,** particularly a reduction in the desire to have sex and to get and keep an erection. These problems should last for a short while only, and normal function should return as treatment continues. Explain that if side effects are problematic, other treatment options for the enlarged prostate may be considered, so further discussions are to be encouraged. Explain that tenderness or growth in the tissue underneath the nipples may occur and should prompt medical review. Usually, these changes are harmless. However, very rarely, men can get breast cancer, and this is slightly more likely with finasteride treatment. Emphasise that women who could become pregnant must not handle the tablets, because they could be harmful to an unborn baby. For the same reason, it is essential to wear a condom during sex with a woman who could become pregnant.
Monitoring and stopping	Schedule a follow-up appointment in 3–6 months to review changes in lower urinary tract symptoms (or hair growth if used for androgenetic alopecia) and the development of adverse effects. Continue check-ups every 6–12 months while treatment continues. Treatment should be stopped if its benefits are outweighed by adverse effects, and alternative options (such as surgery) considered.
Cost	Non-proprietary forms of finasteride and dutasteride are inexpensive.

Clinical tip—5α-reductase inhibitors suppress serum levels of PSA. This happens progressively over the first 6 months of treatment. It is therefore advisable to obtain a new baseline PSA measurement at 6 months, so that any subsequent changes can be detected and interpreted correctly. If the on-treatment baseline PSA is not known, a useful rule of thumb is to double the value to account for the effect of long-term treatment with a 5α-reductase inhibitor.

Acetylcholinesterase inhibitors

CLINICAL PHARMACOLOGY

Common indications	❶ Mild-to-moderate **Alzheimer's disease** ❷ Mild-to-moderate **dementia in Parkinson's disease** (rivastigmine)
Mechanisms of action	Acetylcholine is an important central nervous system (CNS) neurotransmitter, which is essential to many brain functions including learning and memory. A decrease in activity of the brain's cholinergic system is seen in Alzheimer's disease and in the form of dementia associated with Parkinson's disease. These drugs **inhibit** the **cholinesterase enzymes** that break down acetylcholine in the CNS. It is thought that by increasing the availability of acetylcholine for neurotransmission, they improve cognitive function and reduce the rate of cognitive decline. However, recovery of function in people with these conditions on starting treatment is modest and not universal.
Important adverse effects	**GI upset** is the most common adverse effect, arising from increased cholinergic activity in the peripheral nervous system. This may resolve over time. People with asthma or COPD may experience an exacerbation of **bronchospasm.** Less common, but serious, peripheral effects include **peptic ulcers** and **bleeding, bradycardia,** and **heart block**. Central cholinergic effects may induce **hallucinations** and **altered/aggressive behaviour**. These resolve with reduction of dose or discontinuation of therapy. There is a small risk of **extrapyramidal symptoms** and **neuroleptic malignant syndrome**. These are discussed more fully in **Antipsychotics (first generation)**.
Warnings	Acetylcholinesterase inhibitors should be used with caution in people with ▲ **asthma** and ▲ **COPD** and those at risk of developing ▲ **peptic ulcers**. They should be avoided in people with ✖ **heart block** or ✖ **sick sinus syndrome**. Rivastigmine may worsen tremor in those with ▲ **Parkinson's disease**.
Important interactions	Concomitant therapy with ▲ **NSAIDs** and ▲ **systemic corticosteroids** may increase the risk of peptic ulceration. Use alongside ▲ **antipsychotics** may increase the risk of neuroleptic malignant syndrome. Bradycardia and/or heart block may occur when prescribed alongside other rate-limiting medications (e.g. ▲ β-blockers). Drugs with **prominent anticholinergic effects** (e.g. **antimuscarinic drugs**, **tricyclic antidepressants**) can additively worsen cognitive function and antagonise the effects of acetylcholinesterase inhibitors.

PRACTICAL PRESCRIBING

Prescription	Acetylcholinesterase inhibitors should be prescribed by, or on the advice of, clinicians with experience in managing dementia or Parkinson's disease. When commencing treatment, a low dose should be used to reduce the risk of adverse effects. The starting dose is 5 mg daily for donepezil and 1.5 mg 12-hrly for rivastigmine. The dosage may be titrated up after 2–4 weeks.
Administration	Generally, these drugs are available as tablets, capsules or liquid. In addition, rivastigmine is available as a patch, which may be useful for people with swallowing difficulties. Donepezil should be taken at night, before bed. However, if they experience vivid dreams as a problematic side effect, advise them to take the drug in the morning instead.
Communication	You should explain to the person and their family or caregiver that this treatment improves memory and brain function for some people and may delay deterioration. Explain that recovery of brain function is modest and it is not a cure for dementia. Discuss the adverse effects and explain that some may resolve with prolonged use. Ask them to report any abnormal movements or agitated/aggressive behaviour to their doctor. Explain that if these effects occur, they are reversible by reducing the dose or stopping treatment.
Monitoring and stopping	Review for **adverse effects** 2–4 weeks after initiation of treatment or dosage adjustment. At 3 months, repeat the cognitive assessment to assess **treatment efficacy**. Continue treatment only if there is worthwhile improvement in cognitive, functional or behavioural symptoms. Involve the person and those close to them in any decisions to change or cease treatment.
Cost	Non-proprietary formulations of acetylcholinesterase inhibitors are widely available. There are no clinically relevant differences between agents in terms of efficacy or safety. The drug with the lowest cost should therefore be prescribed.

Clinical tip—No new treatment for Alzheimer's disease has been approved by regulators in the two decades since acetylcholinesterase inhibitors emerged. Aducanumab, one of several monoclonal antibodies designed to target amyloid beta protein, has shown some promise, based primarily on its effects on a surrogate endpoint (amyloid plaques). Its approval in the US based on these early results sparked some controversy, because it is not yet known whether they will translate into meaningful clinical benefits. At the time of writing, it is not available in the UK or Europe.

Acetylcisteine and carbocisteine

CLINICAL PHARMACOLOGY

Common indications	❶ IV acetylcysteine is the antidote for **paracetamol poisoning.** ❷ Oral carbocisteine and acetylcysteine are used as **mucolytics** to reduce the viscosity of respiratory secretions associated with chronic cough and sputum. Nebulised acetylcysteine is an alternative for people in hospital.
Mechanisms of action	In therapeutic doses, **paracetamol** is metabolised mainly by conjugation with glucuronic acid and sulfate. A small amount is converted **to N-acetyl-p-benzoquinone imine (NAPQI),** which is hepatotoxic. Normally, this is quickly detoxified by conjugation with glutathione. However, in paracetamol poisoning, the body's supply of glutathione is overwhelmed, and NAPQI is left free to cause liver damage. Acetylcysteine works mainly by **replenishing** the body's supply of **glutathione.** If carbocisteine or acetylcysteine are brought into contact with mucus, they **break disulfide bonds,** degrading the three-dimensional mucus matrix and reducing its viscosity. This may aid sputum clearance if respiratory secretions are tenacious.
Important adverse effects	When administered IV in paracetamol poisoning, acetylcysteine can cause an **anaphylactoid reaction.** This is similar to an anaphylactic reaction (presenting with nausea, tachycardia, rash, and wheeze) but involves histamine release independent of immunoglobulin E (IgE) antibodies. Therefore once the reaction has settled (by stopping the acetylcysteine and giving an **antihistamine** ± a bronchodilator, e.g. **salbutamol**), it is usually safe to restart acetylcysteine, but at a lower rate of infusion. Oral carbocisteine and acetylcysteine uncommonly cause **GI upset**. Carbocisteine can disrupt the gastric mucosal barrier and has been reported to cause **GI bleeding**. When administered in nebulised form as a mucolytic, acetylcysteine may cause **bronchospasm.** Therefore a bronchodilator should usually be given immediately beforehand.
Warnings	History of an anaphylactoid reaction to IV acetylcysteine does not contraindicate its use in future if it is required. It is important that such reactions are not erroneously labelled as 'allergic', which may lead to effective treatment for paracetamol poisoning being inappropriately denied. However, it is essential to obtain specialist advice if there is any doubt. Oral carbocisteine and acetylcysteine should be used with caution in people with ▲ **peptic ulcer disease.**
Important interactions	If administered simultaneously, acetylcysteine can increase the vasodilatory effects of **glyceryl trinitrate**, causing hypotension. There is also potential for oral acetylcysteine to inactivate oral antibiotics, so doses should be separated by at least 2 hours.

PRACTICAL PRESCRIBING

Prescription	In the treatment of **paracetamol poisoning**, weight-adjusted doses of acetylcysteine are given in three consecutive IV infusions (total infusion time 21 hours). For use as a **mucolytic**, oral carbocisteine is initiated at a dosage of 750 mg three times daily, reducing to twice daily as the condition improves. Acetylcysteine is prescribed for oral administration at a dosage of 600 mg once daily. Acetylcysteine is not a licensed for administration by nebulisation, so should only be prescribed under specialist guidance.
Administration	Acetylcysteine is diluted in glucose 5% for IV infusion. The three separate components are complicated to prepare as each requires a different amount of acetylcysteine, different fluid volume, and different infusion time, so an up-to-date protocol should always be followed. Oral carbocisteine is available as capsules or oral solution, which comes in different flavours, including rum! Effervescent oral acetylcysteine tablets should be dissolved in water before swallowing.
Communication	In the treatment of **paracetamol poisoning,** explain that you are offering an antidote to prevent serious damage to the liver. Advise that the treatment is given slowly through a drip over 21 hours and that they *must* receive the entire treatment to get the full benefit. Ask them to alert staff immediately if they notice a rash, nausea or wheeziness, as these could indicate a serious adverse reaction that can be managed easily if identified. When using these medicines orally as **mucolytics,** explain that the aim of treatment is to loosen secretions and help them clear their sputum. Advise that treatment is additional to other measures to improve sputum clearance, such as maintaining hydration and doing regular chest clearance exercises.
Monitoring and stopping	In the treatment of **paracetamol poisoning,** monitor efficacy of IV acetylcysteine by measuring international normalised ratio (INR), serum alanine aminotransferase, and creatinine concentrations at presentation and on completion of treatment to track the trajectory of liver injury. Monitor safety by observing regularly for symptoms or signs of an anaphylactoid reaction. When used as a **mucolytic,** monitor efficacy of oral carbocisteine or acetylcysteine by enquiry about frequency of cough and sputum production. Stop treatment if there is no improvement in symptoms; if unacceptable side effects develop; or if sputum production is no longer a problem.
Cost	Prescribe by generic name, as branded products vary in price.

Clinical tip—Acetylcysteine is also available as *eye drops* (artificial tears). It reduces the viscosity and tenacity of mucus in the eye and is of potential benefit in the treatment of dry eye syndromes. However, as acetylcysteine drops are many times more expensive than formulations of other **ocular lubricants** (e.g. hypromellose), it is probably best reserved as an option only if these are ineffective.

Aldosterone antagonists

CLINICAL PHARMACOLOGY

Common indications	❶ **Ascites and oedema due to liver cirrhosis:** spironolactone is the first-line diuretic in this indication. ❷ **Chronic heart failure:** of at least moderate severity or arising within 1 month of a myocardial infarction, usually as an addition to a **β-blocker** and an **angiotensin-converting enzyme (ACE) inhibitor/angiotensin receptor blocker**. ❸ **Primary hyperaldosteronism:** while awaiting surgery, or if surgery is not an option.
Mechanisms of action	Aldosterone is a mineralocorticoid that is produced in the adrenal cortex. It acts on mineralocorticoid receptors in the distal tubules of the kidney to increase the activity of luminal epithelial sodium (Na^+) channels (ENaC). This increases the reabsorption of sodium and water, elevating blood pressure, with a corresponding increase in potassium excretion. Aldosterone antagonists inhibit the effect of aldosterone by **competitive inhibition** at **mineralocorticoid receptors.** This increases sodium and water *excretion* and potassium *retention*. Their effect is greatest when circulating aldosterone is increased, e.g. in primary hyperaldosteronism or cirrhosis.
Important adverse effects	An important adverse effect of aldosterone antagonists is **hyperkalaemia,** which can lead to muscle weakness, arrhythmias, and even cardiac arrest. Spironolactone causes **gynaecomastia** (enlargement of male breast tissue), which can have a significant impact on adherence in men (see Communication). Eplerenone is less likely to cause endocrine side effects. Aldosterone antagonists can cause liver impairment and jaundice and spironolactone is a cause of Stevens–Johnson syndrome (a T-cell-mediated hypersensitivity reaction) that causes a bullous skin eruption.
Warnings	Aldosterone antagonists are contraindicated in ✖ **severe renal impairment,** ✖ **hyperkalaemia,** and ✖ **adrenal insufficiency**. Aldosterone antagonists can cross the placenta during pregnancy and appear in breast milk so should be avoided where possible in ▲ **pregnant or lactating women.**
Important interactions	The combination of an aldosterone antagonist with other ▲ **potassium-elevating drugs,** including ▲ **ACE inhibitors** and ▲ **angiotensin receptor blockers (ARBs)**, increases the risk of hyperkalaemia. Nevertheless, when supported by appropriate monitoring, this may be a beneficial combination in the context of heart failure. Aldosterone antagonists should not be combined with ✖ **potassium** supplements except in specialist practice.

PRACTICAL PRESCRIBING

Prescription	Spironolactone is used for all indications, whereas eplerenone is licensed for the treatment of heart failure only. Aldosterone antagonists should be prescribed for regular administration, to be taken orally, generally as a single daily dose. You should tailor the dose to the specific indication as, for example, much higher doses are used to treat ascites secondary to cirrhosis than are used in heart failure. A typical starting dose of spironolactone is 100 mg daily for ascites compared with 25 mg daily for heart failure. Spironolactone is also available as a combined preparation with a **thiazide** or **loop diuretic**.
Administration	Spironolactone should generally be taken with food.
Communication	When starting treatment with spironolactone, particularly in high doses, it is important to warn men about the possibility of growth and tenderness of tissue under the nipples and impotence. Reassure them that such effects are benign and reversible, but acknowledge that they may be uncomfortable and embarrassing. Ask them to return if they have troublesome side effects, as these may respond to dose reduction or, in heart failure, substitution with eplerenone. Advise that aldosterone antagonists can cause the potassium level to rise and reinforce the importance of attending for blood tests.
Monitoring and stopping	**Efficacy** should be monitored by symptoms and clinical findings, e.g. reduction in ascites, oedema, and/or blood pressure. **Safety** should be monitored by checking renal function and serum potassium concentration due to the risk of renal impairment and hyperkalaemia. Except in the treatment of primary hyperaldosteronism prior to surgery (where treatment should be withdrawn after surgery), aldosterone antagonist treatment is usually required indefinitely due to the chronic nature of the underlying condition. However, development of renal impairment or hyperkalaemia (particularly if persistent or recurrent) should prompt consideration of dose reduction and/or stopping of treatment.
Cost	Spironolactone and eplerenone are available in non-proprietary form and cost less than £10 per month.

Clinical tip—Spironolactone is a relatively weak diuretic that takes several days to start having an effect. It is therefore usually prescribed in combination with a **loop** or **thiazide diuretic**, where it both counteracts potassium wasting and potentiates the diuretic effect. For example, in the treatment of ascites due to chronic liver failure, spironolactone and furosemide are generally used together in a ratio of about 5:1 (e.g. spironolactone 200 mg with furosemide 40 mg).

Alginates and antacids

CLINICAL PHARMACOLOGY

Common indications	❶ **Gastro-oesophageal reflux disease (GORD):** for symptomatic relief of heartburn. ❷ **Dyspepsia:** for short-term relief of indigestion.
Mechanisms of action	These drugs are most often taken as compound preparations containing an alginate with one or more antacids, such as sodium bicarbonate, calcium carbonate, magnesium or aluminium salts. *Antacids* work by **buffering stomach acid.** *Alginates* act to increase the **viscosity** of the stomach contents, which reduces the reflux of acid into the oesophagus. After reacting with stomach acid they form a floating **'raft',** which separates the gastric contents from the gastro-oesophageal junction to prevent mucosal damage. There is some evidence that they also inhibit **pepsin production.** Antacids alone (usually aluminium or magnesium compounds) can be used for the short-term relief of dyspepsia.
Important adverse effects	Compound alginates cause few side effects, which vary depending on their constituents and the dose taken. Magnesium salts can cause **diarrhoea,** whereas aluminium salts can cause **constipation.**
Warnings	Compound alginates are well tolerated and are safe in pregnancy. Sodium- and potassium-containing preparations should be used with caution in people with fluid overload or hyperkalaemia (e.g. ▲ **renal failure**). Some preparations contain sucrose, which can worsen hyperglycaemia in people with diabetes mellitus.
Important interactions	The **divalent cations** (e.g. Ca^{2+}, Mg^{2+}) in compound alginates can bind to other drugs, reducing their absorption. Antacids can reduce serum concentrations of many drugs, so doses should be separated by 2 hours. This applies to **angiotensin-converting enzyme (ACE) inhibitors,** some antibiotics (e.g. **cephalosporins, ciprofloxacin,** and **tetracyclines**), **bisphosphonates, digoxin, levothyroxine,** and **proton pump inhibitors (PPIs).** By increasing the alkalinity of urine, antacids can increase the excretion of **aspirin** and lithium. Compound alginates are incompatible with ▲ **thickened infant milk** products, as they can lead to excessively thick stomach contents that cause bloating and abdominal discomfort.

alginic acid compound preparations, sodium bicarbonate

PRACTICAL PRESCRIBING

Prescription	Compound alginates are available as oral suspensions or chewable tablets. They are available over the counter without prescription. When prescribed, a brand name may be stated, as they are proprietary compound products without approved compound generic names. They are usually taken on an as-required basis for symptomatic relief. Check the constituents of the brand chosen, particularly if prescribing for people with renal impairment or diabetes mellitus.
Administration	They should be taken following meals, before bedtime and/or when symptoms occur. For infants, oral powder can be mixed with feeds or water.
Communication	Explain that the medicine should relieve the symptoms of heartburn and acid indigestion within about 20 minutes, and for several hours afterwards. Explain that compound alginates should be taken after mealtimes and before bed, and if relevant, that a **gap of at least 2 hours** is required between these medicines and other drugs that they may interact with (see INTERACTIONS). Advise that these medicines are only a temporary measure, and long-term use is not recommended. Discuss lifestyle measures that can reduce reflux, such as eating smaller meals more often, identifying and avoiding food and drink triggers, stopping smoking and raising the head of the bed. Ask them to return for review if symptoms persist.
Monitoring and stopping	Efficacy is monitored by symptom response. If there are persistent symptoms or 'red flags', such as bleeding, vomiting, dysphagia, or weight loss, further investigation and specialist review are required. When symptoms are controlled or an underlying cause has been treated, stop treatment. Drugs that may cause dyspepsia, such as **antimuscarinics**, **aspirin**, **bisphosphonates**, **corticosteroids,** and **non-steroidal antiinflammatory drugs,** should be reviewed to check that they are required and, if so, the lowest effective dose is being used.
Cost	Compound alginates are inexpensive. They can be purchased over the counter. If prescribing, prefer low-cost products.

Clinical tip—Compound alginates are a useful treatment in the armamentarium of the paediatrician. Around 10%–20% of children suffer from GORD, and compound alginates have been shown to reduce the frequency of symptoms. Note, however, the interaction with thickened milk products (see INTERACTIONS).

Allopurinol

CLINICAL PHARMACOLOGY

Common indications	❶ To prevent recurrent attacks of **gout,** particularly in people with two or more attacks per year or with signs of joint damage or renal impairment. ❷ To prevent uric acid and calcium oxalate **renal stones.** ❸ To prevent **hyperuricaemia** and **tumour lysis syndrome** due to chemotherapy.
Mechanisms of action	Allopurinol is a purine analogue that **inhibits xanthine oxidase.** Xanthine oxidase metabolises xanthine (produced from purines) to uric acid. Inhibition of xanthine oxidase lowers plasma uric acid concentrations and reduces precipitation of uric acid in the joints or kidneys.
Important adverse effects	Allopurinol is generally well tolerated. However, starting allopurinol can **trigger or worsen an acute attack of gout,** possibly through effects on preformed crystals. The risk of triggering an attack may be reduced by co-prescription of an **NSAID** or colchicine in the initiation phase (see PRESCRIPTION). The most common side effect is a **skin rash,** which may be mild or may indicate a more serious hypersensitivity reaction such as **Stevens–Johnson syndrome** or **toxic epidermal necrolysis. Allopurinol hypersensitivity syndrome** is a rare, life-threatening reaction to allopurinol that can include fever, eosinophilia, lymphadenopathy, and involvement of other organs, such as the liver and skin. If allopurinol is not tolerated or is contraindicated, febuxostat (a *non-purine* xanthine oxidase inhibitor) is an alternative second-line therapy. However, a prior history of hypersensitivity to allopurinol is associated with potential hypersensitivity to febuxostat.
Warnings	Allopurinol should not be started during an ✖ **acute attack of gout,** but can be continued if already established, to avoid sudden fluctuations in serum uric acid levels. ✖ **Recurrent skin rash** or signs of more ✖ **severe hypersensitivity** to allopurinol are contraindications to therapy. Allopurinol is metabolised in the liver and excreted by the kidney. The dose should therefore be reduced in severe ▲ **renal impairment** or ▲ **hepatic impairment.**
Important interactions	The active metabolite (mercaptopurine) of the pro-drug ▲ azathioprine is metabolised by xanthine oxidase. Concurrent administration with allopurinol increases the risk of azathioprine toxicity. Co-prescription of allopurinol with ▲ **angiotensin-converting enzyme (ACE) inhibitors** or **thiazides** increases the risk of hypersensitivity reactions, and with **amoxicillin** increases the risk of skin rash.

PRACTICAL PRESCRIBING

Prescription	For **gout,** start at a low dose (e.g. 100 mg orally daily) and titrate up according to serum uric acid concentrations to usual maintenance of 200–600 mg daily in 1–2 divided doses. Also prescribe an **NSAID** (e.g. naproxen 250 mg 12-hrly) or colchicine on a short-term basis (until 1 month after serum uric acid levels normalise) to avoid triggering an acute gout attack. Although allopurinol should not be started during an acute attack of gout, it may be continued if already established. Where allopurinol is used to prevent **hyperuricaemia,** it should be started before chemotherapy.
Administration	Allopurinol is best taken after meals, and good hydration with a fluid intake of 2–3 L daily should be encouraged.
Communication	In gout, advise that the purpose of treatment is to reduce risk of attacks (or formation of kidney stones). Ask them to seek medical advice if they develop a rash. Explain that this is a common side effect, which is usually mild and goes away on stopping the drug, but it can be a sign of a more serious allergy. Advise that if they have an attack of gout, they should continue allopurinol but may need additional treatment for the acute symptoms.
Monitoring and stopping	Check serum uric acid concentrations 4 weeks after starting allopurinol or changing the dose. Aim to lower uric acid concentrations to less than 300 µmol/L where possible, by increasing the dose of allopurinol as needed. Allopurinol treatment should be stopped if a rash develops. For mild skin rashes, treatment can be reintroduced cautiously once the rash resolves. Recurrence of the rash or signs of more severe hypersensitivity to allopurinol are contraindications to further therapy. Prevention of gout or renal stones with allopurinol is usually lifelong. However, if serum uric acid levels have been normal for many years and clinical response has been achieved (e.g. no acute attacks, tophi resolved), the dose can be reduced or even stopped completely. In particular, this should be considered where modifiable risk factors have been addressed.
Cost	Allopurinol is available in a non-proprietary form and is inexpensive.

Clinical tip—Treatment with **thiazide** or **loop diuretics** increases serum uric acid concentrations and can cause gout. Low-dose **aspirin** inhibits renal excretion of uric acid and can trigger acute attacks of gout. Always consider drug-induced gout as a cause of new-onset joint pain if these medicines are being taken.

α-blockers

CLINICAL PHARMACOLOGY

Common indications	❶ As a first-line medical option to improve **lower urinary tract symptoms (LUTS)** in **benign prostatic enlargement,** when lifestyle changes are insufficient or voiding symptoms are moderate to severe. **5α-reductase inhibitors** may be added in selected cases. Surgical treatment is also an option, particularly if there is evidence of urinary tract damage (e.g. hydronephrosis). ❷ As an add-on treatment in **resistant hypertension,** when other medicines (e.g. **calcium channel blockers, angiotensin-converting enzyme (ACE) inhibitors, thiazide diuretics**) are insufficient.
Mechanisms of action	Although often described using the broad term 'α-blocker', most drugs in this class (including doxazosin, tamsulosin, and alfuzosin) are highly selective for α_1-adrenoceptors. These are found mainly in smooth muscle, including in blood vessels and the urinary tract (the bladder neck and prostate in particular). Stimulation induces contraction; blockade induces relaxation. **Inhibiting** the **α_1-adrenoceptor** therefore causes vasodilation and a fall in blood pressure (BP) and reduces resistance to urine outflow from the bladder.
Important adverse effects	Predictably from their effects on vascular tone, α-blockers can cause **postural hypotension, dizziness,** and **syncope.** This is particularly prominent after the **first dose.**
Warnings	Avoid α-blockers in people with existing ▲ **postural hypotension.**
Important interactions	In general, combining antihypertensive drugs results in additive BP-lowering effects (this may well be the therapeutic aim). To avoid pronounced first-dose hypotension, it may be prudent to omit doses of one or more existing antihypertensive drugs on the day the α-blocker is started. This is particularly the case for **β-blockers**, which inhibit the reflex tachycardia that forms part of the compensatory response to **vasodilation.** α-blockers can also lead to symptomatic hypotension in combination with **phosphodiesterase type 5 (PDE-5) inhibitors** (e.g. sildenafil). People with benign prostatic enlargement (typically older men) may also suffer from erectile dysfunction, so this combination is not uncommon. Ideally α-blocker treatment should be stabilised before starting a PDE-5 inhibitor.

PRACTICAL PRESCRIBING

Prescription	Doxazosin and tamsulosin are the most commonly prescribed α-blockers in the UK. Doxazosin is licensed both for **benign prostatic enlargement** and **hypertension;** it is typically started at a dose of 1 mg orally daily and increased at 1–2-week intervals according to response. Tamsulosin is licensed for **benign prostatic enlargement** only. It also has a BP-lowering effect, but this is probably less pronounced than for doxazosin. It is given at a dose of 400 micrograms orally daily.
Administration	Given the pronounced BP-lowering effect of doxazosin, it is best to take this at bedtime, at least initially.
Communication	As appropriate, advise that you are offering them a treatment for urinary symptoms and/or their blood pressure. Explain that it may cause dizziness on standing, particularly after the first dose. Advise them to start by taking the medicine at bedtime to minimise the impact of this (and warn that if they need to get up in the night, they should rise from bed slowly).
Monitoring and stopping	The best guide to **efficacy** is the improvement in symptoms and/ or BP, as applicable. For **tolerability** and **safety,** adverse effects are identified from symptoms and lying and standing BP. Treatment is usually required long-term, provided its benefits continue to outweigh its adverse effectives. However, in **benign prostatic enlargement,** it may be stopped if a 'definitive' intervention, such as surgery or long-term catheterisation, has been performed and is successful. Likewise, for **resistant hypertension,** blood pressure targets should be reviewed at regular intervals and may be eased in people aged over 80 years or who develop frailty or multimorbidity. Relaxing treatment targets may allow dose reduction or even discontinuation.
Cost	Non-proprietary forms of doxazosin and tamsulosin are inexpensive. Both drugs are also available in modified-release (MR) forms which, as brand name products, are more expensive. There is little evidence that the MR forms are any more effective than standard-release forms, and since they are all taken at the same frequency (daily), they do not improve convenience. They are not recommended.

Clinical tip—Although α-blockers are usually reserved for hypertension resistant to other drug classes, many men with hypertension also have benign prostatic enlargement. Discovering that a man with hypertension also has benign prostatic enlargement may prompt you to introduce doxazosin at an earlier stage in the treatment pathway. In doing so, you may be able to improve both conditions with a single drug. This exemplifies why the 'review of systems' is an important part of history taking.

Aminoglycosides

CLINICAL PHARMACOLOGY

Common indications	Systemic aminoglycosides (gentamicin, amikacin) are used to treat severe infections, particularly those caused by Gram-negative aerobes (including *Pseudomonas aeruginosa*): ❶ **Sepsis,** including cases where the source is unidentified. ❷ **Pyelonephritis** and **complicated urinary tract infection.** ❸ **Intraabdominal infection.** ❹ **Endocarditis.** ❺ Topical neomycin is an option for **otitis externa.**
Spectrum of activity	The main activity of aminoglycosides that is clinically relevant is against **Gram-negative aerobic bacteria.** They also have some activity against staphylococci and mycobacteria, but other agents are preferred. They are inactive against streptococci and anaerobes, so are often used as part of combination treatment (e.g. with a **penicillin** and **metronidazole**).
Mechanisms of action	Aminoglycosides **bind irreversibly to bacterial ribosomes** (30S subunit) and **inhibit protein synthesis.** They are bactericidal (they kill bacteria), an effect that probably involves other, incompletely understood, mechanisms. Aminoglycosides enter bacterial cells via an oxygen-dependent transport system. Streptococci and anaerobic bacteria do not have this transport system, so have innate aminoglycoside resistance. Other bacteria acquire resistance through reduced cell membrane permeability to aminoglycosides or acquisition of enzymes that modify aminoglycosides to prevent them from reaching the ribosomes. As penicillins weaken bacterial cell walls, they may enhance aminoglycoside activity by increasing penetration into bacterial cells.
Important adverse effects	The most important adverse effects of systemic treatment are **nephrotoxicity** and **ototoxicity.** Aminoglycosides accumulate in renal tubular epithelial cells and cochlear and vestibular hair cells where they trigger apoptosis and cell death. Nephrotoxicity presents as reduced urine output and rising serum creatinine and is potentially reversible. Ototoxicity may cause hearing loss, tinnitus (cochlear damage) and/or vertigo (vestibular damage) and is more likely to be irreversible.
Warnings	Aminoglycosides are renally excreted. In systemic therapy, careful dose adjustment based on plasma drug concentrations is essential to prevent renal, cochlear, and vestibular damage, particularly in ▲ **neonates,** ▲ **older people** and those with ▲ **renal impairment.** Aminoglycosides can impair neuromuscular transmission and so should not be given to people with ▲ **myasthenia gravis** unless unavoidable.
Important interactions	▲ **Ototoxicity** and ▲ **nephrotoxicity** are more likely if aminoglycosides are co-prescribed with **loop diuretics** or **glycopeptide antibiotics.** ▲ **Nephrotoxicity** is more likely if aminoglycosides are co-prescribed with **cephalosporins, NSAIDs,** and other nephrotoxic drugs.

PRACTICAL PRESCRIBING

Prescription	Aminoglycosides are highly polarised, so do not cross lipid membranes and are not absorbed from the gut. Systemic therapy must therefore be given parenterally. In **severe infection**, aminoglycosides are given by intermittent IV infusion, usually once daily. Dose is calculated from body weight (see CLINICAL TIP) and renal function. The dose interval (time between doses) is determined by drug level monitoring, with subsequent doses being administered only when plasma concentrations have fallen to a safe level (see MONITORING). The dose interval is usually 24 hours for people with normal renal function and longer (e.g. 36–48 hours) in renal impairment.
Administration	For IV administration, aminoglycosides are infused slowly (e.g. over 30 min). This limits exposure of the ear to high peak concentrations (a potential hazard of impatience during IV injection).
Communication	Explain that the aim of treatment is to get rid of infection and improve symptoms. Enquire daily about change in hearing, ringing in the ears or dizziness. Ensure that the prescription clearly indicates that dosing depends on plasma concentrations and that measurement and recording of these have been organised, particularly if this is required at weekends or overnight.
Monitoring and stopping	For **efficacy,** monitor symptoms, signs and blood markers (e.g. CRP) to ensure resolution of infection. For **safety,** measure renal function before (to guide dosing) and during (to detect toxicity) parenteral aminoglycoside therapy. Follow local protocols for **plasma drug concentration** measurement. Levels may be taken 18–24 hours after a dose *(trough level),* and the next dose administered if this has fallen to a safe level (e.g. gentamicin <1 mg/mL). Alternatively, a *mid-interval concentration* (6–14 hours after the dose) may be compared to a nomogram to determine when the next dose is given. Treatment duration should be as short as possible to limit toxicity: usually less than 7 days, and often just a single dose.
Cost	Cost is not usually a consideration when prescribing aminoglycosides for life-threatening infection. Short courses are inexpensive.

Clinical tip—Aminoglycosides have a narrow therapeutic index, meaning that there is little 'safety margin' between the clinically effective dose and the toxic dose. One means of tailoring the dose to the individual is to base it on body weight. This is complicated in obesity, as the 'excess weight' contains disproportionately more fat than water. Since aminoglycosides distribute only through body water (not fat), only a proportion of the excess weight is included in dosage calculation. This is achieved by basing the dose on adjusted body weight, typically calculated as [ideal body weight] + 0.4 × ([actual body weight] − [ideal body weight]).

Aminosalicylates

CLINICAL PHARMACOLOGY

Common indications	❶ Mesalazine is a first-line option for mild-moderate **ulcerative colitis (UC);** sulfasalazine is an alternative but has largely been replaced by mesalazine for this indication. **Corticosteroids** are also used. ❷ Sulfasalazine is one of several options for **rheumatoid arthritis,** in which it is used as a disease-modifying antirheumatic drug (DMARD), usually as part of combination therapy.
Mechanisms of action	In ulcerative colitis, mesalazine and sulfasalazine both exert their therapeutic effects by releasing **5-aminosalicylic acid (5-ASA).** The precise mechanism of action of 5-ASA is unknown, but it has both **antiinflammatory** and **immunosuppressive** effects and appears to act topically on the gut rather than systemically. For this reason, 5-ASA preparations are designed to delay delivery of the active ingredient to the colon. The oral form of mesalazine comprises a tablet with a coating that resists gastric breakdown, instead releasing 5-ASA further down the gut. Sulfasalazine consists of a molecule of 5-ASA linked to sulfapyridine. In the colon, bacterial enzymes break this link and release the two molecules. Sulfapyridine does not contribute to its therapeutic effect in ulcerative colitis, but it does cause side effects, and for this reason it has largely been replaced by mesalazine for this indication. By contrast, sulfapyridine is probably the active component of sulfasalazine in rheumatoid arthritis, though its mechanism is unclear. Mesalazine has no role in rheumatoid arthritis.
Important adverse effects	Mesalazine generally causes fewer side effects than sulfasalazine. Most commonly, these are **GI upset** (e.g. nausea, dyspepsia) and **headache.** Both drugs can cause rare but serious blood abnormalities (e.g. **leukopenia, thrombocytopenia**) and **renal impairment.** In men, sulfasalazine may induce a reversible decrease in the number of sperm (**oligospermia**). It can also cause a **serious hypersensitivity reaction,** comprising fever, rash, and liver abnormalities.
Warnings	Mesalazine and sulfasalazine are salicylates, like **aspirin.** They are contraindicated in people with ✖ **aspirin hypersensitivity.**
Important interactions	Mesalazine tablets with a pH-sensitive coating (e.g. Asacol® MR) may interact with drugs that alter gut pH. For example, **proton pump inhibitors** increase gastric pH and so may cause the coating to be broken down prematurely. **Lactulose** lowers stool pH and may prevent 5-ASA release in the colon.

PRACTICAL PRESCRIBING

Prescription

For mild-moderate rectal or rectosigmoid **ulcerative colitis,** a mesalazine enema or suppository is generally used first-line. In an acute attack, this is taken once daily or 12-hrly for 4–6 weeks to induce remission. If preferred, or if disease is more proximal, an oral formulation may be used. Drug choice (and therefore dosage regimen) is likely to be dictated by local policies. Decisions regarding choice of therapy in **rheumatoid arthritis** should be taken by a specialist.

Administration

The Asacol® foam enema, a common mesalazine preparation, requires thorough mixing before administration. The can should be shaken vigorously for two 15-second periods. An applicator is then attached and inserted as far as possible into the rectum. The can is held upside-down and the dome is pressed and released to deliver a dose. The applicator should then be removed and disposed of cleanly, and hands washed. For suppositories, the person should empty their bowels first, insert the suppository, and then avoid opening their bowels for at least an hour if possible. Tablet forms of mesalazine should be swallowed whole (so as not to damage the modified-release coating).

Communication

Explain the aim of treatment, as appropriate for the indication, and how to take the medicine—particularly if it is a rectal preparation (see ADMINISTRATION). If taking the medicine orally, advised that any unexplained bleeding, bruising or infective symptoms should prompt urgent medical review, as this could be a sign of a potentially serious blood count abnormality.

Monitoring and stopping

Symptoms are the best guide to **efficacy** in ulcerative colitis. In rheumatoid arthritis, this may be supplemented by disease activity scores and measurement of acute phase reactant concentrations (CRP, erythrocyte sedimentation rate). Treatment should be stopped or switched if there is inadequate response. For **safety,** oral mesalazine therapy should be accompanied by renal function monitoring, and sulfasalazine supported by full blood count (FBC) and liver profile monitoring. Aminosalicylates may be continued long-term provided the balance of efficacy and safety remains favourable. Stopping should be guided by a specialist, based on disease activity.

Cost

Mesalazine is available in several branded forms which vary in price. Choice is likely to be dictated by local formulary agreements.

Clinical tip—Administration of mesalazine rectally is not easy, particularly for people with active proctitis. Provide written advice and explain it. For those using a foam enema, supply (or advise them to obtain) a water-based lubricant to facilitate insertion of the applicator. Similarly, insertion of suppositories can be made easier by greasing their tip with a little petroleum jelly.

Amiodarone

CLINICAL PHARMACOLOGY

Common indications	Amiodarone is used in a wide range of tachyarrhythmias, including **atrial fibrillation** (AF), **atrial flutter, supraventricular tachycardia** (SVT), **ventricular tachycardia** (VT) and refractory **ventricular fibrillation** (VF). It is generally used only if other treatments (drugs or electrical cardioversion) are ineffective or contraindicated.
Mechanisms of action	Amiodarone has many effects on myocardial cells, including **blockade** of **sodium, calcium and potassium channels,** and **antagonism** of α- **and** β-**adrenergic receptors.** These effects reduce spontaneous depolarisation (automaticity), slow conduction velocity and increase resistance to depolarisation (refractoriness), including in the atrioventricular (AV) node. By interfering with AV node conduction, amiodarone reduces the ventricular rate in AF and atrial flutter. Through its other effects, it may also increase the chance of conversion to, and maintenance of, sinus rhythm. In SVT involving a self-perpetuating ('re-entry') circuit that includes the AV node, amiodarone may break the circuit and restore sinus rhythm. Amiodarone's effects in suppressing spontaneous depolarisations make it an option for both treatment and prevention of VT and for improving the chance of successful defibrillation in refractory VF.
Important adverse effects	In acute use, compared with other antiarrhythmic drugs, amiodarone causes relatively little myocardial depression. It can cause **hypotension** during IV infusion, although this is probably an effect of the solvent rather than the drug itself. When taken chronically, amiodarone has many side effects, several of which are serious. These include effects on the lungs (**pneumonitis**), heart (**bradycardia, AV block**), liver (**hepatitis**) and skin (**photosensitivity** and **grey discolouration**). Due to its iodine content (am*IOD*arone) and structural similarities to thyroid hormone, it may cause **thyroid abnormalities,** including hypo- and hyperthyroidism. Amiodarone has an extremely long half-life. After discontinuation, it may take months to be completely eliminated.
Warnings	Amiodarone is a potentially dangerous drug that should be used only when the risk–benefit balance justifies it. It should generally be avoided in ▲ **severe hypotension,** ▲ **heart block,** and ▲ **active thyroid disease.**
Important interactions	Amiodarone interacts with many drugs—too many to list here— and certain foods. Notably, it increases plasma concentrations of ▲ **digoxin,** ▲ **diltiazem,** and ▲ **verapamil**. This may increase the risk of bradycardia, AV block, and heart failure. The doses of these drugs should be halved if amiodarone is started. Grapefruit juice, by down-regulating cytochrome P450 3A4, can increase exposure to amiodarone, so should be avoided. Due to its long half-life (25–100 days), interactions can occur after stopping the drug.

PRACTICAL PRESCRIBING

Prescription	A decision to prescribe amiodarone, whether for acute or long-term use, always requires senior involvement and should not be taken independently by inexperienced or non-specialist prescribers. One exception is in **cardiac arrest,** in which it is given for VF or pulseless VT immediately after the third shock in the Advanced Life Support (ALS) algorithm. The dose is 300 mg IV, followed by 20 mL of 0.9% sodium chloride or 5% glucose as a flush. In this instance, it should be administered first and prescribed later.
Administration	In cardiac arrest, amiodarone is given as a bolus injection. It is often provided in a pre-filled syringe to facilitate easy administration. It should be given through the 'best' IV cannula available. Outside cardiac arrests, if continuous or repeated IV infusions are anticipated, these should be given via a **central line.** This is because peripheral IV administration can cause significant phlebitis.
Communication	As appropriate, explain that you are offering a treatment for a fast or irregular heart rhythm. Explain that it has several important and potentially serious side effects, and it is being used only because their condition is serious and no other treatments are suitable or effective. In long-term use, ask them to report any symptoms of breathlessness, persistent cough, jaundice, restlessness, weight loss, tiredness or weight gain. Advise them not to drink grapefruit juice, as this can increase the risk of side effects, and to minimise direct sunlight exposure due to the risk of photosensitivity.
Monitoring and stopping	Heart rate and rhythm are the best guides to treatment **efficacy**. For **safety,** IV infusion should be accompanied by continuous cardiac monitoring. In long-term therapy, baseline tests should include renal, liver and thyroid profiles, and a chest X-ray. The liver and thyroid profiles should then be repeated 6 monthly. Acute treatment should usually be stopped once the underlying cause of rhythm disturbance has resolved. In long-term treatment, stopping should be guided by a specialist, taking account of cardiac rhythm control, alternative treatment options and the cumulative risks of long-term therapy.
Cost	Amiodarone is inexpensive.

Clinical tip—While non-specialist prescribers should never initiate amiodarone independently, they may need to rewrite prescriptions for ongoing therapy. Always confirm whether it is appropriate to continue amiodarone and, if in any doubt, seek expert advice. Do not blindly copy the preceding dose, because this may have been a loading dose (which seeks to achieve therapeutic concentrations rapidly), whereas you may need to prescribe a maintenance dose. Again, never hesitate to seek advice. If you find yourself prescribing amiodarone on a discharge prescription, always question whether this is appropriate. If the acute problems have resolved, it may be possible to stop it.

Anaesthetics, general

CLINICAL PHARMACOLOGY

Common indications	❶ To induce reversible unconsciousness, allowing interventional (e.g. surgical) procedures to be performed without awareness or interaction **(general anaesthesia)**. ❷ Some drugs in this group (e.g. propofol) may be used at sub-anaesthetic doses to reduce discomfort from procedures that do not require full general anaesthesia, or as an infusion to improve tolerability of invasive ventilation in critical illness **(sedation)**.
Mechanisms of action	General anaesthetics are a family of diverse compounds, pragmatically grouped by their route of administration. *Intravenous* anaesthetics include propofol, thiopental, and ketamine, while *inhalational* anaesthetics include volatile liquids (e.g. sevoflurane) and simple gases (nitrous oxide). To access the central nervous system (CNS), anaesthetics must be lipid soluble, and this is a strong determinant of their potency. Possible molecular mechanisms of their effects include **disruption of neuronal cell membranes** and interactions with specific ion channels. For example, a family of two-pore **potassium channels (K_{2P})**, which are widely distributed in the CNS and regulate membrane resting potential, are sensitive to volatile anaesthetics. Anaesthetics may interact with K_{2P} channels directly or indirectly by **disrupting crystallin lipids** ('lipid rafts') that surround them. Collectively, these molecular effects enhance the inhibitory action of **γ-aminobutyric acid (GABA)**, particularly via $GABA_A$ receptor activation, and/or antagonise excitatory **N-methyl-D-aspartate (NMDA)** and nicotinic cholinergic receptors. This decreases cortical and thalamic activity, leading to varying degrees of unconsciousness, analgesia, and muscle relaxation. The balance of effects varies between drugs. For example, nitrous oxide and ketamine have useful analgesic effects, whereas most other general anaesthetics do not.
Important adverse effects	CNS depression causes **suppression of airway reflexes and respiratory drive,** usually necessitating airway management (e.g. endotracheal intubation) and ventilation. Most anaesthetics cause **bradycardia, vasodilation,** and **hypotension** (ketamine is an exception, more often causing tachycardia and hypertension). **Nausea and vomiting** are common on emergence from anaesthesia, though this is likely multifactorial. Propofol may cause **pain on injection.**
Warnings	General anaesthesia and sedation should only be undertaken by expert clinicians in appropriate facilities. Assessment of 'fitness for anaesthesia' is complex and beyond the scope of this book. Risk is often classified using the American Society of Anesthesiologists (ASA) Physical Status Classification system, based on the severity of systemic disease.
Important interactions	General anaesthetics predictably enhance the effects of other drugs that suppress consciousness and cardiorespiratory function (e.g. **benzodiazepines**, **opioids**). This may be used to therapeutic effect.

PRACTICAL PRESCRIBING

Prescription	For general anaesthesia, anaesthesia is commonly *induced* with an IV anaesthetic (e.g. propofol), together with a **strong opioid** (e.g. fentanyl) for analgesia, and a muscle relaxant (e.g. rocuronium) if paralysis is required. Anaesthesia may then be *maintained* with an infusion of an IV agent (total IV anaesthesia, TIVA) or by introducing an inhalational anaesthetic (e.g. sevoflurane) into the breathing circuit. Doses of analgesic, muscular relaxant and antiemetic drugs are repeated as necessary during the procedure, and in anticipation of emergence. In critical illness requiring invasive ventilation, a sedative (e.g. propofol or a **benzodiazepine**) and strong opioid are usually given by continuous IV infusion, with doses titrated to maintain comfort and cooperation. Standard hospital templates are not well suited to the prescription and administration of general anaesthetics, and most hospitals will have tools (charts or electronic systems) specifically for this.
Administration	IV anaesthetics are given by bolus injection to induce anaesthesia, and infusion to maintain anaesthesia (or sub-anaesthetic sedation). Inhalational anaesthetics are administered by blending them with the gaseous mixture in the breathing circuit. For volatile anaesthetics, this requires the liquid first to be vaporised using a device that allows the concentration of anaesthetic vapour to be precisely controlled.
Communication	The nature of the discussion will vary according to the clinical context. For planned surgery, an important element of preoperative counselling and informed consent is a discussion about the benefits and risks of general anaesthesia, and any alternative options available (e.g. regional anaesthesia). This discussion should be led by an anaesthetist.
Monitoring and stopping	General anaesthesia requires continuous supervision by an anaesthetist. Physiological monitoring should include cardiac rhythm, blood pressure, oxygen saturations, and the waveform of carbon dioxide in exhaled breath (capnography). Sub-anaesthetic sedation may be administered by non-anaesthetists who have adequate training and expertise. It requires similar monitoring, though capnography may be omitted if the patient is verbally responsive.
Cost	Drug costs contribute substantially to the cost of providing general anaesthesia and critical care services. At a system level, this is taken into account when determining care pathways and the drugs that are available. It is not a major consideration at the bedside.

Clinical tip—If you care for patients who may receive general anaesthesia or sedation, you should be familiar with preoperative fasting requirements. In general, patients must stop eating 6 hours before their procedure, but may drink clear fluids until 1–2 hours before. Clear fluids include water, fruit juice without pulp, and hot beverages without milk.

Anaesthetics, local

CLINICAL PHARMACOLOGY

Common indications	❶ **Surface anaesthesia** to facilitate urinary catheterisation (lidocaine gel), venepuncture (lidocaine with prilocaine cream) or to treat pain arising from a small, well-defined area of skin (lidocaine plasters). ❷ Subcutaneously to provide **local anaesthesia** for procedures such as suturing, vascular access or lumbar puncture (predominantly lidocaine). ❸ To provide **regional anaesthesia/analgesia**, for example spinal or epidural analgesia (bupivacaine, lidocaine, prilocaine). ❹ Lidocaine is a second-line option for **ventricular tachycardia.**
Mechanisms of action	Local anaesthetics **reversibly inhibit voltage-gated sodium channels** on plasma membranes. In neurons, this prevents initiation and propagation of action potentials, inducing local anaesthesia in the area supplied by the blocked nerve fibres. The pharmacokinetics of local anaesthetics determines their speed of onset and duration of effect, and this in turn guides drug choice. For example, lidocaine is readily absorbed through epithelia and has a rapid onset, making it a good choice for topical anaesthesia or medicated plasters. Bupivacaine has high affinity for binding sites, providing a longer duration of action and making it a good choice for regional anaesthesia for surgery. Sodium channel blockade in cardiac conductive tissue slows conduction and reduces automatic firing. This explains lidocaine's antiarrhythmic effect and the adverse cardiac effects of local anaesthetics in overdose.
Important adverse effects	The most common side effect is an initial **stinging** sensation during administration. Systemic adverse effects are uncommon provided care is taken to avoid excessive dosing or intravenous administration. Where this does occur, it may lead to neurological (**drowsiness, restlessness, tremor,** and **fits**) and cardiovascular (**hypotension and arrhythmias)** effects. Adverse effects in spinal/epidural anaesthesia include complications of the insertion procedure (e.g. bleeding, infection). In addition, inadvertent infiltration or tracking of the drug higher than the intended anaesthetic level, or at high doses, may lead to hypotension and bradycardia (due to blockade of sympathetic fibres) and weakness or paralysis (blockade of motor fibres). Skin reactions can occur with use of medicated plasters.
Warnings	Used appropriately, local anaesthetics are generally safe. They are metabolised by the liver, so lower doses should be considered in significant ▲ **liver disease**. Lidocaine has a high *hepatic extraction ratio* (about 70% of drug entering the liver is removed in one pass), meaning that its clearance is particularly influenced by hepatic blood flow. Lower doses should therefore also be considered in ▲ **cardiac failure**.
Important interactions	As duration of action depends on how long the drug stays in contact with the neurons, co-administration with a vasoconstrictor (e.g. **adrenaline**) produces a desirable interaction that may prolong the effect.

PRACTICAL PRESCRIBING

Prescription	For **urinary catheterisation,** lidocaine is formulated as a gel with the antiseptic agent chlorhexidine (e.g. Instillagel®) in pre-filled syringes. For **subcutaneous local anaesthesia,** the 1% (10 mg/mL) solution of lidocaine hydrochloride is a common choice. The maximum dose is 3 mg/kg or 200 mg, whichever is lower (or if combined with **adrenaline**, 7 mg/kg or 500 mg). Maximum doses are calculated using *ideal body weight.* In practice, you draw up the dose you think you will need (not exceeding the maximum dose), then administer enough to produce adequate anaesthesia. For **topical anaesthesia** prior to venepuncture, a cream containing lidocaine and pilocaine (e.g. Emla 5%) is a common choice. When prescribing **medicated plasters**, specify an 'on' and 'off' time, with a 12-hour plaster-free interval to minimise skin reactions.
Administration	In **urinary catheterisation,** to administer Instillagel®, remove the cap, press the plunger gently to free it and expel air, then slowly inject the gel into the urethra. For **subcutaneous local anaesthesia,** initially infiltrate the skin and superficial layers using a fine (orange (25G)) needle, then step up to a larger needle (blue (23G) or green (21G)) as necessary for deeper layers. Briefly retract the plunger before each injection to ensure the tip has not entered a vessel (look for a flash of blood). New/inexperienced prescribers do not administer regional anaesthesia, but may look after patients receiving **patient-controlled epidural analgesia**. This may involve a continuous epidural infusion, supplemented by 'booster' doses when the patient presses a button.
Communication	Explain that you are offering treatment with a local anaesthetic to numb the area. Warn that it may sting initially, but this will disappear. They will feel pushing and pulling, but should not feel pain. Ask them to tell you if they do.
Monitoring and stopping	Quality of anaesthesia is monitored clinically. In epidural anaesthesia, the level (dermatome) of analgesia should be checked regularly. This is usually done by checking similarly inhibited temperature sensation. Where the level is higher than intended, or there are other adverse effects (e.g. hypotension or excessive motor blockade), seek advice from an experienced colleague as the dose may need to be reduced, treatment stopped or further investigations undertaken to detect complications (see ADVERSE EFFECTS).
Cost	Lidocaine solution is cheap. Instillagel® costs about 10–20p per tube.

Clinical tip—A common mistake is not waiting for local anaesthesia to reach maximal effect. The practitioner infiltrates the area and then, 30 seconds later, pricks the skin while saying 'Can you feel this?' The patient jumps and promptly loses confidence in the quality of anaesthesia. *Be patient.* Administer the local anaesthetic early, then complete any other preparatory work for your procedure. Wait 5 minutes before testing the effect.

Angiotensin receptor blockers (ARBs)

CLINICAL PHARMACOLOGY

Common indications	❶ **Hypertension:** for first- or second-line treatment of hypertension, to reduce the risk of stroke, myocardial infarction, and death from cardiovascular disease. ❷ **Chronic heart failure:** for first-line treatment of all stages of heart failure, to improve symptoms and prognosis. ❸ **Secondary prevention of major adverse cardiovascular events** in people with ischaemic heart disease, cerebrovascular disease or peripheral vascular disease. ❹ **Diabetic nephropathy** and **chronic kidney disease (CKD) with proteinuria:** to reduce proteinuria and progression of nephropathy.
Mechanisms of action	ARBs have similar effects to **angiotensin-converting enzyme (ACE) inhibitors**, but instead of inhibiting the conversion of angiotensin I to angiotensin II, ARBs block the action of **angiotensin II** on the **angiotensin type 1 (AT$_1$) receptor.** Angiotensin II is a vasoconstrictor and stimulates aldosterone secretion. Blocking its action reduces peripheral vascular resistance (afterload), which lowers blood pressure. It particularly dilates the efferent glomerular arteriole, which reduces intraglomerular pressure and slows the progression of CKD. Reducing aldosterone concentration promotes sodium and water excretion. This can help to reduce venous return (preload), which has a beneficial effect in heart failure.
Important adverse effects	ARBs can cause **hypotension** (particularly after the **first dose**), **hyperkalaemia,** and **renal failure.** The mechanism is the same as for **ACE inhibitors.** Renal artery stenosis presents a particular risk, as constriction of the efferent glomerular arteriole is required to maintain glomerular filtration. ARBs are less likely than **ACE inhibitors** to cause cough and angioedema, as they do not inhibit ACE, so do not affect bradykinin metabolism. They may therefore preferred in Black people of African or Caribbean origin, who are at higher risk of angioedema.
Warnings	ARBs should be avoided in ✖ **renal artery stenosis** and ✖ **acute kidney injury;** in women who are, or could become, ▲ **pregnant;** or who are ▲ **breastfeeding.** ARBs are valuable in the treatment of ▲ **CKD,** but lower doses should be used, and renal function monitored closely (see MONITORING).
Important interactions	Due to the risk of hyperkalaemia, avoid prescribing ARBs with other ▲ **potassium-elevating drugs,** including **potassium** supplements, **aldosterone antagonists** and potassium-sparing diuretics, except under specialist advice for advanced heart failure. In combination with other diuretics they may be associated with profound first-dose hypotension. The combination of **NSAIDs** with ARBs increases the risk of nephrotoxicity.

PRACTICAL PRESCRIBING

Prescription	The starting dose varies according to the indication, generally being lower in heart failure than in other indications. A common choice is losartan 12.5 mg orally daily in heart failure or 50 mg orally daily in other indications. This is titrated up to the maximum recommended dose over a period of weeks, according to therapeutic response, side effects and renal function.
Administration	ARBs can be taken with or without food. It is best to take the first dose before bed to reduce symptomatic hypotension.
Communication	As applicable, explain that you are offering treatment with a medicine to improve blood pressure control, reduce strain on the heart and/or to slow the rate of kidney damage. If they were unable to tolerate an ACE inhibitor due to cough, explain that the new treatment does not cause this. Warn about dizziness due to low blood pressure, particularly after the first dose. Make sure they understand the need for blood test monitoring, explaining that ARBs can upset potassium balance. Advise them to avoid taking over-the-counter 'antiinflammatories' (**NSAIDs**) due to the risk of kidney damage. Advise that if they develop diarrhoea or vomiting, to maintain their fluid intake, and stop the ACE inhibitor until their symptoms resolve. These 'sick day rules' reduce the risk of dehydration, low blood pressure, and kidney damage.
Monitoring and stopping	Monitor **efficacy** clinically, for example, severity of breathlessness in heart failure and blood pressure in hypertension. For **safety,** check electrolytes and renal function before starting treatment. Repeat this 1–2 weeks into treatment and after increasing the dose. Biochemical changes can be tolerated provided they are within certain limits. ARBs should generally be stopped if the serum creatinine concentration rises more than 30% or the estimated glomerular filtration rate (eGFR) falls more than 25%. If serum potassium rises above 5.0 mmol/L, stop other potassium-elevating and nephrotoxic drugs (see INTERACTIONS). If, despite this, it remains above 5.0 mmol/L, reduce the ARB dose. If it exceeds 6.0 mmol/L, stop the ARB and seek expert advice. ARBs may be required indefinitely, but treatment aims should be reviewed regularly. For example, easing of blood pressure targets in those aged over 80 years, or who develop frailty or multimorbidity, may allow dose reduction or discontinuation.
Cost	ARBs are available in inexpensive non-proprietary forms.

Clinical tip—Sacubitril valsartan (Entresto®) is an additional treatment option for symptomatic heart failure with reduced ejection fraction. It combines sacubitril, a neprilysin inhibitor, with the ARB valsartan. It should be initiated by specialists only. Be alert to the risk of inadvertent co-prescription with an **ACE inhibitor** or another ARB.

Angiotensin-converting enzyme (ACE) inhibitors

CLINICAL PHARMACOLOGY

Common indications	❶ **Hypertension:** for first- or second-line treatment of hypertension, to reduce the risk of stroke, myocardial infarction, and death from cardiovascular disease. ❷ **Chronic heart failure:** for first-line treatment of all grades of heart failure, to improve symptoms and prognosis. ❸ **Secondary prevention of major adverse cardiovascular events** in people with ischaemic heart disease, cerebrovascular disease, or peripheral vascular disease. ❹ **Diabetic nephropathy** and **chronic kidney disease (CKD) with proteinuria:** to reduce proteinuria and progression of nephropathy.
Mechanisms of action	ACE inhibitors **inhibit** the action of **angiotensin-converting enzyme (ACE),** reducing conversion of angiotensin I to angiotensin II. Angiotensin II is a vasoconstrictor and stimulates aldosterone secretion. Blocking its action reduces peripheral vascular resistance (afterload), which lowers blood pressure (BP). It particularly dilates the efferent glomerular arteriole, which reduces intraglomerular pressure and slows the progression of CKD. Reducing aldosterone concentration promotes sodium and water excretion. This can help to reduce venous return (preload), which has a beneficial effect in heart failure.
Important adverse effects	Common side effects include **hypotension** (particularly after the **first dose**), and **hyperkalaemia** (because a lower aldosterone level promotes potassium retention). They can cause or worsen **renal failure.** Renal artery stenosis presents a particular risk, as constriction of the efferent glomerular arteriole is required to maintain glomerular filtration. If detected early, these adverse effects are usually reversible on stopping the drug. **Dry cough** is also common and caused by increased levels of bradykinin (which is inactivated by ACE). An **angiotensin receptor blocker** is an alternative if this occurs. Rare but important side effects of ACE inhibitors include **angioedema** and other **anaphylactoid reactions.**
Warnings	ACE inhibitors should be avoided in ✖ **renal artery stenosis** and ✖ **acute kidney injury;** in women who are, or could become, ▲ **pregnant;** or who are ▲ **breastfeeding.** ACE inhibitors are valuable in the treatment of ▲ **CKD,** but lower doses should be used, and renal function monitored closely (see MONITORING).
Important interactions	Due to the risk of hyperkalaemia, avoid prescribing ACE inhibitors with other ▲ **potassium-elevating drugs,** including **potassium** supplements, **aldosterone antagonists** and potassium-sparing diuretics, except under specialist advice for advanced heart failure. In combination with diuretics they may be associated with profound first-dose hypotension. The combination of an ▲ **NSAID** and an ACE inhibitor particularly increases the risk of nephrotoxicity.

PRACTICAL PRESCRIBING

Prescription	The starting dose varies according to the indication, generally being lower in heart failure than in other indications. A common choice is ramipril 1.25 mg orally daily in heart failure or nephropathy, or 2.5 mg orally daily in most other indications. This is titrated to a maximum of 10 mg orally daily over several weeks, according to therapeutic response, side effects, and renal function.
Administration	ACE inhibitors can be taken with or without food. It is best to take the first dose before bed to reduce symptomatic hypotension.
Communication	As applicable, explain that the treatment is intended to improve blood pressure control, reduce strain on the heart, and/or to slow the rate of kidney damage. Advise about common side effects such as a dry cough, and dizziness due to low blood pressure, particularly after the first dose. Mention that, very rarely, this medicine can cause effects similar to severe allergic reactions; they should stop taking it and seek urgent medical advice if they develop facial swelling or stomach pains. Emphasise the need for blood test monitoring, explaining that ACE inhibitors can upset potassium balance. Advise them to avoid taking over-the-counter 'antiinflammatories' (**NSAIDs**) due to the risk of kidney damage. Advise that if they develop diarrhoea or vomiting, to maintain their fluid intake, and stop the ACE inhibitor until their symptoms resolve. These 'sick day rules' reduce the risk of dehydration, low blood pressure, and kidney damage.
Monitoring and stopping	Monitor **efficacy** clinically; for example, severity of breathlessness in heart failure, and blood pressure in hypertension. For **safety,** check electrolytes and renal function before starting treatment. Repeat these 1–2 weeks into treatment and after increasing the dose. Biochemical changes can be tolerated provided they are within certain limits. The ACE inhibitor should generally be stopped if serum creatinine rises more than 30% or the estimated glomerular filtration rate (eGFR) falls more than 25%. If serum potassium rises above 5.0 mmol/L, stop other potassium-elevating and nephrotoxic drugs (see INTERACTIONS). If, despite this, it remains above 5.0 mmol/L, reduce the ACE inhibitor dose. If it exceeds 6.0 mmol/L, stop the ACE inhibitor and seek expert advice. ACE inhibitors may be required indefinitely, but treatment aims should be reviewed regularly. For example, easing of blood pressure targets in those aged over 80 years, or who develop frailty or multimorbidity, may allow dose reduction or discontinuation.
Cost	ACE inhibitors are available as inexpensive non-proprietary products.

Clinical tip—Concomitant use of diuretics can increase the risk of profound first-dose hypotension with an ACE inhibitor. You should start at a low dose and consider omitting the diuretic dose that precedes the first dose of the ACE inhibitor.

Antidepressants, selective serotonin reuptake inhibitors

CLINICAL PHARMACOLOGY

Common indications	❶ As first-line treatment for **moderate-to-severe depression,** and in **mild depression** if psychological treatments alone are insufficient. ❷ **Panic disorder.** ❸ **Obsessive compulsive disorder.**
Mechanisms of action	Selective serotonin reuptake inhibitors (SSRIs) preferentially **inhibit neuronal reuptake of 5-hydroxytryptamine (serotonin) (5-HT)** from the synaptic cleft, thereby increasing its availability for neurotransmission. This appears to be the mechanism by which SSRIs improve mood and physical symptoms in depression and relieve symptoms of panic and obsessive disorders. SSRIs differ from **tricyclic antidepressants** in that they do not inhibit noradrenaline uptake and cause less blockade of other receptors. The efficacy of the two drug classes in the treatment of depression is similar. However, SSRIs are generally preferred as they have fewer adverse effects and are less dangerous in overdose.
Important adverse effects	Common adverse effects include **GI upset,** changes in **appetite** and **weight** (loss or gain), and **hypersensitivity** reactions, including skin rash. **Hyponatraemia** is an important adverse effect, particularly in older people, and may present with confusion and reduced consciousness. **Suicidal thoughts and behaviour** may be associated with SSRIs. They may **lower the seizure threshold,** though the evidence for this is conflicting. Some (e.g. citalopram) can **prolong the QT interval,** predisposing to arrhythmias. SSRIs also increase the risk of **bleeding.** At high doses, in overdose or in combination with other **serotonergic drugs** (e.g. other antidepressants, **tramadol**), SSRIs can cause **serotonin syndrome.** This triad of autonomic hyperactivity, altered mental state, and neuromuscular excitation usually responds to treatment withdrawal and supportive therapy. **Sudden withdrawal** of SSRIs can cause GI upset, neurological and flu-like symptoms, and sleep disturbance.
Warnings	Caution is required in ▲ **epilepsy** and ▲ **peptic ulcer disease.** In ▲ **young people,** SSRIs have poor efficacy and are associated with an increased risk of self-harm and suicidal thoughts, so should be prescribed by specialists only. As SSRIs are metabolised by the liver, dose reduction may be required in people with ▲ **hepatic impairment.**
Important interactions	SSRIs should not be given with ✖ **monoamine oxidase inhibitors** and other ▲ **serotonergic drugs** (e.g. **tramadol**), as together they may precipitate serotonin syndrome. Bleeding risk is increased if SSRIs are taken with **anticoagulants**, **aspirin**, or **NSAIDs**, and gastroprotection should be considered. Citalopram should not be combined with other ▲ **drugs that prolong the QT interval,** such as **antipsychotics.**

PRACTICAL PRESCRIBING

Prescription	SSRIs should be started at a low dose. A typical starting prescription might be for citalopram 20 mg orally daily. The dose is increased as necessary according to response. Lower starting and maximum doses are recommended for older people.
Administration	Citalopram is available as tablets and as oral drops, which can be mixed with water or other drinks. Oral drops have higher bioavailability than tablets, so are not dose-equivalent. For example, one citalopram 20-mg tablet is equivalent to 16 mg in oral drops.
Communication	Advise that treatment should improve symptoms over a few weeks, particularly sleep and appetite. Discuss the possible role of psychological therapy, which may offer more long-term benefits than drug treatment. Explain that treatment should be continued after they feel better to reduce the chance of depression coming back (see Monitoring). Advise that treatment should not be stopped suddenly as this may cause a withdrawal reaction (stomach upset, flu-like symptoms, sleeping difficulty). While the common adverse effects may be unpleasant, people may tolerate them in preference to depressive symptoms. Pre-emptive discussion of side effects may encourage adherence with treatment, at least until the full antidepressant effects are realised.
Monitoring and stopping	Symptoms should be reviewed 1–2 weeks after starting treatment and regularly thereafter. If no effect has been seen at 4 weeks, consider changing the dose or drug; otherwise, the dose should not be adjusted until after 6–8 weeks of therapy. Once established on treatment, the need to continue this should take into account the number of previous episodes of depression, ongoing symptoms, persistent physical health issues, and psychosocial difficulties. Drug treatment is usually continued for at least 6 months after resolution of symptoms (2 years for recurrent depression) to reduce the risk of relapse. To stop SSRI treatment, the dose and/or frequency should be gradually reduced over 4 weeks to minimise withdrawal symptoms and relapse. Fluoxetine can be stopped more quickly (e.g. abruptly at a dose of 20 mg, or over 2 weeks if taking higher doses) as it, and its metabolites, have a longer half-life.
Cost	SSRIs are available in inexpensive non-proprietary forms.

Clinical tip—For women with breast cancer, treatments that suppress ovarian function can cause early menopause or menopausal symptoms. At the same time, **hormonal replacement therapy** must be avoided because of tumour stimulation. In these circumstances, SSRIs are a useful treatment option for menopausal symptoms. However, paroxetine and fluoxetine (which inhibit CYP2D6) should not be prescribed with tamoxifen due to an interaction (see **Hormone agonists and antagonists in prostate and breast cancer**).

Antidepressants, tetracyclic, and serotonin–noradrenaline reuptake inhibitors

CLINICAL PHARMACOLOGY

Common indications	❶ As an option for **major depression,** if first-line **selective serotonin reuptake inhibitor** (SSRI) treatment is ineffective or not tolerated. ❷ **Generalised anxiety disorder** (venlafaxine, duloxetine). ❸ **Diabetic neuropathy** (duloxetine)
Mechanisms of action	Venlafaxine and duloxetine are a **serotonin–noradrenaline reuptake inhibitors (SNRIs),** interfering with uptake of these neurotransmitters from the synaptic cleft. Mirtazapine is a **tetracyclic antidepressant.** It **antagonises** inhibitory **pre-synaptic α_2-adrenoceptors.** All three drugs increase availability of **monoamines** for neurotransmission, which appears to be the mechanism whereby they improve mood and physical symptoms in moderate-to-severe (but not mild) depression. Duloxetine is also used in neuropathic pain, where it may act by increasing synaptic noradrenaline concentration in descending spinal inhibitory pathways. Venlafaxine and duloxetine are weaker antagonists of muscarinic and histamine (H_1) receptors than **tricyclic antidepressants,** whereas mirtazapine is a potent antagonist of histamine (H_1) but not muscarinic receptors. They therefore have fewer antimuscarinic side effects than tricyclic antidepressants, although mirtazapine commonly causes sedation.
Important adverse effects	Common adverse effects of both drugs include **GI upset** (e.g. nausea, change in weight, and diarrhoea or constipation), **dry mouth,** and **neurological effects** (e.g. headache, abnormal dreams, insomnia, confusion, and convulsions). Less common but serious adverse effects include **hyponatraemia** and **serotonin syndrome** (see **Antidepressants, selective serotonin reuptake inhibitors**). **Suicidal thoughts and behaviour** may increase. Venlafaxine prolongs the QT interval and can increase the risk of ventricular arrhythmias. **Sudden drug withdrawal** can cause GI upset, neurological and flu-like symptoms, and sleep disturbance. Venlafaxine is associated with a greater risk of withdrawal effects than other antidepressants. Mirtazepine may cause **bone marrow suppression.**
Warnings	As with many centrally acting medications, ▲ **older people** are more at risk of adverse effects. Dose reduction should be considered in ▲ **hepatic** or ▲ **renal impairment,** and duloxetine avoided in severe renal impairment. Venlafaxine should be avoided, or otherwise used with caution, in people at risk of ▲ **arrhythmias** (e.g. due to ischaemic heart disease).
Important interactions	The combination of these drugs with drugs from other antidepressant classes can increase the risk of adverse effects (including serotonin syndrome, see **Antidepressants, selective serotonin reuptake inhibitors**) and should, in general, be avoided.

PRACTICAL PRESCRIBING

Prescription	In the treatment of **depression,** these drugs should be reserved for use when SSRIs are ineffective, and prescribed only by those with relevant expertise. They should be used in conjunction with psychological therapies. They are taken orally and the dose varies by indication. Treatment is started at a low dose and titrated up according to response. In **peripheral neuropathic pain,** a typical starting dose of duloxetine is 60 mg orally daily.
Administration	Mirtazapine should be taken at night to mitigate (or benefit from) its sedative effects.
Communication	Advise that treatment should improve symptoms over a few weeks, particularly sleep and appetite. Discuss the potential role of psychological therapy, which may offer more long-term benefits than drug treatment. Explain that they should continue treatment after they feel better, to reduce the chance of depression coming back (see MONITORING). Outline common side effects, including drowsiness, which may impair their ability to drive. While the common adverse effects may be unpleasant, people may tolerate them in preference to depressive symptoms. Pre-emptive discussion of these may encourage adherence with treatment, at least until the full antidepressant effects are realised. Advise that treatment should not be stopped suddenly as this may cause a withdrawal reaction (stomach upset, flu-like symptoms, sleeping difficulty). For mirtazapine, explain that if they develop symptoms of infection, such as sore throat, they should seek medical attention as this could be the early sign of a serious side effect (bone marrow suppression).
Monitoring and stopping	Review symptoms 1–2 weeks after starting treatment and regularly thereafter. If no effect has been seen at 4 weeks, consider changing the dose or drug; otherwise, the dose should not be adjusted until after 6–8 weeks of therapy. Once established, the need to continue treatment should take account of number of previous episodes of depression, ongoing symptoms, persistent physical health issues, and psychosocial difficulties. Drug treatment is usually continued for at least 6 months after resolution of symptoms (2 years for recurrent depression) to reduce the risk of relapse. To stop the drugs, taper the dose over several weeks (the risk of withdrawal is highest with venlafaxine).
Cost	These drugs are available as inexpensive non-proprietary products.

Clinical tip—Counterintuitively, some evidence suggests that mirtazapine's sedative effects are *less* severe at *higher* doses. This may be because at low dose its (sedating) antihistamine effect predominates, while at higher doses this is counteracted by increased monoaminergic effect. However, this is not proven in clinical dosage ranges, so we do not advise increasing the dose to overcome sedation.

Antidepressants, tricyclics, and related drugs

CLINICAL PHARMACOLOGY

Common indications	❶ As second-line treatment for moderate-to-severe **depression** where first-line **selective serotonin reuptake inhibitors** (SSRIs) are ineffective. ❷ **Neuropathic pain,** particularly if this is interfering with sleep. ❸ **Irritable bowel syndrome,** if abdominal pain persists despite an antispasmodic (e.g. an **antimuscarinic** or mebeverine). ❹ Amitriptyline is an option to prevent frequent **migraine** attacks.
Mechanisms of action	Tricyclic antidepressants **inhibit neuronal reuptake of 5-hydroxytryptamine (serotonin) (5-HT) and noradrenaline** from the synaptic cleft, increasing their availability for neurotransmission. This is likely the mechanism by which they improve mood and physical symptoms in depression. Increasing synaptic noradrenaline concentration in descending spinal inhibitory pathways probably accounts for their effect in modifying **neuropathic pain** and reducing abdominal pain associated with **irritable bowel syndrome** (where reduction in gut transit time may also reduce diarrhoea) and **migraine**. Tricyclic antidepressants block an array of receptors, including muscarinic, histamine (H₁), α-adrenergic (α₁ and α₂), and dopamine (D₂) receptors. This accounts for the extensive adverse effect profile.
Important adverse effects	Blockade of *antimuscarinic receptors* causes **dry mouth, constipation, urinary retention,** blurred vision and can cause and exacerbate **cognitive impairment,** particularly in older people. Blockade of *histamine (H₁)-* and *adrenergic (α₁)-receptors* causes **sedation** and **hypotension.** Through multiple mechanisms, cardiac adverse effects include **arrhythmias** and **electrocardiogram (ECG) changes** (including prolongation of the QT and QRS durations). In the brain, serious effects include **seizures, hallucinations,** and **mania.** Blockade of *dopamine (D₂) receptors* can cause **breast changes** and **sexual dysfunction,** and rarely **extrapyramidal symptoms** (tremor and dyskinesia). Tricyclic antidepressants are **dangerous in overdose,** causing life-threatening hypotension, arrhythmias, seizures, coma, and respiratory failure. **Sudden withdrawal** can cause GI upset, neurological and flu-like symptoms, and sleep disturbance.
Warnings	Caution is required in ▲ **older people** and those with ▲ **epilepsy** or ▲ **cardiovascular disease.** Due to their antimuscarinic effects, these drugs may worsen ▲ **constipation,** ▲ **glaucoma,** and urinary symptoms due to ▲ **prostatic enlargement.**
Important interactions	Tricyclic antidepressants should not be given with ✖ **monoamine oxidase inhibitors** as both drug classes increase 5-HT and noradrenaline levels at the synapse and together they can precipitate hypertension and hyperthermia or serotonin syndrome (see **Antidepressants, selective serotonin reuptake inhibitors**). Tricyclic antidepressants can augment antimuscarinic, sedative or hypotensive adverse effects of other drugs.

PRACTICAL PRESCRIBING

Prescription	For **depression,** tricyclic antidepressants have similar efficacy to other antidepressants (e.g. SSRIs), but more severe adverse effects, particularly in overdose. They should be reserved for use when SSRIs are ineffective, and only under specialist direction. A second SSRI is often trialled *before* switching to tricyclic antidepressants. Lofepramine appears to have fewer side effects, including sedation, than other tricyclics. For **neuropathic pain** and **irritable bowel syndrome,** amitriptyline is used at much lower doses (e.g. starting dose 10 mg orally at night) than in depression (typical starting dose 75 mg daily).
Administration	Tricyclic antidepressants are available as tablets and in oral solution. When prescribing for depression, particularly for people at risk of suicide, it is good practice to supply a small quantity at a time (e.g. enough for 2 weeks) to reduce the risk of serious overdose.
Communication	Advise that treatment should improve symptoms over a few weeks, particularly sleep and appetite. Discuss the potential role of psychological therapy, which may offer more long-term benefits than drug treatment. Explain that they should continue treatment after they feel better, to reduce the chance of depression coming back (see Monitoring). Outline common side effects, including drowsiness, which may impair their ability to drive. While the common adverse effects may be unpleasant, people may tolerate them in preference to depressive symptoms. Pre-emptive discussion of these may encourage adherence with treatment, at least until the full antidepressant effects are realised. Advise that treatment should not be stopped suddenly as this may cause a withdrawal reaction (stomach upset, flu-like symptoms, sleeping difficulty).
Monitoring and stopping	Review symptoms 1–2 weeks after starting treatment and regularly thereafter. If no effect is seen at 4 weeks, consider changing the dose or drug; otherwise, the dose should not be adjusted until after 6–8 weeks of therapy. Once treatment for depression is established, the need to continue it should take into account the number of previous episodes of depression, ongoing symptoms, persistent physical health issues, and psychosocial difficulties. Drug treatment is usually continued for at least 6 months after resolution of symptoms (2 years for recurrent depression) to reduce the risk of relapse. To stop, taper the dose over 4 weeks to reduce risk of withdrawal symptoms.
Cost	Non-proprietary forms of tricyclic antidepressants are inexpensive.

Clinical tip—In our experience, people admitted to hospital may have their antidepressants stopped abruptly, either because they are thought erroneously to be contributing to their presentation or because they are overlooked. Take care not to do this without good reason (e.g. if serotonin toxicity is suspected), to avoid precipitating a withdrawal reaction.

Antiemetics, dopamine D₂-receptor antagonists

CLINICAL PHARMACOLOGY

Common indications	Prophylaxis and treatment of **nausea and vomiting** in a wide range of conditions, but particularly in the context of **reduced gut motility.**
Mechanisms of action	Nausea and vomiting are triggered by gut irritation, drugs, motion, vestibular disorders, and higher stimuli (sights, smells, emotions). The pathways converge on a 'vomiting centre' in the medulla, which receives inputs from the chemoreceptor trigger zone (CTZ), the vagus nerve, the vestibular system, and higher centres. Dopamine is relevant in two respects. First, the dopamine D_2 receptor is the main receptor in the CTZ, which senses emetogenic substances (e.g. drugs) in blood. **Antagonism** of the **D_2-receptor** is therefore useful in nausea and vomiting caused by CTZ stimulation. Second, dopamine is an important neurotransmitter in the gut, where it promotes relaxation of the stomach and lower oesophageal sphincter and inhibits gastroduodenal coordination. D_2-receptor antagonists (particularly metoclopramide, which is augmented with enteric 5-HT_4 agonist activity) therefore have a **prokinetic effect.** This contributes to their antiemetic action in states of reduced gut motility (e.g. due to **opioids** or diabetic gastroparesis). D_2-receptor antagonists are classified as *benzamides* (e.g. metoclopramide, domperidone) and *phenothiazines* (e.g. prochlorperazine).
Important adverse effects	**Diarrhoea** is common. Metoclopramide and prochlorperazine can induce **extrapyramidal effects** (movement abnormalities) by the same mechanism as **antipsychotics**. Domperidone does not, as it does not cross the blood–brain barrier (note the CTZ is largely outside the blood–brain barrier). It causes **QT interval prolongation** and **arrhythmias**. Prochloperazine causes drowsiness (see **Antipsychotics, first generation**).
Warnings	Metoclopramide should be avoided in ✖ **neonates,** ▲ **children,** and ▲ **young adults.** Domperidone is contraindicated in ▲ **severe hepatic impairment** and ✖ **cardiac conduction defects.** It is not licensed for ✖ **children under 12 years** or people ✖ **weighing less than 35 kg.** Prokinetics are contraindicated in ▲ **intestinal obstruction** and ✖ **perforation.** D_2-antagonists are avoided in ▲ **Parkinson's disease,** but domperidone may be used as it does not cross the blood–brain barrier.
Important interactions	Extrapyramidal side effects are more likely if metoclopramide is prescribed with ▲ **antipsychotics.** It should not be combined with ✖ **dopaminergic agents for Parkinson's disease,** as it will antagonise their effects. Domperidone should not be prescribed with other ▲ **drugs that prolong the QT interval,** such as antipsychotics, **quinine,** and **selective serotonin reuptake inhibitors,** or ▲ **drugs that inhibit cytochrome P450 (CYP) enzymes** (e.g. **amiodarone, diltiazem, macrolides, fluconazole, protease inhibitors**) as these increase the risk of adverse effects.

PRACTICAL PRESCRIBING

Prescription	Due to their adverse effects, D_2-receptor antagonists should be used for short-term treatment only (maximum 5–7 days). The starting dose for both metoclopramide and domperidone is 10 mg orally 8-hrly. Metoclopramide can also be prescribed for IM or IV injection at the same dose. The route of administration, and whether it is prescribed on a regular or as-required basis, depends on the clinical situation. For example, the oral route is clearly inappropriate in active vomiting. When treating gastroparesis, metoclopramide is preferred because of its better safety profile. Due to its tendency to cause drowsiness, prochlorperazine is reserved as a second-line agent in severe cases, when it may be given by IM injection.
Administration	IV injections of metoclopramide should be given slowly (over at least 3 minutes for a standard 10-mg dose).
Communication	Explain that you are offering an antisickness medicine. As appropriate, explain that only short-term use is recommended (but see CLINICAL TIP). Explain that although most individuals are able to take it without significant side effects, a minority experience movement abnormalities, which can be significant. Advise them to stop taking the medicine and seek medical attention if they notice any side effects of this type.
Monitoring and stopping	Resolution of symptoms is the best guide to efficacy and stopping. Prolonged use is not recommended (see CLINICAL TIP), but if unavoidable, monitor carefully for extrapyramidal features. These may be subtle (e.g. an increased tendency to fall) and their relationship to the drug may not be obvious.
Cost	Non-proprietary preparations of these drugs are inexpensive.

Clinical tip—Despite general recommendations to limit duration of D_2-receptor antagonist therapy, gastroparesis may require long-term prokinetic treatment (i.e. greater than 5 days). To minimise exposure to metoclopramide, it should be used at the lowest effective dose (e.g. 5 mg 8-hrly). It may be alternated with erythromycin, which also has prokinetic properties. It is also good practice to have regular trials of treatment suspension ('drug holidays') to ensure it is still needed.

Antiemetics, histamine H₁-receptor antagonists

CLINICAL PHARMACOLOGY

Common indications	Prophylaxis and treatment of **nausea and vomiting,** particularly in the context of **motion sickness** or **vertigo.** Other drugs in this class are used in the treatment of allergies (see **Antihistamines (H₁-receptor antagonists)**).
Mechanisms of action	Nausea and vomiting are triggered by gut irritation, drugs, motion, vestibular disorders, and higher stimuli (sights, smells, emotions). The pathways converge on a 'vomiting centre' in the medulla, which receives inputs from the chemoreceptor trigger zone, the vagus nerve (via the solitary tract nucleus), the vestibular system, and higher centres. Histamine H₁ and muscarinic acetylcholine receptors predominate in the **vomiting centre** and in its communication with the **vestibular system.** Drugs such as cyclizine block both receptors. This makes them useful treatments for nausea and vomiting in a wide range of conditions (e.g. drug-induced, postoperative, radiotherapy), particularly when associated with motion or vertigo.
Important adverse effects	The most common adverse effect is **drowsiness.** Cyclizine is the least sedating drug in this class and is therefore usually preferred. Due to their anticholinergic effects they may cause **dry throat and mouth.** This is usually undesirable, but in people with copious mucosal secretions it may be beneficial. After IV injection they may cause transient **tachycardia,** which may be experienced as **palpitations.** Along with their central anticholinergic effects (excitation or depression) this may make for a rather unpleasant experience.
Warnings	Due to their sedating effect, these drugs should be avoided in people at risk of ▲ **hepatic encephalopathy.** They should also be avoided in people susceptible to anticholinergic side effects, such as those with ▲ **prostatic enlargement** (who may develop urinary retention).
Important interactions	Sedation may be greater when combined with other sedative drugs (e.g. **benzodiazepines**, **opioids**). Anticholinergic effects may be more pronounced in people taking **ipratropium** or **tiotropium.**

PRACTICAL PRESCRIBING

Prescription	A typical prescription might be for cyclizine 50 mg 8-hrly as required. It may be given orally, IV or IM at the same dose. The route of administration, and whether it is prescribed on a regular or as-required basis, depends on the clinical situation. For example, the oral route is clearly inappropriate if there is active vomiting. As IM injections are painful and rapid IV injections are unpleasant (see ADVERSE EFFECTS), *slow* IV injection is the best choice when oral administration is inappropriate.
Administration	Intravenous injections of cyclizine should be given slowly (over about 2 minutes).
Communication	Explain that you are offering an anti-sickness medicine. Although it is generally effective, it does not work for everyone and a second or different medicine may be necessary. Ask them to let you know if they do not achieve satisfactory relief. Advise that the medicine may cause drowsiness and impair the ability to perform tasks such as driving, which they should therefore avoid.
Monitoring and stopping	Resolution of symptoms is the best guide to efficacy. Antiemetics may be taken on an as-required basis, in which case treatment will naturally stop when the underlying cause has resolved. If taken regularly on a pre-emptive basis, periodic interruption of treatment is advisable to determine whether it is still needed.
Cost	Oral antihistamine antiemetics are inexpensive.

Clinical tip—H_1-receptor antagonists are commonly used in the prevention and treatment of motion sickness. Hyoscine hydrobromide (an **antimuscarinic** drug) is a useful alternative. It is widely used as an over-the-counter remedy for this indication and is effective. It can also be usefully administered transdermally using a patch, applied behind the ear a few hours before departure. One 1.5-mg patch can be left in place for up to 72 hours, over which time the average amount absorbed is 1 mg.

Antiemetics, serotonin 5-HT₃-receptor antagonists

CLINICAL PHARMACOLOGY

Common indications	Prophylaxis and treatment of **nausea and vomiting,** particularly in the context of general anaesthesia and chemotherapy.
Mechanisms of action	Nausea and vomiting are triggered by gut irritation, drugs, motion, vestibular disorders, and higher stimuli (sights, smells, emotions). The pathways converge on a 'vomiting centre' in the medulla, which receives inputs from the **chemoreceptor trigger zone (CTZ),** the vagus nerve, the vestibular system and higher centres. **Serotonin (5-hydroxytryptamine (5-HT))** plays an important role in two of these pathways. First, there is a high density of 5-HT₃ receptors in the CTZ, which are responsible for sensing emetogenic substances in the blood (e.g. drugs). Second, 5-HT is the key neurotransmitter released by the gut in response to emetogenic stimuli. Acting on 5-HT₃ receptors, it stimulates the vagus nerve, which in turn activates the vomiting centre via the solitary tract nucleus. Of note, 5-HT is not involved in communication between the vestibular system and the vomiting centre. Thus 5-HT₃ antagonists are effective against nausea and vomiting as a result of CTZ stimulation (e.g. drugs) and visceral stimuli (gut infection, radiotherapy), but not in motion sickness.
Important adverse effects	**Constipation, headache,** and **flushing** are common. Serious adverse effects are rare. There is a small risk that 5-HT₃ antagonists may **prolong the QT interval,** although this is usually evident only at high doses (e.g. >16 mg ondansetron).
Warnings	5-HT₃ antagonists should be used with caution in people with ▲ **prolonged QT interval.** If there is a risk factor for this, review an electrocardiogram (ECG) before prescribing. Ondansetron is not recommended in the first trimester of ▲ **pregnancy,** as it has been linked in epidemiological studies to an increased risk of cleft lip and palate.
Important interactions	Avoid 5-HT₃ antagonists in people taking ▲ **drugs that prolong the QT interval,** such as **antipsychotics**, **quinine,** and **selective serotonin reuptake inhibitors**.

PRACTICAL PRESCRIBING

Prescription	A typical starting dose for ondansetron is 4–8 mg 12-hrly, orally or IV. The dosing regimens differ for each indication, with higher doses generally reserved for chemotherapy-induced nausea and vomiting. Oral, rectal, and injectable preparations are available. The route of administration, and whether it is prescribed on a regular or as-required basis, depends on the clinical indication. As IM injections are painful, the IV route is usually preferable if oral/rectal administration is inappropriate. Where drugs are used to prevent nausea (e.g. before an anaesthetic), oral doses should be taken an hour before symptoms are anticipated. IV doses can be given immediately before the treatment or procedure.
Administration	There are no special considerations in relation to oral administration. IV injections should be given slowly (over about 30 seconds).
Communication	Explain that you are offering an anti-sickness medicine. Generally it is a very safe medicine, although constipation and headache can be troublesome for some people. Although it is generally effective, it does not work for everyone and a second or different medicine may be necessary. Request that they let you know if they do not obtain satisfactory relief.
Monitoring and stopping	Resolution of symptoms is the best guide to efficacy. Antiemetics may be taken on an as-required basis, in which case treatment will naturally stop when the underlying cause has resolved. If taken regularly on a pre-emptive basis, periodic interruption of treatment is advisable to determine whether it is still needed.
Cost	Non-proprietary tablet and injectable formulations of ondansetron are available and relatively inexpensive. Branded ondansetron products, orodispersible tablets and oral solutions, are expensive. Granisetron is expensive.

Clinical tip—Nausea and vomiting of pregnancy, and its more severe form, hyperemesis gravidarum, can be difficult to treat as drugs administered during the first trimester of pregnancy may cause spontaneous abortion and fetal abnormalities. Studies suggest that **histamine H1-receptor antagonists** (e.g. promethazine and cyclizine) and **phenothiazines** (e.g. prochlorperazine) are safe and effective, so these are usually recommended as first-line drug treatments. Other possible treatments include **metoclopramide** or a combination of the antihistamine doxylamine and vitamin pyridoxine. There is less safety data for these, but the information that is available does not suggest they are harmful. Ondansetron can be considered for women with ongoing symptoms despite use of other antiemetics. However, there is a possible link between ondansetron use in early pregnancy and cleft lip/palate and heart defects. A useful source of up-to-date information on the use of medicines in pregnancy is the 'Best use of medicines in pregnancy' (BUMPS) website.

Antifungal drugs

CLINICAL PHARMACOLOGY

Common indications	❶ Treatment of **local fungal infections,** including of the oropharynx, vagina or skin. They may be applied topically (nystatin, clotrimazole) or taken orally (fluconazole). ❷ Systemic treatment of **invasive or disseminated fungal infections.** Specialist treatment is required for these infections, which will not be discussed further in this book.
Mechanisms of action	Fungal cell membranes contain ergosterol. As ergosterol is not found in animal or human cells it is a target for antifungal drugs. **Polyene antifungals** (e.g. nystatin) bind to ergosterol in fungal cell membranes, creating a polar pore which allows intracellular ions to leak out of the cell. This can kill or slow growth of the fungi. **Imidazole** (e.g. clotrimazole) and **triazole antifungals** (e.g. fluconazole) inhibit ergosterol synthesis, impairing cell membrane synthesis, cell growth, and replication. Resistance to antifungals is relatively infrequent but can occur during long-term treatment in people with immune suppression. Mechanisms include alteration of membrane synthesis to exclude ergosterol, changes in target enzymes or increased drug efflux.
Important adverse effects	Nystatin and clotrimazole are used topically at the site of infection, so have few adverse effects apart from occasional **local irritation** where applied. Fluconazole is taken orally and so has systemic adverse effects. The most common are **GI upset** (including nausea, vomiting, diarrhoea, and abdominal pain), **headache, increase in liver enzymes,** and **hypersensitivity** causing skin rash. Rare but potentially life-threatening reactions include **severe hepatic toxicity; prolonged QT interval** predisposing to **arrhythmias;** and severe hypersensitivity, including **cutaneous reactions** and **anaphylaxis.**
Warnings	Topically administered nystatin and clotrimazole have no major contraindications. Fluconazole should be prescribed with caution in ▲ **liver disease** and ▲ **QT interval prolongation**. A dose reduction is required in ▲ **moderate renal impairment.** It should be avoided in ✖ **pregnancy** due to the risk of fetal malformation.
Important interactions	There are no significant drug interactions with topical nystatin or clotrimazole. Fluconazole inhibits cytochrome P450 (CYP) enzymes, causing an increase in plasma concentrations and risk of adverse effects when prescribed with ▲ **drugs metabolised by CYP enzymes,** including **carbamazepine**, phenytoin, **warfarin, diazepam, simvastatin,** and **sulphonylureas**. It may reduce the antiplatelet actions of **clopidogrel,** a pro-drug which requires activation by liver metabolism. It also increases the risk of serious arrhythmias if prescribed with ▲ **drugs that prolong the QT interval,** such as **amiodarone, antipsychotics, quinine, quinolone** and **macrolide** antibiotics and **selective serotonin reuptake inhibitors (SSRIs).**

PRACTICAL PRESCRIBING

Prescription	Nystatin is administered topically for **oropharyngeal candidiasis** (thrush) at a dose of 100,000 units (1 mL) of oral suspension dropped into the mouth four times daily for 7 days or until 48 hours after lesions have resolved. Clotrimazole is used to treat fungal infections of the skin and genital tract, such as **tinea** (ringworm, including athlete's foot) and **candida** (thrush). For skin or mucosal infections, the dose of clotrimazole 1% (1 g in 100 g) cream is one application two or three times daily until 1–2 weeks after infection has resolved. Clotrimazole is also formulated as a pessary for vaginal candidiasis. Fluconazole is prescribed as a single dose of 150 mg orally for **vaginal candidiasis.** For **other mucosal infections,** e.g. of the oropharynx, oesophagus, and airways, the dose is 50 mg orally daily for a more prolonged course (e.g. 1–2 weeks). Treatment duration may be longer for **fungal skin infections.** Fluconazole is also available as an IV preparation for invasive or disseminated fungal infection.
Administration	Oral nystatin should be administered after food and held in the mouth to allow good contact with the lesions. Dentures should be removed to expose affected areas to treatment.
Communication	Advise that, with correct application, treatment should improve symptoms. For skin infections, encourage them to continue treatment for 1–2 weeks after symptoms resolve. If prescribing fluconazole for a prolonged course, advise that they should seek medical advice if they experience any unusual symptoms such as nausea, loss of appetite, lethargy, or dark urine, as these could indicate liver damage.
Monitoring and stopping	**Efficacy** is monitored clinically. Where prolonged courses of fluconazole are required, **safety** should be monitored by measurement of liver enzymes before and during treatment to monitor for hepatic toxicity, particularly where high doses are used. Antifungals are generally prescribed for short courses, which may include a recommendation to continue treatment for a short period once infection has resolved. Make sure the treatment duration and cessation instructions are clear on the prescription.
Cost	Nystatin, clotrimazole, and fluconazole are inexpensive in standard formulations.

Clinical tip—Older people admitted to hospital are particularly susceptible to oral candida infection. They are commonly treated with **antibiotics** and systemic or inhaled **corticosteroids**, which predispose to oral candidiasis, and with **antimuscarinic** drugs that reduce saliva (anatural defence mechanism). A sore mouth can reduce appetite and delay recovery. Take a pen torch on your ward round to check for oral candida infection. Encourage mouth care and prescribe nystatin to promote recovery.

Antihistamines (H₁-receptor antagonists)

CLINICAL PHARMACOLOGY

Common indications	❶ As a first-line treatment for **allergies,** particularly **seasonal allergic rhinitis** (hay fever). ❷ To aid relief of itchiness (**pruritus**) and hives (**urticaria**) due, for example, to insect bites, infections (e.g. chickenpox) and drug allergies. ❸ As symptomatic treatment for skin symptoms in **anaphylaxis,** but only after administration of **adrenaline** and other life-saving measures. Other drugs in this class may be used for **nausea and vomiting** (see **Antiemetics, histamine H₁-receptor antagonists**).
Mechanisms of action	The term 'antihistamine' is generally applied to **antagonists** of the **H₁** receptor. **H₂-receptor antagonists** have different uses and are discussed separately. Histamine is released from storage granules in mast cells in response to antigen binding to IgE on the cell surface. Mainly via H₁ receptors, histamine induces the features of immediate-type (type 1) hypersensitivity: increased capillary permeability causing oedema formation (wheal), vasodilation causing erythema (flare) and itch as a result of sensory nerve stimulation. When histamine is released in the nasopharynx, as in hay fever, it causes nasal irritation, sneezing, rhinorrhoea, congestion, conjunctivitis, and itch. In the skin, it causes urticaria. Widespread histamine release, as in anaphylaxis, produces generalised vasodilation and vascular leakage, with consequent hypotension. Antihistamines work in these conditions by antagonism at the H₁ receptor, blocking the effects of excess histamine. In anaphylaxis, their effect is too slow to be life-saving. They are not recommended in initial emergency treatment (in which **adrenaline** and intravenous fluid resuscitation are the critical components), but they may be used subsequently to treat the skin symptoms.
Important adverse effects	The 'first-generation' antihistamines (e.g. chlorphenamine) cause **sedation.** This is because histamine, via H₁ receptors, has a role in the brain in maintaining wakefulness. Newer 'second-generation' antihistamines (including loratadine, cetirizine, and fexofenadine) do not cross the blood–brain barrier, so tend not to have this effect. They have few adverse effects.
Warnings	Commonly used antihistamines, including those mentioned above, are safe in most people. Sedating antihistamines (e.g. chlorphenamine) should be avoided in ▲ **severe liver disease,** as they may precipitate hepatic encephalopathy.
Important interactions	The antihistamines mentioned here are not subject to any major drug interactions.

PRACTICAL PRESCRIBING

Prescription	Cetirizine (10-mg tablets), loratadine (10-mg tablets) and chlorphenamine (4-mg tablets and 2 mg/5 mL oral solution) may be purchased without prescription. Cetirizine and loratadine are taken orally on a once-daily basis. Chlorphenamine is taken orally every 4–6 hours and can be given intravenously in selected cases.
Administration	There are no special considerations for the administration of cetirizine and loratadine. Although oral chlorphenamine may be taken throughout the day, some people prefer to reserve it for use in the evening when its sedating effect may be desirable.
Communication	As appropriate, explain that you are offering a treatment to help relieve their allergic symptoms or their itchy rash/hives. In hay fever, explain that the tablets improve sneezing, itchiness, and runniness, but tend not to help with nasal congestion. For cetirizine and loratadine, you can say that you do not anticipate any side effects. For chlorphenamine, explain that it may make them feel sleepy or lose concentration. They should therefore avoid taking it if they need to drive or carry out any other activity that requires concentration. They should also avoid combining it with alcohol, which may exacerbate this effect.
Monitoring and stopping	Clinical assessment of allergic symptoms, physical signs (e.g. rash) and enquiry about side effects is the best form of monitoring. Treatment should be stopped if its benefits are outweighed by adverse effects. For allergies with an intermittent or self-limiting time course, treatment should be stopped when the underlying condition resolves or exposure to the allergen reduces (e.g. in hay fever, when atmospheric pollen levels reduce).
Cost	Non-proprietary antihistamines listed here are inexpensive. People who pay for their prescriptions will generally save money if they buy them directly from a pharmacy. There is no reason to use the more expensive brand name products.

Clinical tip—It may be useful to advise that larger pack sizes can be purchased from the pharmacy counter than can be obtained off the shelf or from a non-pharmacy retailer. These may be more convenient and economical.

Antimuscarinics, bronchodilators

CLINICAL PHARMACOLOGY

Common indications	**❶** In **chronic obstructive pulmonary disease (COPD),** short-acting antimuscarinics are used to relieve acute breathlessness associated with, for example, exercise or exacerbations. Long-acting antimuscarinics (LAMAs) are used to prevent breathlessness and exacerbations either (1) in COPD with *no features of asthma or steroid responsiveness,* as first-line regular therapy in combination with a long-acting β₂-agonist (LABA); or (2) in COPD *with features of asthma or steroid responsiveness,* as second-line regular therapy in combination with a LABA and inhaled corticosteroid (see **Corticosteroids, inhaled**). **❷** In **acute severe asthma,** short-acting antimuscarinics may augment the bronchodilator effects of short-acting β₂ agonists (e.g. salbutamol). In **chronic asthma,** LAMAs can be trialled if control is insufficient despite moderate-dose **inhaled corticosteroid** and **LABA** treatment.
Mechanisms of action	Antimuscarinic drugs bind to **muscarinic receptors,** where they act as **competitive inhibitors of acetylcholine.** Stimulation of muscarinic receptors, of which there are various subtypes (designated M_1–M_5), brings about a wide range of parasympathetic 'rest and digest' effects. In blocking the receptors, antimuscarinics have the opposite effects: they increase heart rate and conduction (M_2 receptors); reduce smooth muscle tone, including in the respiratory tract, gut, and urinary tract (M_3 receptors); and reduce secretions from glands in the respiratory tract and gut (M_1 and M_3 receptors). In the eye, they cause relaxation of the pupillary constrictor and ciliary muscles (M_3 receptors), causing pupillary dilation and preventing accommodation, respectively. Inhaled antimuscarinics relieve airway obstruction in COPD and asthma by allowing smooth muscle relaxation, causing bronchodilation, and by reducing respiratory secretions.
Important adverse effects	**Dry mouth** is common. Inhalation may irritate the respiratory tract, causing **cough** or **hoarse voice.** As a class, antimuscarinics can also cause **tachycardia, constipation, urinary retention, and blurred vision.** However, as very little active drug enters the systemic circulation in inhaled therapy, these adverse effects are much less likely than with oral/IV antimuscarinics. This is particularly so for aclidinium, which is hydrolysed rapidly after absorption, and has a low frequency of systemic adverse reactions, including dry mouth.
Warnings	Antimuscarinics should be used with caution in people susceptible to ▲ **angle-closure glaucoma,** in whom they can precipitate a dangerous rise in intraocular pressure, and those with or at risk of ▲ **arrhythmias** or ▲ **urinary retention.** However, in practice, most people can take these drugs by inhalation without major problems.
Important interactions	Interactions are unproblematic, due to the small doses used and the low proportion entering the circulation in active form (low *bioavailability*).

tiotropium, umeclidinium, glycopyrronium, ipratropium

PRACTICAL PRESCRIBING

Prescription

Short-acting antimuscarinics such as ipratropium may be taken regularly or as needed for breathlessness. A typical prescription for stable COPD is ipratropium 40 micrograms inhaled 6-hrly. Higher doses (e.g. 250–500 micrograms nebulised 6-hrly) are used during acute attacks. **Long-acting antimuscarinics** (e.g. tiotropium, glycopyrronium, aclidinium) are taken regularly, once- or twice-daily. They may be prescribed singly or in combination with a **long-acting β₂-agonist** ('dual therapy', LAMA + LABA) or as 'triple therapy', which also includes an **inhaled corticosteroid** (LAMA + LABA + ICS). Inhaler prescriptions should include the brand name so that the same device is dispensed each time, optimising adherence and inhaler technique.

Administration

Inhaled medication comes in a range of inhaler devices, with the choice of medicine often being directed by the device that best suits the individual. Liquid for nebulisation is put into the chamber below a mask covering the mouth and nose. Gas is bubbled through the liquid, vaporising the medicine. In asthma, the driving gas is usually **oxygen**. In people with ▲ **chronic type 2 (hypercapnic) respiratory failure,** who are at risk of carbon dioxide retention, medical air is used.

Communication

Explain that the aim of treatment is to open up the airways, which should reduce shortness of breath. Emphasise that this treats the symptoms, not the disease. Explain clearly how and when to take the inhaler (e.g. for acute symptoms, pre-emptively before exercise, or regularly for long-acting medication). Discuss possible side effects such as dry mouth, and advise them to chew gum or suck sweets (which should be sugar-free; see **Antimuscarinics, genitourinary uses**), or keep a bottle of water with them to relieve these.

Monitoring and stopping

Monitor **efficacy** by asking about symptoms and (for asthma) reviewing peak flow measurements. Monitor **safety** by enquiring about side effects, particularly dry mouth. **Check inhaler technique** at every review, and correct it as necessary to optimise treatment effects. Stop short-acting antimuscarinics if a LAMA is started. Stop LAMAs if they are ineffective, e.g. after a treatment trial in asthma.

Cost

Ipratropium is available in inexpensive non-proprietary forms. LAMAs are newer medicines, with most drugs and inhaler devices remaining under patent protection. They are therefore relatively expensive.

Clinical tip—There is no advantage in prescribing short-acting antimuscarinics more often than 6-hrly, as this increases adverse effects without increasing benefits. By contrast, **β₂ agonists** can be administered more frequently (e.g. 2-hrly) if needed, increasing the bronchodilator effect, albeit at a cost of more intense adverse effects.

Antimuscarinics, cardiovascular and GI uses

CLINICAL PHARMACOLOGY

Common indications	❶ Atropine and glycopyrronium are first-line options in the management of severe or symptomatic **bradycardia,** to increase heart rate. ❷ Antimuscarinics (particularly hyoscine butylbromide) are first-line drug treatment options for **irritable bowel syndrome (IBS),** where they are used for their antispasmodic effect. Mebeverine (a direct-acting smooth muscle relaxant) is an alternative that may be better tolerated. ❸ In **palliative care,** antimuscarinics (e.g. glycopyrronium, hyoscine butylbromide) are used to prevent or reduce copious **respiratory secretions,** which can cause distressing noisy breathing.
Mechanisms of action	Antimuscarinic drugs bind to the muscarinic receptor, where they act as a **competitive inhibitor of acetylcholine.** *Stimulation* of muscarinic receptors, of which there are various subtypes (designated M_1–M_5), brings about a wide range of parasympathetic 'rest and digest' effects. In *blocking* the receptors, antimuscarinics have the opposite effects: they increase heart rate and conduction (M_2 receptors); reduce tone and peristaltic contraction of smooth muscle in the gut and urinary tract (M_3 receptors); and reduce secretions from glands in the respiratory tract and gut (M_1 and M_3 receptors). In the eye, they cause relaxation of the pupillary constrictor and ciliary muscles (M_3 receptors), causing pupillary dilation and preventing accommodation, respectively.
Important adverse effects	Predictably from their antagonism of parasympathetic 'rest and digest' effects, antimuscarinics can cause **tachycardia, dry mouth,** and **constipation.** By reducing detrusor (bladder) muscle activity, they can cause **urinary retention**. Their ocular effects may cause **blurred vision,** especially for near objects. Muscarinic receptors (particularly M_1) are widely distributed in the brain, and lipid-soluble antimuscarinics (the tertiary amines such as atropine) have central effects including **drowsiness** and **confusion,** particularly in older people. Quaternary ammonium compounds such as glycopyrronium and hyoscine butylbromide (but *not* hyoscine hydrobromide—see CLINICAL TIP) are less lipid soluble, and so have fewer central nervous system effects.
Warnings	There are no contraindications to the use of antimuscarinics for life-threatening bradycardia. In other indications, caution should be exercised in people susceptible to ▲ **angle-closure glaucoma,** in whom they can precipitate a dangerous rise in intraocular pressure. They should generally be avoided in people at risk of ▲ **arrhythmias** (e.g. those with significant cardiac disease, unless of course the indication for use is bradycardia). They may precipitate urinary retention in people with ▲ **benign prostatic enlargement.**
Important interactions	Adverse effects are more pronounced when they are combined with other drugs that have antimuscarinic effects, such as **tricyclic antidepressants**.

PRACTICAL PRESCRIBING

Prescription	For **bradycardia,** atropine is given IV in incremental doses (e.g. 500 micrograms every 1–2 minutes, to a maximum of 3 mg) until an acceptable heart rate is restored. Glycopyrronium is an alternative. It does not penetrate the brain so causes less drowsiness, but it tends not to be so readily available on general wards. For **IBS,** an antimuscarinic is taken orally on a regular basis. Hyoscine butylbromide (Buscopan®) 10 mg 8-hrly is a common choice and available without prescription. For the control of **respiratory secretions,** glycopyronnium or hyoscine butylbromide can be given SC, either by injection or as part of a continuous infusion.
Administration	In general, IV administration of atropine should be performed only by, or under direct supervision of, an individual experienced in its use. To facilitate rapid administration in emergencies, atropine is provided in pre-filled disposable syringes. It is a good idea to familiarise yourself with these devices before you need to use them for real. The concentration of atropine in pre-filled syringes may be 100, 200 or 300 micrograms/mL—be sure to check this before administration.
Communication	Depending on the clinical context, it may be appropriate to outline common adverse effects, such as dry mouth and blurred vision.
Monitoring and stopping	When using antimuscarinics to increase heart rate, high-intensity monitoring (including continuous cardiac rhythm monitoring) is required. It is essential that this is continued after restoration of normal heart rate, as the effect of the drug may be transient. For other indications, enquiry about symptoms is the best guide to the effect of treatment and its continued value. The dose is titrated to achieve the optimal balance between beneficial and adverse effects.
Cost	Antimuscarinics are relatively inexpensive.

Clinical tip—Take care not to confuse hyoscine butylbromide and hyoscine hydrobromide. Hyoscine butylbromide is a quaternary amine with few central nervous system effects. Hyoscine hydrobromide is a tertiary amine which crosses the blood–brain barrier and commonly causes drowsiness, dizziness, and (in older people) confusion. Their dosages are also an order of magnitude different. Hyoscine butylbromide is preferred for most indications, but hyoscine hydrobromide has one remaining common use: it is available as a transdermal patch, which is a convenient option for prevention and treatment of motion sickness.

Antimuscarinics, genitourinary uses

CLINICAL PHARMACOLOGY

Common indications	To reduce urinary frequency, urgency and urge incontinence in **overactive bladder,** as a first-line pharmacological treatment if bladder training is ineffective.
Mechanisms of action	Antimuscarinic drugs bind to muscarinic receptors, where they act as a **competitive inhibitor of acetylcholine.** Contraction of the smooth muscle of the bladder is under parasympathetic control. Blocking muscarinic receptors therefore promotes bladder relaxation, increasing bladder capacity. In overactive bladder, this may reduce urinary frequency, urgency, and urge incontinence. Antimuscarinics work in overactive bladder through **antagonism at the M_3 receptor,** which is the main muscarinic receptor subtype in the bladder. Solifenacin is more selective for the M_3 receptor, which may reduce side effects caused by actions on other muscarinic receptor subtypes (see **Antimuscarinics, cardiovascular and GI uses**).
Important adverse effects	Predictably from their antimuscarinic action, **dry mouth** is a very common side effect of these drugs. Other classic antimuscarinic side effects such as **tachycardia, constipation,** and **blurred vision** are also common. **Urinary retention** may occur if there is bladder outflow obstruction. **Cognitive effects** (e.g. drowsiness, confusion) are most problematic with oxybutynin, because it is lipid soluble (so readily crosses the blood–brain barrier) and also acts on the M_1 receptor (which is widely distributed in the brain).
Warnings	Antimuscarinics are contraindicated in ✖ **urinary tract infection.** Urinalysis is therefore an important part of assessment before prescribing treatment for overactive bladder. Cognitive effects can be particularly problematic in ▲ **older people** and those with ▲ **dementia.** Antimuscarinics should be used with caution in people susceptible to ▲ **angle-closure glaucoma,** in whom they can precipitate a dangerous rise in intraocular pressure. They should be used with caution in people at risk of ▲ **arrhythmias** (e.g. those with significant cardiac disease) and, for obvious reasons, those at risk of ▲ **urinary retention.**
Important interactions	Adverse effects are more pronounced when combined with other drugs that have antimuscarinic effects, such as ▲ **tricyclic antidepressants**.

PRACTICAL PRESCRIBING

Prescription	You should prescribe antimuscarinics for **urge incontinence** only after an adequate trial of non-pharmacological treatment, including bladder training, weight loss, and caffeine reduction. Where they are indicated, an immediate-release antimuscarinic medication is recommended for first-line therapy. A typical prescription would be for tolterodine 2 mg orally every 12 hours. Other formulations (e.g. modified-release (MR) tablets, transdermal patches) and other antimuscarinics should be reserved for use when an immediate-release preparation is ineffective or poorly tolerated.
Administration	Immediate-release antimuscarinics should be taken at roughly equal intervals, with or without food. MR forms should be taken at a similar time each day and swallowed whole, not chewed.
Communication	Explain that you are offering a treatment with a medicine that relaxes the bladder. This will hopefully reduce how often they need to pass water, the urgency with which they need to get to the toilet, and the chance of accidents. However, it can take at least 4 weeks, and sometimes substantially longer, for the full benefits to be realised. Explain that dry mouth is a very common side effect, affecting more than 1 in 10 people (see Clinical tip). Explain that there is some uncertainty over whether antimuscarinic medicines have long-term effects on cognitive function. When prescribing for older people, it may be emphasised that the medicine may cause drowsiness and confusion, and to stop taking it if this occurs.
Monitoring and stopping	Review response and side effects within a month of starting therapy. If treatment is not tolerated or not effective (generally after a trial of at least 4 weeks) it should be stopped and alternative options considered (e.g. the β_3 adrenergic agonist, mirabegron).
Cost	Immediate-release tolterodine and oxybutynin are available in non-proprietary products and are relatively inexpensive. Other preparations, such as modified-release formulations, are more expensive and should be reserved for second-line use.

Clinical tip—Dry mouth is a very common side effect of antimuscarinic therapy. Chewing gum or sucking sweets helps to alleviate this. This may be worth mentioning in your consultation, but it is important to emphasise that they should use sugar-free products, because dry mouth increases the risk of tooth decay. For the same reason, good dental care is important in anyone who requires antimuscarinic treatment on a long-term basis.

Antiplatelet drugs, ADP-receptor antagonists

CLINICAL PHARMACOLOGY

Common indications	❶ For treatment of **acute coronary syndrome (ACS)**, usually in combination with **aspirin**, where rapid inhibition of platelet aggregation can prevent or limit arterial thrombosis and reduce subsequent mortality. ❷ To prevent coronary artery **stent occlusion**, usually in combination with **aspirin**. ❸ For **secondary prevention of major adverse cardiovascular events** in people with ischaemic heart disease, cerebrovascular disease or peripheral vascular disease, alone or in combination with **aspirin**.
Mechanisms of action	Thrombotic events occur when platelet-rich thrombus forms in atheromatous arteries and occludes the circulation. ADP-receptor antagonists **prevent platelet aggregation** and reduce the risk of arterial occlusion by binding irreversibly to **adenosine diphosphate (ADP) receptors** (P2Y$_{12}$ subtype) on the surface of platelets. As this process is independent of the cyclooxgenase (COX) pathway, its actions are synergistic with those of aspirin. Clopidogrel and prasugrel are irreversible inhibitors of ADP receptors, whereas ticagrelor acts reversibly. This has important implications for decisions based on their duration of action (see CLINICAL TIP).
Important adverse effects	The most common adverse effect is **bleeding,** which can be serious, particularly if GI or intracranial. **GI upset,** including dyspepsia, abdominal pain, and diarrhoea, is also common. Rarely, antiplatelet agents can affect platelet numbers as well as function, causing **thrombocytopenia.**
Warnings	Antiplatelet drugs should not be prescribed for people with ✖ **active bleeding** and may need to be stopped 7 days before ▲ **elective surgery** and other procedures (see CLINICAL TIP). They should be used with caution in ▲ **renal** and ▲ **hepatic impairment,** especially if there are any other risk factors for bleeding.
Important interactions	Clopidogrel is a **pro-drug,** activated by hepatic cytochrome P450 (CYP) enzymes. Its efficacy may therefore be reduced by ▲ **CYP inhibitors,** which reduce its activation. Examples include **omeprazole, ciprofloxacin, erythromycin,** some **antifungals** and some **selective serotonin reuptake inhibitors,** as well as grapefruit juice. Where a **proton pump inhibitor** is required alongside clopidogrel, lansoprazole or pantoprazole are preferred as they are considered less likely to inhibit clopidogrel activation than omeprazole. Prasugrel is also a pro-drug, but less susceptible to interactions. Ticagrelor is not a pro-drug, but interacts with ▲ **CYP inhibitors** (which may increase toxicity) and **inducers** (which may reduce efficacy). Co-prescription with other ▲ **antiplatelet drugs,** ▲ **anticoagulants** (e.g. **heparin**) or ▲ **NSAIDs** increases bleeding risk.

PRACTICAL PRESCRIBING

Prescription	Clopidogrel is the most commonly used example in this class. It is available only as an oral preparation. Low doses of clopidogrel require up to a week to reach full effect. When rapid effect is needed you should prescribe a *loading dose,* normally a single dose of 300 mg orally for ACS. A regular *maintenance dose* of 75 mg orally daily is started the next day. It is good practice to state the indication and duration of antiplatelet therapy as additional instructions, particularly on the discharge prescription. Following insertion of a drug-eluting coronary stent, dual antiplatelet therapy should be continued for 12 months to reduce the risk of stent thrombosis.
Administration	Clopidogrel, ticagrelor, and prasugrel can be taken with or without food. They should be taken at regular intervals.
Communication	Advise that the purpose of treatment is to reduce the risk of heart attacks, strokes, and other blocked arteries, as applicable, and to prolong life. In those taking treatment following insertion of a drug-eluting stent, emphasise the importance of continuing treatment as directed, usually for 12 months, to make sure the stent does not block and cause a heart attack. Explain that if they have any bleeding, it might take longer than usual to stop, but they should report any unusual or sustained bleeding to their doctor. Advise them not to drink grapefruit juice while taking clopidogrel, as this can make the treatment much less effective.
Monitoring and stopping	Clinical monitoring for adverse effects is most appropriate. Antiplatelet therapy may be required long-term. However, *dual* antiplatelet therapy is usually limited to 12 months, so treatment should be reviewed and reduced to a single antiplatelet drug accordingly. Dual antiplatelet therapy should not be discontinued prematurely without discussion with a cardiologist.
Cost	Clopidogrel and prasugrel are available as inexpensive non-proprietary preparations, whereas ticagrelor remains on patent at the time of writing and is 10–30 times more expensive.

Clinical tip—Clopidogrel and prasugrel act on the ADP receptor *irreversibly,* so their effects persist for the lifespan of platelets (7–10 days). In consultation with relevant specialists, these drugs should be stopped 7 days before elective surgery and invasive procedures. As ticagrelor acts *reversibly*, its antiplatelet effect wears off quicker. It can be stopped 5 days before surgery. In an emergency, platelet transfusion may be needed to reverse the effect of antiplatelet drugs. Decisions should be made by specialists and may be guided by platelet function tests (e.g. thromboelastography). This is helpful because there is significant inter-individual variability, partly due to genetic variation in CYP enzymes which metabolise these drugs. For example, platelet receptor inhibition with clopidogrel can vary from as little as 15% to as much as 100%. People with more than 76% inhibition are 11 times more likely to need transfusion for bleeding.

Antiplatelet drugs, aspirin

CLINICAL PHARMACOLOGY

Common indications	❶ For treatment of **acute coronary syndrome (ACS)** and **acute ischaemic stroke,** where rapid inhibition of platelet aggregation can prevent or limit arterial thrombosis and reduce subsequent mortality. ❷ For **secondary prevention of major adverse cardiovascular events** in ischaemic heart disease, cerebrovascular disease, or peripheral vascular disease. ❸ At higher doses, aspirin can be used in mild-to-moderate **pain** and **fever,** although **paracetamol** and other **NSAIDs** are usually preferred.
Mechanisms of action	Thrombotic events occur when platelet-rich thrombus forms in atheromatous arteries and occludes the circulation. Aspirin **irreversibly inhibits cyclooxygenase** (COX) to reduce production of the pro-aggregatory factor thromboxane from arachidonic acid, reducing platelet aggregation and the risk of arterial occlusion. The antiplatelet effect of aspirin occurs at low doses and lasts for the lifetime of a platelet (7–10 days), as platelets do not have nuclei to allow synthesis of new COX. As a result, the effect of aspirin only wears off as new platelets are made.
Important adverse effects	The most common adverse effect of aspirin is **GI upset.** More serious effects include **peptic ulceration** and **haemorrhage,** and hypersensitivity reactions including **bronchospasm.** In regular high-dose therapy, aspirin can cause **tinnitus.** Aspirin overdose is life-threatening. Features include hyperventilation, hearing changes, metabolic acidosis, and confusion, followed by convulsions, cardiovascular collapse, and respiratory arrest.
Warnings	Aspirin should not be given to ✖ **children aged under 16 years** due to the risk of **Reye's syndrome,** a rare but life-threatening illness that principally affects the liver and brain. It should not be taken by people with ✖ **aspirin hypersensitivity,** i.e. who have had bronchospasm or other allergic symptoms triggered by exposure to aspirin or another **NSAID.** However, aspirin is not *routinely* contraindicated in asthma. Aspirin should be avoided in the ✖ **third trimester of pregnancy** when prostaglandin inhibition may lead to premature closure of the ductus arteriosus. Aspirin should be used with caution in ▲ **peptic ulceration** (consider gastroprotection) and ▲ **gout,** where it may trigger an attack.
Important interactions	Aspirin acts synergistically with other antiplatelet agents which, although therapeutically beneficial, can lead to increased risk of bleeding. So although it may be given with ▲ **antiplatelet drugs** (e.g. **clopidogrel**) and ▲ **anticoagulants** (e.g. **heparin**, **warfarin**) in some situations (e.g. ACS), caution is required.

PRACTICAL PRESCRIBING

Prescription | Aspirin is available for oral or rectal (higher doses) administration. In **ACS,** prescribe aspirin initially as a once-only *loading dose* of 300 mg followed by a regular dose of 75 mg daily. Higher initial daily doses may be used for **acute ischaemic stroke** (e.g. 300 mg daily for 2 weeks), so you should consult local protocols. For **long-term prevention of thrombosis** after an acute event prescribe low-dose aspirin 75 mg daily. Much higher doses of aspirin are required for the treatment of **pain,** with a maximum daily dose of 4 g, taken in divided doses. **Gastroprotection** (e.g. with a **proton pump inhibitor**) should be considered for people taking low-dose aspirin with risk factors for GI complications. These include age >65 years, previous peptic ulcer disease, co-morbidities (such as cardiovascular disease, diabetes), and concurrent therapy with other drugs with GI side effects, particularly **NSAIDs** and **prednisolone**.

Administration | To minimise gastric irritation, aspirin should be taken after food. Enteric-coated tablets may help further, but are associated with slower absorption and are therefore not suitable for use in medical emergencies or for rapid pain relief.

Communication | Advise that the purpose of low-dose aspirin treatment is to reduce risk of heart attacks, strokes, and other blocked arteries, as applicable, and to prolong life. Warn about indigestion and bleeding symptoms and ask the patient to report these to their doctor if they occur.

Monitoring and stopping | Enquiry about side effects is the most appropriate form of monitoring. Antiplatelet therapy may be in indefinite. However, *dual* antiplatelet therapy is usually limited to 12 months, so treatment should be reviewed and reduced to a single antiplatelet drug accordingly. Aspirin is usually preferred as the long-term single agent for coronary artery and peripheral vascular disease, whereas **clopidogrel** is preferred following stroke or transient ischaemic attack (TIA).

Cost | Aspirin is inexpensive, available off-patent and over the counter.

Clinical tip—In the UK, aspirin is not recommended or licensed for use in primary prevention of cardiovascular disease (i.e. in people who have not previously had an event). The reason is that large-scale, randomised controlled trials and meta-analyses have found that the absolute risk of major adverse cardiovascular events in this group is low (around 1/500), and the benefits of preventing a proportion of these with aspirin are offset by the increased risk of serious bleeding (around 1/1000).

Antipsychotics, first-generation (typical)

CLINICAL PHARMACOLOGY

Common indications	❶ **Rapid tranquilisation** in severe psychomotor agitation that is causing dangerous or violent behaviour, or to enable assessment. ❷ **Schizophrenia,** particularly when the metabolic side effects of **second-generation (atypical) antipsychotics** are problematic. ❸ **Bipolar disorder,** particularly in acute mania or hypomania. ❹ **Nausea and vomiting,** particularly in the palliative care setting.
Mechanisms of action	Antipsychotic drugs **block** post-synaptic **dopamine D_2 receptors.** There are three main dopaminergic pathways in the brain. The *mesolimbic/mesocortical pathway* runs between the midbrain and the limbic system/frontal cortex. D_2 blockade in this pathway is probably the main determinant of antipsychotic effect, but this is incompletely understood. The *nigrostriatal pathway* connects the substantia nigra with the corpus striatum of the basal ganglia. The *tuberohypophyseal pathway* connects the hypothalamus with the pituitary gland. Activity in these pathways explains some of the drugs' adverse effects. D_2 receptors are also found in the *chemoreceptor trigger zone,* where blockade accounts for their use in nausea and vomiting. All antipsychotics, but particularly chlorpromazine, have some sedative effect. This may be beneficial in acute psychomotor agitation.
Important adverse effects	**Extrapyramidal effects**—movement abnormalities that arise from D_2 blockade in the *nigrostriatal pathway*—are the main drawback of first-generation antipsychotics. They take several forms: **acute dystonic reactions** are involuntary parkinsonian movements or muscle spasms; **akathisia** is a state of inner restlessness; and **neuroleptic malignant syndrome** is a rare but life-threatening side effect characterised by rigidity, confusion, autonomic dysregulation, and pyrexia. These tend to occur early in treatment. By contrast, **tardive dyskinesia** is a late adverse effect (*tardive,* late), occurring after months or years. This comprises movements that are pointless, involuntary, and repetitive (e.g. lip smacking). It is disabling and may not resolve on stopping treatment. Other adverse effects include **drowsiness, hypotension, QT interval prolongation** (and consequent **arrhythmias**), **erectile dysfunction,** and symptoms arising from **hyperprolactinaemia** due to *tuberohypophyseal* D_2 blockade (e.g. menstrual disturbance, galactorrhoea, and breast pain).
Warnings	▲ **Older people** are particularly sensitive to antipsychotics, so start with lower doses. Antipsychotics should ideally be avoided in ▲ **dementia,** as they may increase the risk of death and stroke. They should be avoided if possible in ▲ **Parkinson's disease** due to their extrapyramidal effects.
Important interactions	Consult the BNF when prescribing antipsychotics as there is an extensive list of interactions. Prominent among these are ▲ **drugs that prolong the QT interval** (e.g. **amiodarone, macrolides**).

PRACTICAL PRESCRIBING

Prescription	Regular treatment is required to treat schizophrenia and should be started and adjusted under the guidance of a psychiatrist. A single dose may be used to control acute or violent behaviour. Haloperidol is a common first-line choice. The dosage depends on the clinical context and you may require guidance from a clinician experienced in its use. For example, older people may be markedly sedated by as little as 0.5 mg IM, whereas a young adult with extreme agitation may need 5–10 mg, or more, to achieve adequate response. For the control of nausea, haloperidol is used in regular small oral or SC doses (e.g. 1.5 mg at night) or as a component of a continuous SC infusion.
Administration	For regular administration, typical antipsychotics can be taken orally (tablet and liquid) or given by slow-release IM ('depot') injection. For rapid tranquilisation, haloperidol is usually given by rapid-acting IM injection and occasionally IV, although it is not licensed by this route. IV haloperidol should only be administered by clinicians capable of managing its acute adverse effects, including arrhythmias such as torsade de pointes (a form of ventricular tachycardia), which are more likely when antipsychotics are given by injection or in high dose.
Communication	Adherence is a significant issue when treating psychiatric disorders, both because of the underlying disease and adverse effects of treatment. Good communication about the aims and benefits of treatment, as well as its potential side effects, is therefore very important. Emphasise that if another healthcare professional is prescribing or advising them about medicines, it is important that they know about the antipsychotic medicine, due to the risk of interactions.
Monitoring and stopping	Antipsychotic effects may take weeks to establish and the dose may need to be adjusted to obtain the optimum balance between beneficial and adverse effects. If adverse effects are problematic, a **second-generation antipsychotic** may be considered. Prolactin concentration should be measured at the start of therapy, at 6 months, and then yearly, particularly if the person reports breast symptoms. When using high doses in rapid tranquilisation, the dose–response relationship is unpredictable. Close monitoring is required to detect adverse effects.
Cost	Typical antipsychotics are relatively old drugs and are available in inexpensive non-proprietary forms. Branded products, including oral solutions and depot injections, are more expensive.

Clinical tip—Chlorpromazine and haloperidol are also licensed for the treatment of intractable hiccups, as is metoclopramide. This can be a very distressing condition which is difficult to treat. A variety of non-pharmacological manoeuvres (e.g. Valsalva manoeuvre, breath holds, sipping ice-cold water) may be tried first. In our experience, these rarely work in intractable cases, but chlorpromazine (e.g. 25 mg orally) is sometimes effective.

Antipsychotics, second-generation (atypical)

CLINICAL PHARMACOLOGY

Common indications	❶ **Schizophrenia,** particularly when extrapyramidal side effects have complicated the use of **first-generation (typical) antipsychotics,** or when negative symptoms are prominent. Clozapine is more effective than other antipsychotics in refractory schizophrenia. ❷ **Bipolar disorder,** particularly in acute mania or hypomania.
Mechanisms of action	Like first-generation antipsychotic drugs, second-generation antipsychotics **block** post-synaptic **dopamine D₂ receptors.** Blockade in the *mesolimbic/mesocortical pathway* (between the midbrain and the limbic system/frontal cortex) probably accounts for at least part of the drugs' antipsychotic effects, and activity in the *nigrostriatal pathway* (between the substantia nigra and the corpus striatum of the basal ganglia) and *tuberohypophyseal pathway* (hypothalamus to pituitary gland) probably accounts for some of their adverse effects. However, second-generation antipsychotics have greater activity at other receptors (particularly 5-HT$_{2A}$ antagonism), and a characteristic of 'looser' binding to D₂ receptors (in the case of clozapine and quetiapine). This may explain why the second-generation agents are more efficacious in 'treatment-resistant' schizophrenia (particularly clozapine) and against negative symptoms, and why they have a lower risk of extrapyramidal symptoms.
Important adverse effects	Second-generation antipsychotics are generally better tolerated than first-generation agents. **Extrapyramidal effects** (see **Antipsychotics, first-generation**), in particular, are less common, and drowsiness and cognitive impairment are less marked. However, **metabolic disturbances,** including weight gain, diabetes mellitus, and lipid changes, are common with second-generation antipsychotics. Antipsychotics can **prolong the QT interval** and thus cause **arrhythmias.** Risperidone has particular effects on dopaminergic transmission in the *tuberohypophyseal pathway,* which regulates secretion of prolactin. This can cause **breast symptoms** (in both women and men) and **sexual dysfunction.** Clozapine causes a severe deficiency of neutrophils **(agranulocytosis)** in about 1% of individuals, which can lead to severe infections. Rarely, it causes **myocarditis.**
Warnings	Antipsychotics should be used with caution in ▲ **cardiovascular disease.** Clozapine must not be used in ✖ **severe heart disease** or people with a history of ✖ **neutropenia.**
Important interactions	Sedation may be more pronounced when used with other sedating drugs. They should not be combined with other ▲ **antiemetics that block dopamine D2 receptors** or ▲ **drugs that prolong the QT interval** (e.g. **amiodarone, quinine, macrolides, selective serotonin reuptake inhibitors**).

PRACTICAL PRESCRIBING

Prescription	Decisions to start a second-generation antipsychotic drugs should be taken by specialists. They may be used both for treatment of acute symptoms and for prevention of subsequent attacks. Options include daily oral treatment or intermittent slow-release IM ('depot') injections. Clozapine is considered when other agents have proved ineffective or intolerable. You are most likely to encounter these drugs as part of established treatment: for example, when the person is admitted to hospital with a concurrent problem. In this situation, you should not usually stop the antipsychotic, but must check carefully that the acute illness is not caused or compounded by it (see CLINICAL TIP). Check also for interactions with newly-started treatments.
Administration	Oral second-generation antipsychotics should generally be taken at the same time every day. In once-daily administration, if drowsiness is an issue, some people may prefer to take the dose in the evening.
Communication	Good communication about the aims and benefits of treatment, as well as its potential side effects, is important. If the person has previously taken a **first-generation antipsychotic**, explain that the side effects they may have experienced with these are less likely with second-generation antipsychotics. On the other hand, other side effects, such as high blood sugars and weight gain, may be more likely. Monitoring for these will be important. Special counselling is necessary for people starting clozapine. They should be informed about the need for regular blood tests and to report infective symptoms immediately.
Monitoring and stopping	Treatment **efficacy** is best monitored clinically. Prolactin concentration should be measured at the start of therapy, at 6 months, and then yearly, particularly if the person reports breast symptoms. **Safety** monitoring for metabolic and cardiovascular side effects is important for second-generation antipsychotics. This includes body weight, lipid profile, and fasting blood glucose at baseline and intermittently during treatment. An intensive monitoring programme is required for **clozapine** due to the risk of agranulocytosis, and stopping criteria are clearly set out in the BNF. In other situations, antipsychotic drugs should generally be tapered rather than stopped abruptly, with close monitoring for acute withdrawal syndromes or early relapse.
Cost	Non-proprietary forms of quetiapine, olanzapine, and risperidone are available and are less expensive than their brand name counterparts.

Clinical tip—If you admit a person on clozapine to hospital, liaise with psychiatry on its dosing during the acute illness and the need for plasma concentration monitoring. Acute illnesses are associated with reduced clozapine metabolism by cytochrome P450 (CYP) 1A2 enzymes, and a corresponding increase in the risk of toxicity. Additionally, substances in tobacco smoke induce CYP1A2 enzymes, so cessation of smoking (including switching to e-cigarettes) can also cause clozapine concentrations to rise.

Antiviral drugs, aciclovir

CLINICAL PHARMACOLOGY

Common indications	❶ Treatment of **acute episodes of herpesvirus infections,** including herpes simplex (e.g. cold sores, genital ulcers, encephalitis) and varicella-zoster (e.g. chickenpox, shingles). ❷ Suppression of **recurrent herpes simplex attacks** where these are occurring at a frequency of 6 or more per year.
Mechanisms of action	The herpesvirus family includes herpes simplex 1 and 2 and varicella-zoster. These viruses contain double-stranded deoxyribonucleic acid (DNA), which requires a herpes-specific DNA polymerase for the virus to replicate. Aciclovir enters herpes-infected cells and **inhibits the herpes-specific DNA polymerase**, stopping further viral DNA synthesis and therefore replication.
Important adverse effects	Common adverse effects of aciclovir include **headache, dizziness, GI upset,** and **skin rash**. IV aciclovir can cause inflammation or **phlebitis** at the injection site. Aciclovir is relatively water insoluble. During high-dose IV therapy, delivery of a high concentration of aciclovir into the renal tubules can cause precipitation, leading to crystal-induced **acute renal failure.** The risk of this can be minimised by ensuring good hydration and slowing the rate of infusion.
Warnings	Aciclovir has no major contraindications. It does cross the placenta and is expressed in breast milk, so caution is advised in ▲ **pregnant women** and women who are ▲ **breastfeeding**. However, infections such as viral encephalitis, varicella pneumonia, and genital herpes carry significant risks to the mother and fetus, so the benefits of treatment in such circumstances are likely to outweigh its risks. Aciclovir is **excreted by the kidneys**; the dose and/or frequency of administration should therefore be reduced in ▲ **severe renal impairment** to prevent accumulation of the drug and subsequent toxicity.
Important interactions	Aciclovir can increase the plasma concentration of theophylline and aminophylline, increasing the risk of adverse effects. Renal function should be monitored when aciclovir is prescribed with other drugs that can also increase the risk of nephrotoxicity, including **NSAIDs**, antibiotics (**aminoglycosides, cephalosporins, trimethoprim, vancomycin**) and **methotrexate.**

PRACTICAL PRESCRIBING

Prescription	**Acute episodes of oral and genital herpes simplex** are treated with aciclovir 200 mg orally five times a day. Treatment should ideally be started during the prodromal phase. In **recurrent infections**, suppressive treatment (400 mg orally 12-hrly) may be given. **Herpes simplex encephalitis** requires high-dose therapy (10 mg/kg IV 8-hrly). Treatment should be started urgently if the presentation is suggestive, then later stopped if analysis of cerebrospinal fluid (CSF) shows no evidence of herpesviruses. In confirmed cases, or if clinical suspicion is high in the absence of CSF analysis, treatment should be continued for 14–21 days.
Administration	Tablets are taken with water, with or without food, and are available in dispersible form if swallowing is difficult. IV aciclovir should be given by infusion over at least 1 hour to minimise tubular precipitation. Care should be taken to ensure the cannula is properly sited in a vein, as extravasation causes tissue damage.
Communication	Explain that aciclovir is an antiviral medicine that works by stopping the virus from reproducing. It does not clear the virus from the body completely, so a risk of recurrent infection will remain. This is particularly true for cold sores and genital infections, but these usually become less frequent and less severe after a couple of years. Where aciclovir is prescribed as episodic treatment (taken if an attack occurs), advise them to start treatment as soon as they notice symptoms such as tingling or numbness. When prescribed for **suppressive treatment,** explain that while aciclovir may reduce the frequency of infections and the **risk of passing on the virus** to sexual partners, it does not prevent these altogether. Warn about common side effects such as headache, dizziness, and stomach upset.
Monitoring and stopping	Efficacy can be monitored clinically. In high-dose IV treatment, renal function should be monitored for safety. Suppressive treatment should be stopped after a year to assess continuing need, but can be restarted if recurrence is still frequent.
Cost	Aciclovir is inexpensive. Topical aciclovir should not be routinely prescribed but can be bought over the counter if people find it helpful.

Clinical tip—Advise about **self-care options** for herpetic lesions, including keeping hydrated, and using barrier preparations, topical **anaesthetics**, oral **paracetamol,** and/ or **NSAIDs** to reduce pain. Explain that there is **risk of transmission** to others and auto-inoculation of the eye when using contact lenses. This is minimised by washing hands with soap and water after touching lesions, and avoiding kissing and sex until the lesions have healed.

Antiviral drugs, other

CLINICAL PHARMACOLOGY

Common indications	❶ Acute treatment of certain **viral infections,** e.g. influenza or SARS-CoV-2 (the cause of COVID-19), to reduce illness duration and severity. ❷ **Pre-exposure prophylaxis (PrEP),** to reduce the risk of human immunodeficiency virus (HIV) infection in people at high risk (e.g. those whose partner has HIV) and **post-exposure prophylaxis (PEP),** e.g. for influenza in unvaccinated adults, or HIV after needle-stick injury. ❸ Chronic treatment to suppress (and if possible, eliminate) viral load in **hepatitis B, C or HIV infection,** to reduce morbidity, mortality, and onward transmission.
Mechanisms of action	Viruses consist of nucleic acid (RNA or DNA), encapsulated in a protein coat. They attach to and invade host cells, then use cell machinery to synthesise new viral nucleic acids and proteins. These are assembled and released as whole virions. Antiviral drugs target key stages of viral replication. For treatment of influenza A and B, oseltamivir and zanamivir **inhibit neuraminidases,** viral surface enzymes important for entry into and release from host cells. For SARS-CoV-2, molnupiravir and remdesivir are nucleotide analogues that block **viral RNA synthesis,** and nirmatrelvir (with ritonavir) is a protease inhibitor that **inhibits viral replication.** Antiretroviral drugs used in the treatment of HIV and hepatitis B include **nucleoside/nucleotide** (e.g. emtricitabine, tenofovir) and **non-nucleoside** (e.g. efavirenz) **reverse transcriptase inhibitors** (NRTIs and NNRTIs, respectively). These inhibit synthesis of DNA from viral RNA. **Protease inhibitors** (e.g. atazanavir) inhibit the enzyme which cleaves inert polyproteins into structural and functional viral proteins. Drugs used for hepatitis C include **RNA-dependent RNA polymerase inhibitors** (e.g. sofosbuvir).
Important adverse effects	These include **GI upset**, **skin reactions**, **dizziness,** and **sleep problems,** which are usually mild and self-limiting. Inhaled zanamivir may cause **bronchospasm. Immune-mediated effects** include hypersensitivity reactions, hepatitis, blood dyscrasias, and severe cutaneous reactions. Long-term treatment can cause **dyslipidaemia, hyperglycaemia, hypertension,** and **weight gain,** increasing cardiovascular risk.
Warnings	People with ▲ **asthma or COPD** are at increased risk of bronchospasm with inhaled zanamivir. NNRTIs and protease inhibitors are contraindicated in ✖ **acute porphyria** and should be used with caution in those at risk of ▲ **QT prolongation.**
Important interactions	Interactions are common and important: check for these (e.g. hiv-druginteractions.org) and seek specialist advice. Ritonavir and cobicistat have a beneficial interaction with protease inhibitors. By inhibiting enzymes that metabolise them, they smooth peaks and troughs in antiviral drug concentration and reduce dosing frequency (**'pharmacokinetic boosting'**).

PRACTICAL PRESCRIBING

Prescription	For **influenza**, oseltamivir is prescribed at a dose of 75 mg by mouth (reduced in children and small adults), or zanamivir 10 mg by inhalation. Doses are taken twice daily for 5 days for treatment of infection, or once daily for 10 days for prevention. Duration may be extended during epidemics or for people with immune suppression. The use of antivirals for **COVID-19** continues to evolve, and you should consult current guidelines. Treatment or PrEP of **HIV or viral hepatitis** should be initiated and adjusted by a specialist. **PEP** is most likely to be effective if started as soon as possible, so should be prescribed immediately after risk assessment, guided by local protocols.
Administration	Antivirals should be administered at equal dosage intervals, to avoid periods of subtherapeutic drug concentration. A short-acting bronchodilator (e.g. β_2 **agonist**) should be available in case of bronchospasm when administering inhaled zanamivir to people with airways disease.
Communication	Where antivirals are prescribed for **acute viral infections**, advise that the aim of therapy is to speed recovery and reduce severity. Where antivirals are used as **influenza prophylaxis**, emphasise the need to take the full course as prescribed, and discuss future seasonal vaccination with them. Key messages for people taking antiretroviral medicines for **HIV** include: treatment keeps the virus under control, allowing them to live a long and healthy life; it is not a cure, so needs to be taken long term; when treatment achieves an undetectable viral load, the virus is considered untransmissible to sexual partners (undetectable=untransmissible, 'U=U'); and it is very important that they don't miss or skip doses, as the virus can quickly change and become resistant to the drugs.
Monitoring and stopping	No specific monitoring is required during short-term treatment with antivirals for acute infections beyond that required to monitor the underlying disease. Monitoring of HIV and viral hepatitis treatment is a specialist area. In simple terms, viral load is the best marker of virological response to treatment, while CD4 count (in HIV) tracks subsequent reconstitution of the immune system. Drug choice is crucially guided by viral genotypic resistance testing.
Cost	The cost of antivirals varies widely. Decisions about their value and cost-effectiveness are usually made at a national level.

Clinical tip—Abacavir, a nucleoside reverse transcriptase inhibitor, is associated with a severe hypersensitivity reaction in a minority of people. It is strongly linked to carriage of the human leukocyte antigen (HLA) allele HLA-B*57:01. By testing for this allele, and avoiding abacavir in those who carry it, the risk of abacavir hypersensitivity syndrome is greatly reduced. This is a notable early example of a pharmacogenetic test that has made an important impact on practice.

Benzodiazepines

CLINICAL PHARMACOLOGY

Common indications	❶ First-line in the management of **status epilepticus.** ❷ First-line in the management of **alcohol withdrawal reactions.** ❸ Sedation in **palliative care, for interventional procedures** (if general anaesthesia is unnecessary or undesirable) or for **rapid tranquilisation**. ❹ For *short-term* treatment of severe, disabling or distressing **anxiety** or **insomnia,** although non-pharmacological treatment (or treatment of the underlying cause, if applicable) is invariably preferable.
Mechanisms of action	The target of benzodiazepines is the **γ-aminobutyric acid type A (GABA$_A$) receptor.** The GABA$_A$ receptor is a chloride channel that opens in response to binding by gamma-aminobutyric acid (GABA), the main inhibitory neurotransmitter in the brain. Opening the channel allows chloride to flow into the cell, making the cell more resistant to depolarisation. Benzodiazepines change the shape of the receptor to **facilitate and enhance binding of GABA** to the GABA$_A$ receptor (allosteric modulation). This has a widespread depressant effect on synaptic transmission. The clinical manifestations of this include reduced anxiety, sleepiness, sedation, and anticonvulsive effects. Ethanol ('alcohol') also acts on the GABA$_A$ receptor, and in chronic excessive use, *tolerance* develops. Abrupt cessation then provokes the excitatory state of alcohol withdrawal. This can be treated by introducing a benzodiazepine, which can then be withdrawn in a gradual and more controlled way.
Important adverse effects	Predictably, benzodiazepines cause dose-dependent **drowsiness, sedation,** and **coma.** There is relatively little cardiorespiratory depression in **benzodiazepine overdose** (in contrast to **opioid** overdose), but loss of airway reflexes can lead to **airway obstruction** and **death.** If used repeatedly for more than a few weeks, a state of **dependence** can develop. Abrupt cessation then produces a **withdrawal reaction** similar to that seen with alcohol.
Warnings	▲ **Older people** are more susceptible to the effects of benzodiazepines and so should receive a lower dose. Benzodiazepines are best avoided in significant ▲ **respiratory impairment** or ▲ **neuromuscular disease** (e.g. myasthenia gravis). Benzodiazepines should also be avoided in ▲ **liver failure** as they may precipitate hepatic encephalopathy. If their use is essential (e.g. for alcohol withdrawal), lorazepam may be the best choice, as it depends less on the liver for its elimination.
Important interactions	The effects of benzodiazepines are additive to those of other sedating drugs, including alcohol and **opioids**. Most depend on cytochrome P450 (CYP) enzymes for elimination, so concurrent use with ▲ **CYP inhibitors** (e.g. **amiodarone**, **diltiazem**, **macrolides**, **fluconazole**, **protease inhibitors**) may increase their effects.

PRACTICAL PRESCRIBING

Prescription	The *effects* of the drugs in this class are similar. What distinguishes them is their *duration of action*, and this determines how they are used. For **seizures,** a long-acting drug is preferred, usually lorazepam (initial dose 4 mg IV) or diazepam (10 mg IV). Oromucosal midazolam is an alternative if IV access in unavailable, although its effect is short-lived. For **alcohol withdrawal,** oral chlordiazepoxide (long-acting) is the traditional choice, but diazepam and lorazepam are equally acceptable; dosage regimens depend on symptom severity and alcohol intake. For **procedural sedation,** midazolam is preferred, because its short duration allows rapid recovery after completion of the procedure or inadvertent over-sedation. It should be used only by individuals skilled in safe sedation, and in an appropriate clinical environment. For **insomnia** and **anxiety,** an intermediate-acting drug at the lowest effective dose (e.g. temazepam 10 mg orally) is used for the shortest possible period (usual maximum 2 weeks).
Administration	Diazepam is available as a water-based solution and an oil-in-water emulsion. The solution is more irritant to veins. IV administration of benzodiazepines, whether for seizures or sedation, should be undertaken only where facilities and expertise exist to deal with over-sedation (including airway management). An oromucosal formulation of midazolam is presented in pre-filled syringes, for administration into the buccal cavity.
Communication	When treating **insomnia** and **anxiety,** advise that pharmacological therapy is only a short-term measure. Discuss the risk of dependence, advising that this can be minimised by avoiding daily use if possible and taking the drug for the shortest possible period. Advise that they should not drive or operate complex or heavy machinery after taking the drug, noting that sometimes sleepiness may persist to the next day.
Monitoring and stopping	Close monitoring of clinical status and vital signs is essential following IV or high-dose oral administration of a benzodiazepine, including the settings of seizures, alcohol withdrawal, and sedation. In insomnia and anxiety, enquiry about symptoms and side effects is the best form of monitoring. Treatment should be for no longer than 4 weeks, with dosage reduction starting at 2 weeks. If taken for longer than this, gradual tapering is important to avoid a withdrawal reaction.
Cost	Benzodiazepines are generally inexpensive.

Clinical tip—Flumazenil is a specific antagonist of benzodiazepines. However, use of this drug is rarely indicated. Specifically, it should *not* be given to reverse sedation caused by benzodiazepines as part of a mixed or uncertain overdose. In this context, flumazenil may precipitate seizures which—having now blocked the benzodiazepine receptor—will be difficult to treat.

β₂-agonists

CLINICAL PHARMACOLOGY

Common indications	**❶ Asthma:** short-acting β₂-agonists (SABAs) are used to relieve bronchospasm during acute asthma attacks, and for intermittent breathlessness or wheeze in chronic asthma. Long-acting β₂-agonists (LABAs) are *added* to **inhaled corticosteroids** (ICS) in chronic asthma if symptoms are uncontrolled by an ICS alone. **❷ Chronic obstructive pulmonary disease (COPD):** SABAs are used to relieve breathlessness and exercise limitation. If a SABA is insufficient, a LABA is recommended as first-line regular therapy. Depending on whether the person does, or does not, have features of asthma or steroid responsiveness, the LABA is combined with either a **long-acting antimuscarinic** (LAMA) or an **inhaled corticosteroid**, respectively.
Mechanisms of action	**β₂-receptors** are found in smooth muscle of the bronchi, gut, uterus, and blood vessels. **Stimulation** of these G protein-coupled receptors activates a signalling cascade that leads to smooth muscle relaxation and bronchodilation. This improves airflow, reducing breathlessness. Like **insulin**, β₂-agonists also stimulate Na^+/K^+-adenosine triphosphatase (ATPase) pumps on cell membranes, shifting K^+ from the extracellular to intracellular compartment. This can cause the adverse effect of hypokalaemia, but may also have therapeutic benefit as an *adjunct* to other treatments for hyperkalaemia, particularly if IV access is difficult. β₂-agonists are classified as *short-acting* (SABAs, e.g. salbutamol, terbutaline) or *long-acting* (LABAs, e.g. salmeterol, formoterol) according to their duration of effect. SABAs, which have a fast onset of action (within 5 minutes), are used to relieve acute breathlessness. LABAs are used as maintenance (preventer) therapy. Taken regularly for COPD, LABAs also reduce exacerbations.
Important adverse effects	Activation of β₂-receptors in diverse tissues accounts for the common 'fight or flight' adverse effects of **tachycardia, palpitations, anxiety, tremor,** and **headache.** β₂-agonists can cause **hypokalaemia** and elevate serum **lactate**, particularly at high doses. They promote glycogenolysis, so may cause hyperglycaemia. LABAs can cause **muscle cramps**.
Warnings	LABAs should be used in asthma only if an **inhaled corticosteroid** is also part of therapy. This is because, without a steroid, LABAs are associated with increased asthma deaths. Care should be taken when prescribing β₂-agonists in ▲ **cardiovascular disease,** as tachycardia may provoke angina or arrhythmias, particularly at high doses.
Important interactions	**β-blockers** may reduce the effectiveness of β₂-agonists. Concomitant use of high-dose nebulised β₂-agonists with theophylline and **corticosteroids** increases the risk of hypokalaemia, so serum potassium concentrations should be monitored.

PRACTICAL PRESCRIBING

Prescription	A common choice of **SABA** in adults is salbutamol 100–200 micrograms *inhaled* as required. In asthma and COPD exacerbations requiring hospital treatment, regular *nebulised* therapy is used acutely (e.g. salbutamol 2.5 mg nebulised 4-hrly), although inhalation via a spacer (e.g. 10 doses of salbutamol 100 micrograms inhaled) is reasonable if the exacerbation is not life threatening. **LABAs** are prescribed regularly for maintenance therapy, usually as a combination inhaler with an **inhaled corticosteroid** (LABA + ICS), a **long-acting antimuscarinic** (LABA + LAMA) or both (LABA + LAMA + ICS). Many permutations of drug, device type, and doses are available in combination inhalers, so the brand name should be included in prescriptions for clarity and consistency.
Administration	The inhaler type should be selected according to the needs and capabilities of the individual. Aerosol (metered dose) inhalers (MDIs) require coordination, while dry powder inhalers (DPIs) require forceful inspiration. Training on inhaler technique is essential and should be checked at every visit.
Communication	Advise people who require a reliever inhaler to carry this with them and take it when breathless or 10 minutes before exercise. Explain that this will open the airways, reducing breathlessness within minutes, and that the effect should last for several hours. Advise those taking a preventer (LABA) to use it regularly, but to take their reliever in addition if breathlessness still occurs. Outline common side effects such as tremor and palpitations and state the maximum number of inhalations (usually 8) they should take in 24 hours. Advise that these inhalers treat symptoms, not the disease, and if they need increased doses of their reliever inhaler or it becomes less effective, they should seek medical advice, or if applicable, follow the steps on their written action plan.
Monitoring and stopping	For **asthma**, disease severity is monitored by symptoms and serial peak expiratory flow rate (PEFR) measurements. LABA treatment may be 'stepped down' once disease has been controlled for at least 3 months. For **COPD**, symptom severity and exacerbation rates are the main indicators of effect. LABAs will usually only be withdrawn if they are ineffective or causing problematic side effects.
Cost	Inhalers account for 3% of NHS carbon emissions, mainly due to propellant in MDIs. A move to lower carbon DPIs is part of the NHS plan to move to 'net zero' and reduce its cost to the environment.

Clinical tip—A **spacer** (or valved holding chamber) can improve airway deposition and therefore treatment efficacy with MDIs. Spacers also reduce oropharyngeal deposition and therefore oral adverse effects. They are a good option for people who find it difficult to coordinate inhaler actuation with inhalation (e.g. children).

β-blockers

CLINICAL PHARMACOLOGY

Common indications	❶ **Ischaemic heart disease (IHD):** to improve symptoms and prognosis in **angina** and **acute coronary syndrome (ACS).** ❷ **Chronic heart failure:** to improve prognosis. ❸ **Atrial fibrillation (AF):** to reduce the ventricular rate and, in paroxysmal AF, to maintain sinus rhythm. ❹ **Supraventricular tachycardia (SVT):** to restore sinus rhythm. ❺ **Resistant hypertension:** as a fourth-line treatment option. ❻ **Prophylaxis of migraine:** other options are **amitriptyline, valproate,** and drugs targeting calcitonin gene-related peptide (e.g. galcanezumab). ❼ **Thyrotoxicosis:** for symptoms caused by sympathetic stimulation.
Mechanisms of action	Via β_1-adrenoreceptors, which are located mainly in the heart, β-blockers reduce force of cardiac contraction and speed of conduction. In **IHD,** this reduces cardiac work and oxygen demand and increases myocardial perfusion. In **chronic heart failure,** it improves prognosis probably by 'protecting' the heart from chronic sympathetic stimulation. In **AF,** it reduces ventricular rate by prolonging the refractory period of the atrioventricular (AV) node, and therefore the proportion of fibrillation waves that are conducted. By the same effect, β-blockers may terminate **SVT** if this is due to a self-perpetuating ('re-entry') circuit. The **blood pressure-lowering** effect of β-blockers is complex, likely involving reduced β_1-mediated renin secretion from the kidney. Their action in **migraine** is thought to be via modulation of neuronal excitability in the brain, perhaps through reduced firing in noradrenergic neurons. In **thyrotoxicosis,** they offset the effect of β-adrenoreceptor upregulation, which causes symptoms such as tremor and palpitations. An additional effect (particularly with propranolol) is inhibition of monodeiodinase, reducing conversion of thyroxine (T_4) to triiodothyronine (T_3), but the clinical importance of this is doubtful.
Important adverse effects	**Fatigue, cold extremities, headache,** and **GI upset** are common. β-blockers can also cause **sleep disturbance**, **nightmares,** and **impotence**.
Warnings	In ✖ **asthma,** β-blockers can cause life-threatening bronchospasm and should be avoided. This effect is mediated via β_2-adrenoreceptors located in smooth muscle of the airways. β-blockers are usually safe in **COPD,** but it is prudent to choose a relatively β_1-selective option (e.g. bisoprolol, metoprolol). In ▲ **heart failure,** β-blockers should be started at a low dose and increased slowly, as they may initially impair cardiac function. They are contraindicated in ✖ **heart block** and severe ✖ **hypotension** and generally require dosage reduction in significant ▲ **hepatic failure.**
Important interactions	β-blockers must not be used with ✖ **non-dihydropyridine calcium channel blockers** (e.g. verapamil, diltiazem), except in specialist practice, as this can cause heart failure, bradycardia, and even asystole.

PRACTICAL PRESCRIBING

Prescription	Choice of drug and dosage varies by indication. For example, in **heart failure,** bisoprolol and carvedilol are preferred, whereas in **migraine** and **thyrotoxicosis,** propranolol may be preferred due to its increased lipid solubility. In general, it is best to start at the lowest dosage listed in the BNF for the relevant indication. The dosage used in heart failure is considerably lower than that used in other indications. IV preparations (e.g. of metoprolol) are available for when rapid effect is necessary, such as in acute treatment of **SVT** and **AF.**
Administration	Orally administered β-blockers should be taken at equal intervals (e.g. roughly the same time each day for once-daily drugs such as bisoprolol); the exact time is not important. IV preparations should be prescribed and administered only by those experienced in their use, and only in a well-monitored environment.
Communication	Explain the rationale for treatment as appropriate for the situation. Discuss common side effects, including impotence where relevant. In **heart failure,** warn about the risk of initial deterioration in symptoms, and advise them to seek medical advice if this occurs. Warn those with obstructive airways disease to stop treatment and seek medical advice if they develop any breathing difficulty.
Monitoring and stopping	Symptoms (e.g. chest pain) and heart rate are the best guide to dosage adjustment. In **ischaemic heart disease,** aim for a resting heart rate of around 55–60 beats/min. During initiation and titration of a β-blocker in **heart failure,** daily measurement of body weight can be useful. Progressively increasing body weight suggests fluid accumulation, which may provide an opportunity to slow the titration schedule and avert more severe deterioration. In established treatment, if the β-blocker needs to be stopped (e.g. due to intolerable adverse effects) the dose should be reduced gradually over 1–2 weeks. This is because in long-term treatment, β-adrenoreceptors are upregulated, increasing sensitivity to circulating catecholamines. Abrupt withdrawal can lead to a surge of sympathetic stimulation, which can precipitate myocardial ischaemia.
Cost	The commonly used β-blockers are available in non-proprietary forms, which are generally inexpensive.

Clinical tip—When starting a β-blocker acutely, such as in ACS, it is usually best to select a drug with a relatively short half-life, e.g. oral metoprolol (typical starting dose 12.5 mg 8-hrly; later increased to 25 mg 8-hrly). This will be more responsive to dosage adjustment and can be stopped quickly if necessary. Once stability is achieved, it can be converted to a once-daily preparation (e.g. bisoprolol), which will be more convenient for long-term use.

Bisphosphonates

CLINICAL PHARMACOLOGY

Common indications	❶ Alendronic acid and risedronate sodium are first-line drug treatment options to reduce risk of **osteoporotic fragility fractures.** ❷ Pamidronate and zoledronic acid are used in the treatment of **severe hypercalcaemia** of malignancy, after appropriate IV rehydration. ❸ In **myeloma** and **breast cancer with bone metastases,** pamidronate and zoledronic acid reduce the risk of pathological fractures, cord compression, and the need for radiotherapy or surgery. ❹ Bisphosphonates are used first-line in the treatment of metabolically active **Paget's disease,** with the aim of reducing bone turnover and pain.
Mechanisms of action	Bisphosphonates reduce bone turnover by **inhibiting** the action of **osteoclasts,** the cells responsible for bone resorption. Bisphosphonates have a similar structure to naturally occurring pyrophosphate, and therefore are readily incorporated into bone. As bone is resorbed, bisphosphonates accumulate in osteoclasts, where they inhibit activity and promote apoptosis. The net effect is reduction in bone loss and improvement in bone mass.
Important adverse effects	Common side effects include **oesophagitis** (when taken orally) and **hypophosphataemia.** A rare but serious adverse effect of bisphosphonates is **osteonecrosis of the jaw,** which is more likely with high-dose IV therapy. Good dental care is important to minimise the risk of this. Another rare but important adverse effect is **atypical femoral fracture,** particularly in long-term treatment.
Warnings	Bisphosphonates are renally excreted and should be avoided in ✖ **severe renal impairment.** They are contraindicated in ✖ **hypocalcaemia,** so calcium and vitamin D levels should be checked before starting treatment and, if necessary, corrected. Oral administration is contraindicated in active ✖ **upper GI disorders.** Because of the risk of jaw osteonecrosis, care should be exercised in prescribing bisphosphonates for ▲ **smokers** and people with major ▲ **dental disease.**
Important interactions	Bisphosphonates bind calcium. Their absorption is therefore reduced if taken with **calcium** salts (including milk), as well as **antacids** and **iron** salts (see Administration).

PRACTICAL PRESCRIBING

Prescription	For **osteoporosis,** alendronic acid may be prescribed at a dosage of 10 mg orally daily. A 70 mg oral *weekly* dosage is an alternative in women, but not licensed in men. For severe **hypercalcaemia** and **bone metastases,** pamidronate or zoledronic acid is prescribed as slow IV infusions, in single or divided doses. Calcium-lowering effects may not become apparent for 3–4 days, and are maximal at 7–10 days, so re-prescription should not be considered before 1 week. For **Paget's disease,** risedronate is given orally and pamidronate as an IV infusion.
Administration	Oral bisphosphonates are poorly absorbed, but this can be enhanced by correct administration. For example, alendronic acid tablets should be swallowed whole at least 30 minutes before breakfast or other medications, and taken with plenty of water. The person should remain upright for 30 minutes after taking to reduce oesophageal irritation.
Communication	Explain that you are recommending a medicine to help strengthen the bones to prevent fractures and/or lower calcium levels in the blood to improve symptoms. Explain that the tablets can cause inflammation of the oesophagus ('throat'). To minimise this risk, give clear advice on how to take the tablets and ask them to report any symptoms of oesophageal irritation (e.g. retrosternal pain). Advise them to see their dentist before and during bisphosphonate treatment. Emphasise the dose and frequency of bisphosphonate treatment to avoid overdosing errors, especially for those taking tablets weekly.
Monitoring and stopping	In **osteoporosis,** efficacy is monitored by dual-energy X-ray absorptiometry (DEXA) scans every 3–5 years, to check whether bone mineral density (BMD) is stable or increasing. For people at high risk of osteoporotic fragility factures (age over 75 years, previous hip or vertebral facture), alendronic acid should be continued for up to 10 years or risedronate for up to 7 years. For people at low risk, treatment can be stopped if the BMD T-score is greater than −2.5. Safety monitoring is by vigilance for symptoms of oesophagitis, osteonecrosis of the jaw and atypical femoral fractures, and serum calcium monitoring. For **hypercalcaemia,** efficacy is seen in calcium concentration and associated symptoms. For **myeloma, bone metastases,** and **Paget's disease,** clinical monitoring of symptoms (e.g. pain) and bone complications (e.g. fracture) is most informative.
Cost	Alendronic acid is the cheapest bisphosphonate; non-proprietary preparations cost around £1 a month. IV bisphosphonates are substantially more expensive.

Clinical tip—Fragility fractures cause significant morbidity and mortality. After hip fracture, 30% die within 1 year and 50% have reduced function. Bisphosphonates reduce recurrent fracture by 50%. You can assume a diagnosis of osteoporosis in women aged >75 years who have had a fragility fracture and start treatment with a bisphosphonate without further tests for osteoporosis (i.e. there is no need to do a DEXA scan).

Calcium and vitamin D

CLINICAL PHARMACOLOGY

Common indications	❶ Calcium and vitamin D are used in **osteoporosis** to ensure positive calcium balance when dietary intake and/or sunlight exposure are insufficient. Other treatments, such as **bisphosphonates,** may be given to reduce the risk of fragility fractures. ❷ Calcium and vitamin D are used in **chronic kidney disease (CKD)** to treat and prevent secondary hyperparathyroidism and renal osteodystrophy. ❸ Calcium (usually as calcium gluconate) is used in **severe hyperkalaemia** to prevent life-threatening arrhythmias. Other treatments, e.g. **insulin** with glucose, are given to lower the potassium concentration. ❹ Calcium is used in **hypocalcaemia** that is symptomatic (e.g. paraesthesia, tetany, seizures) or severe (<1.9 mmol/L). ❺ Vitamin D is used in the prevention and treatment of **vitamin D deficiency,** including rickets (in children) and osteomalacia (adults).
Mechanisms of action	Calcium is essential for normal function of muscle, nerves, bone, and clotting. Calcium homeostasis is controlled mainly by parathyroid hormone and vitamin D, which elevate serum calcium levels by increasing its intestinal absorption and renal reabsorption, and promote bone resorption. In **osteoporosis** there is a loss of bone mass, which increases the risk of fracture. Restoring positive calcium balance, either by dietary means or with calcium and vitamin D supplements, may reduce the rate of bone loss; whether this prevents fractures is less clear. In severe **CKD,** impaired phosphate excretion and reduced activation of vitamin D cause hyperphosphataemia and hypocalcaemia. This stimulates secondary hyperparathyroidism, which leads to a range of bone changes called renal osteodystrophy. Treatment may include oral calcium to bind phosphate in the gut, and alfacalcidol to provide vitamin D that does not depend on renal activation. In **hyperkalaemia,** calcium raises the myocardial threshold potential, reducing excitability and the risk of arrhythmias (it has no potassium-lowering effect). The rationale for giving calcium in **hypocalcaemia** and vitamin D in **vitamin D deficiency** is self-explanatory.
Important adverse effects	Oral calcium is usually well tolerated, but may cause **dyspepsia** and **constipation.** When administered IV for the treatment of hyperkalaemia, calcium gluconate can cause **hypotension** if administered too fast, and **local tissue damage** if accidentally given into subcutaneous tissue.
Warnings	Calcium and vitamin D should be avoided in ✖ **hypercalcaemia.**
Important interactions	Oral calcium reduces the absorption of many drugs, including **iron, bisphosphonates, tetracyclines,** and **levothyroxine.** Administered IV, calcium must not be allowed to mix with ✖ **sodium bicarbonate** due to the risk of precipitation.

colecalciferol, alfacalcidol, calcium carbonate, calcium gluconate

PRACTICAL PRESCRIBING

Prescription
In **osteoporosis,** if calcium intake is inadequate, you should aim to supplement dietary intake with 1–1.2 g of calcium and 400–800 units of vitamin D per day. Combined preparations of calcium and vitamin D are available. Vitamin D_3 is usually derived from animal fat, so vitamin D_2 is recommended for strict vegans as it comes from plant sources. Other preparations are also available for those with halal or kosher diets. In **severe hyperkalaemia,** prescribe 30 mL of calcium gluconate 10% (see CLINICAL TIP) for slow IV injection. Repeat doses may be required if electrocardiogram (ECG) changes persist. Given the urgency of the situation, it is acceptable to give the treatment first and write the prescription later. **Seek expert guidance** for the use of calcium and vitamin D in other indications.

Administration
Oral calcium preparations should usually be chewed then swallowed. Doses should be separated from potentially interacting medicines (see INTERACTIONS) by about 4 hours. They may also interact with certain foods, including spinach, bananas, and whole cereals; about 2 hours' separation is required if these have been consumed. **Calcium gluconate** should be administered by slow IV injection over 5–10 minutes into a large vein. Make sure the cannula is working by first flushing it with sodium chloride 0.9%, to avoid accidental subcutaneous administration ('extravasation').

Communication
Explain the rationale for treatment as appropriate for the clinical indication. Advise that they should seek medical advice if they develop side effects such as abdominal pain and limb pain, as these may be a sign of high calcium levels, requiring a blood test.

Monitoring and stopping
Continuous cardiac monitoring is required in severe hyperkalaemia. Repeat a 12-lead ECG after administration of calcium gluconate to confirm resolution of initial ECG abnormalities (e.g. normalisation of PR interval and QRS duration). In other indications for calcium or vitamin D supplements, check serum calcium levels at regular intervals or if the person develops symptoms of hypercalcaemia. Most people continue calcium and vitamin D lifelong unless the underlying cause for deficiency is corrected (e.g. dietary change, treatment for malabsorption). After 3–6 months of vitamin D treatment the dose can be reduced to a lower maintenance dose.

Cost
Oral calcium and vitamin D preparations are inexpensive on a per-patient basis, but at a population level they account for substantial healthcare spending.

Clinical tip—When dosed according to mass of the compound, calcium chloride contains three times as much elemental calcium as calcium gluconate, so the doses are not equivalent. In hyperkalaemia, to give the 6.8 mmol of calcium initially recommended, you require 30 mL of calcium gluconate 10%, or 10 mL of calcium chloride 10%.

Calcium channel blockers

CLINICAL PHARMACOLOGY

Common indications	❶ Amlodipine and, to a lesser extent, nifedipine are used for the first- or second-line treatment of **hypertension,** to reduce the risk of stroke, myocardial infarction, and death from cardiovascular disease. ❷ All calcium channel blockers can be used to control angina in people with **ischaemic heart disease; β-blockers** are the main alternative. ❸ Diltiazem and verapamil are used to control heart rate in people with **supraventricular arrhythmias,** including supraventricular tachycardia, atrial flutter, and atrial fibrillation.
Mechanisms of action	Calcium channel blockers decrease calcium ion (Ca^{2+}) entry into vascular and cardiac cells, **reducing intracellular calcium concentration.** This causes relaxation and vasodilation in arterial smooth muscle, lowering arterial pressure. In the heart, calcium channel blockers reduce myocardial contractility. They suppress cardiac conduction, particularly across the atrioventricular (AV) node, slowing ventricular rate. Reduced ventricular rate, contractility, and afterload reduce myocardial oxygen demand, preventing angina. Calcium channel blockers can broadly be divided into two classes. *Dihydropyridines*, including amlodipine and nifedipine, are relatively selective for the vasculature, whereas *non-dihydropyridines* are more selective for the heart. Of the *non-dihydropyridines*, verapamil is the most cardioselective, whereas diltiazem also has some effects on blood vessels.
Important adverse effects	Common adverse effects of amlodipine and nifedipine include **ankle swelling, flushing, headache,** and **palpitations,** which are caused by vasodilation and compensatory tachycardia. Verapamil commonly causes **constipation** and less often, but more seriously, **bradycardia, heart block,** and **cardiac failure.** As diltiazem has mixed vascular and cardiac actions, it can cause any of these adverse effects.
Warnings	Verapamil and diltiazem should be used with caution in ▲ **impaired left ventricular function,** as they can precipitate or worsen heart failure. They should generally be avoided in ▲ **AV nodal conduction delay,** as they may provoke complete heart block. Amlodipine and nifedipine should be avoided in ✖ **unstable angina** as vasodilation causes a reflex increase in contractility and tachycardia, which increases myocardial oxygen demand. In ✖ **severe aortic stenosis,** amlodipine and nifedipine should be avoided as they can cause collapse.
Important interactions	Non-dihydropyridine calcium channel blockers (verapamil and diltiazem) should not be prescribed with ✖ **β-blockers** except under close specialist supervision. Both drug classes are negatively inotropic and chronotropic, and together may cause heart failure, bradycardia, and even asystole.

PRACTICAL PRESCRIBING

Prescription	Calcium channel blockers are generally taken orally; of the examples listed, only verapamil is available for IV administration in the acute management of arrhythmias. Amlodipine has a plasma half-life of 35–50 hours and is suitable for once-daily administration. By contrast, the half-lives of nifedipine (2–3 hours), verapamil (2–8 hours) and diltiazem (6–8 hours) are relatively short. Diltiazem and nifedipine are available in standard-release and modified-release (MR) preparations. These may need to be prescribed by brand name to avoid unanticipated changes in effect (see CLINICAL TIP). Example treatment regimens are: for **hypertension,** amlodipine 5–10 mg orally daily; for **angina,** diltiazem MR 90 mg orally 12-hrly; and for **supraventricular arrhythmias,** verapamil 40–120 mg orally 8-hrly.
Administration	MR and long-acting preparations should be **swallowed whole.** Crushing or chewing these tablets will result in more rapid absorption.
Communication	Explain why the calcium channel blocker has been prescribed, as appropriate for the indication. Discuss other measures to **reduce cardiovascular risk,** including smoking cessation. Highlight **common side effects,** particularly ankle oedema if relevant.
Monitoring and stopping	Treatment efficacy can be judged by regular blood pressure monitoring for hypertension, enquiry about chest pain for angina, and by pulse rate and rhythm from examination or electrocardiogram (ECG) for arrhythmias. Continuous ECG recording may be useful for intermittent (paroxysmal) arrhythmias. Depending on the indication and whether it can be definitively treated, calcium channel blockers may need to be taken lifelong, but treatment aims should be reviewed regularly. For example, easing of blood pressure targets in those aged over 80 years, or who develop frailty or multimorbidity, may allow dose reduction or discontinuation. Stopping suddenly can cause withdrawal angina, so reducing the dose and frequency over a period of weeks may be advisable.
Cost	Amlodipine is available in non-proprietary form and is inexpensive. For diltiazem and nifedipine, only the longer-acting preparations are licensed to treat hypertension. These are more expensive.

Clinical tip—The different longer-acting preparations of nifedipine and diltiazem may not be 'bioequivalent' (i.e. pharmaceutically interchangeable). You should therefore request a specific brand when prescribing either of these drugs.

Carbamazepine

CLINICAL PHARMACOLOGY

Common indications	❶ Seizure prophylaxis in **epilepsy.** Specifically, carbamazepine is a second-line option for prophylaxis of focal seizures (with or without secondary generalisation). It is *not* recommended in absence or myoclonic seizures. ❷ **Trigeminal neuralgia,** as a first-line option to control pain and reduce frequency and severity of attacks.
Mechanisms of action	The mechanism of action of carbamazepine is incompletely understood. It **inhibits neuronal sodium channels,** stabilising resting membrane potentials and inhibiting repetitive neuronal firing. This may inhibit spread of seizure activity in epilepsy and control neuralgic pain by blocking synaptic transmission in the trigeminal nucleus.
Important adverse effects	The most common dose-related adverse effects are **GI upset** (e.g. nausea and vomiting) and **neurological effects** (particularly dizziness and ataxia). Other adverse effects include **oedema** and **hyponatraemia** due to an antidiuretic hormone-like effect, and **skin rashes.** More severe **hypersensitivity reactions** affect around 1 in 5000 people taking carbamazepine, and rarely there is cross-sensitivity with other antiepileptic drugs. Clinical features include severe skin reactions (e.g. Stevens–Johnson syndrome, toxic epidermal necrolysis), fever, and lymphadenopathy with systemic (e.g. haematological, hepatic, renal) involvement. These severe reactions are life-threatening.
Warnings	Carbamazepine exposure *in utero* is associated with neural tube defects, cardiac and urinary tract abnormalities and cleft palate. Women with epilepsy planning ▲ **pregnancy** should discuss treatment with a specialist and start taking high-dose **folic acid** supplements before conception. The risk of Stevens–Johnson syndrome is strongly associated with ▲ **carriage of the HLA-B*1502 allele**. This is most prevalent in people of Han Chinese and Thai origin, who should be tested for this allele before starting treatment. Caution is also required in ▲ **hepatic,** ▲ **renal** or ▲ **cardiac disease,** due to an increased risk of toxicity.
Important interactions	Carbamazepine induces cytochrome P450 (CYP) enzymes, reducing plasma concentration and efficacy of ▲ **drugs that are metabolised by CYP enzymes** (e.g. **warfarin, oestrogens,** and **progestogens**). Carbamazepine is itself metabolised by these enzymes, so 'auto-induces' its own metabolism over the first 2–3 weeks. Its concentration and adverse effects are increased by ▲ **CYP inhibitors** (e.g. **macrolides**). Complex interactions occur with ▲ **other antiepileptic drugs** (e.g. see **lamotrigine**), due to altered drug metabolism. The efficacy of antiepileptic drugs is reduced by ▲ **drugs that lower the seizure threshold** (e.g. **antipsychotics, tramadol**).

PRACTICAL PRESCRIBING

Prescription	Carbamazepine can be prescribed for oral or rectal administration. It is usually **started at a low dose,** e.g. 100–200 mg orally once or twice daily, to limit dose-related adverse effects. As tolerance develops to adverse effects, the dose is **increased gradually** to a usual maximum of 1.6 g/day in divided doses. Modified-release preparations are available and may be better tolerated.
Administration	Carbamazepine tablets should be taken at regular intervals, with or without food. Different formulations of carbamazepine may be absorbed differently. For **epilepsy**, you should **avoid brand switching**. This is because loss of seizure control and/or worsening of side effects have been associated with changing brands, due to differing absorption characteristics. Use of rectal suppositories should be limited to short periods when oral administration is not possible, as rectal irritation may occur.
Communication	Explain that the aim of treatment is to reduce seizure frequency, not to 'cure' epilepsy. Warn them about the signs of severe hypersensitivity, including skin rashes; bruising, bleeding, a high temperature or mouth ulcers (blood toxicity); and reduced appetite or abdominal pain (liver toxicity). If any of these occur they should seek urgent medical advice. For women, discuss contraception and pregnancy (see **valproate**). Advise that driving is not allowed unless they have been seizure-free for 12 months, and for 6 months after changing or stopping treatment.
Monitoring and stopping	**Efficacy** is monitored by seizure frequency, and **safety** is monitored by enquiry about new symptoms (as above). Routine measurement of full blood count and liver enzymes is unlikely to coincide with unpredictable hypersensitivity reactions, so is not recommended. **Plasma carbamazepine concentrations** are not routinely measured, but may be useful in selected cases. Blood should be taken immediately before the next dose, when carbamazepine concentrations should be 4–12 mg/L. Time to steady-state plasma concentrations (and appropriate sampling for repeat measurements) is 1–2 weeks after starting treatment or a dose change. Treatment should not be stopped suddenly, due to risk of disease recurrence. It should be withdrawn gradually and under specialist supervision.
Cost	Carbamazepine in oral formulations is inexpensive.

Clinical tip—Neuropathic pain can be difficult to manage, with little evidence to guide choice between agents. Trigeminal neuralgia is, to an extent, an exception. It stands alone in having a clear first-line choice, carbamazepine, the effectiveness of which has been well demonstrated. By contrast, the effectiveness of carbamazepine in other neuropathic pain syndromes has not been well studied. What little evidence there is generally suggests that **gabapentinoids** and **tricyclic antidepressants** are preferable.

Cephalosporins and carbapenems

CLINICAL PHARMACOLOGY

Common indications	❶ Oral cephalosporins are second- and third-line options for treatment of **urinary tract infections, pneumonia,** and other respiratory tract infections (e.g. **epiglottitis**). ❷ Parenteral cephalosporins and carbapenems are reserved for infections that are **very severe** or **complicated,** or caused by **antibiotic-resistant organisms.**
Spectrum of activity	Cephalosporins and carbapenems have a **broad spectrum** of activity. For cephalosporins, structural modification has led to successive 'generations' (first to fifth), with increasing activity against Gram-negative bacteria including *Pseudomonas aeruginosa* and variable activity against Gram-positive bacteria including *Staphylococcus aureus*. Cephalosporins and carbapenems are naturally more **resistant to β-lactamases** than **penicillins,** due to fusion of the β-lactam ring with a dihydrothiazine ring *(cephalosporins)* or a unique hydroxyethyl side chain *(carbapenems).*
Mechanisms of action	Cephalosporins and carbapenems are derived from naturally occurring antimicrobials produced by fungi and bacteria. Like **penicillins,** their **bactericidal** effect is due to their **β-lactam ring**. During bacterial cell growth, cephalosporins and carbapenems inhibit enzymes responsible for cross-linking peptidoglycans in bacterial cell walls. This weakens cell walls, preventing them from maintaining an osmotic gradient, resulting in **bacterial cell swelling, lysis,** and **death.**
Important adverse effects	**GI upset** (e.g. nausea, diarrhoea) is common. Less frequently, disturbance of normal gut flora allows overgrowth of toxin-producing *Clostridioides difficile,* producing **antibiotic-associated colitis**. This can be complicated by perforation and death. Immediate- and delayed-type **hypersensitivity reactions** may occur (see **Penicillins, broad-spectrum**). And as cephalosporins, carbapenems, and penicillins are structurally similar, there is a risk of cross-reactivity in 'true' allergy. This is not a concern for mild, non-allergic reactions (e.g. GI upset). Rarely, in parenteral therapy, cephalosporins and carbapenems can cause **seizures.**
Warnings	Cephalosporins and carbapenems should be used with caution in people ▲ **at risk of *C. difficile* infection,** particularly older people and those in hospital. The main contraindication is ✖ **allergy** to a β-lactam antibiotic, particularly if the history is suggestive of ✖ **immediate-type hypersensitivity.** Dose reduction is required in ▲ **renal impairment.**
Important interactions	Cephalosporins and carbapenems enhance the anticoagulant effect of **warfarin** by killing normal gut flora that synthesise vitamin K. Carbapenems substantially reduce plasma concentration and efficacy of ▲ **valproate.**

cefuroxime, ceftriaxone, cefalexin, meropenem, ertapenem

PRACTICAL PRESCRIBING

Prescription	Most cephalosporins are used intravenously at high dose for severe infections (e.g. ceftriaxone 4 g IV daily for bacterial meningitis). Cefalexin is an orally active example. Carbapenems are only available for IV administration (e.g. meropenem 1–2 g IV 8-hrly). Document indication, review date, and treatment duration on all inpatient antibiotic prescriptions to aid antibiotic stewardship.
Administration	Cephalosporins can be administered orally, as tablets, capsules or oral suspension, or by injection, which can be IV, as bolus injection or infusion or IM. Carbapenems can be administered as IV injection or infusion. Ertapenem is a carbapenem that is administered once daily. This facilitates administration of IV antibiotic therapy outside hospital, to allow prolonged treatment to be continued at home.
Communication	Explain that the aim of treatment is to get rid of infection and improve symptoms. Before prescribing, always check with patients personally (or get collateral history) that they do not have an **allergy** to any β-lactam antibiotic. Warn them to seek medical advice if a rash or other unexpected symptom develops. If an allergic reaction occurs, give written and verbal advice not to take this antibiotic class in the future and make sure that the allergy (including the nature of the reaction) is clearly recorded in the notes.
Monitoring and stopping	Check that infection resolves by symptoms, signs (e.g. resolution of pyrexia) and blood tests (e.g. falling CRP and white cell count). The duration of antibiotic therapy is a balance between ensuring effective treatment of infection and reducing adverse reactions and emergence of antimicrobial resistance. Always set a stop or review date when prescribing antibiotics, referring to local protocols for guidance. For IV antibiotics, oral switch should be considered after 48 hours if the patient is improving and able to take oral medication. However, as later-generation cephalosporins and carbapenems are only available for injection, oral switch is only possible if the infection is sensitive to an alternative orally-active antibiotic.
Cost	The costs of IV antibiotic therapy include drugs, administration time and equipment, complications (e.g. *C. difficile* infection), and need for inpatient stay. Where clinically appropriate, costs can be reduced by limiting duration of antibiotic therapy, IV-to-oral antibiotic switch during recovery and outpatient administration of IV antibiotics.

Clinical tip—Ceftriaxone's spectrum of activity covers the common bacterial causes of infections such as cellulitis and pyelonephritis, and its long half-life (around 8 hours) allows for once-daily dosing. This makes it a valuable option for ambulatory treatment of people who would otherwise have been admitted to hospital for IV treatment. This can provide a better patient experience and produce substantial cost savings.

Chloramphenicol

CLINICAL PHARMACOLOGY

Common indications	❶ **Bacterial conjunctivitis** using *eye drops* or *ointment*. ❷ Chloramphenicol as *ear drops* can be used to treat **otitis externa,** but is considered less suitable than alternative antibiotics. Systemic (*oral or IV*) chloramphenicol is rarely used due to toxicity. In the UK, it is restricted to the treatment of life-threatening infection, and only where other, safer antibiotic classes cannot be used due to allergy or bacterial resistance. This may include occasional cases of epiglottitis (*Haemophilus influenzae*) and typhoid fever (*Salmonella* spp.).
Spectrum of activity	Chloramphenicol has a **broad spectrum** of activity against many Gram-positive, Gram-negative, aerobic, and anaerobic organisms.
Mechanisms of action	Chloramphenicol binds to **bacterial ribosomes,** inhibiting **protein synthesis.** It is thus **bacteriostatic** (stopping bacterial growth), which helps the immune system to clear microorganisms. In high concentrations and with highly susceptible organisms it can be bactericidal (killing). The most common mechanism of bacterial resistance to chloramphenicol is production of acetyltransferase enzymes that directly inactivate the drug. Other mechanisms include target modification, decreased membrane permeability, and increased expression of efflux pumps. Bacteria share antibiotic resistance genes by 'horizontal transfer' in plasmids. Many bacteria remain sensitive to chloramphenicol, probably due to its restricted use over recent decades.
Important adverse effects	The most common adverse effects of *topical* administration are transient **stinging, burning,** and **itching.** *Systemic* administration, which is unusual in high-income countries, carries a significant risk of bone marrow toxicity. **Dose-related bone marrow suppression** is more likely with high-dose therapy, or when the drug accumulates due to impaired metabolism. It occurs during treatment and improves on withdrawal. **Aplastic anaemia** is a rare, idiosyncratic reaction to systemic therapy. It has an unpredictable relationship with dose and may be delayed. **Grey baby syndrome** is circulatory collapse occurring in exposed **neonates,** who are unable to metabolise and excrete the drug. **Optic and peripheral neuritis** may occur with prolonged use.
Warnings	Chloramphenicol is contraindicated in people with previous ✘ **hypersensitivity reactions** or a personal or family history of ✘ **bone marrow disorders**. *Systemic* chloramphenicol is contraindicated in the ✘ **third trimester of pregnancy,** ✘ **breastfeeding,** and ✘ **children** **<2 years** because of the risk of grey baby syndrome. *Topical* preparations should also be avoided in these groups unless essential. Chloramphenicol is metabolised by the liver, so dose adjustment and monitoring are required in ▲ **hepatic impairment** when used systemically.
Important interactions	Chloramphenicol has no important interactions when administered *topically*.

PRACTICAL PRESCRIBING

Prescription	For **superficial eye infections,** chloramphenicol is prescribed for topical administration as eye drops or ointment. In these preparations, the amount of chloramphenicol is expressed as a percentage, which refers to the mass in grams of drug in 100 mL of diluent (e.g. 0.5 g per 100 mL for a 0.5% solution). Drug application to the eye needs to be frequent as tears and blinking remove the drug. Eye drops (0.5%) should be prescribed initially as 1 drop every 2 hours (when awake), with frequency reduced to three to four times daily as infection is controlled. Eye ointment (1%) stays in the eye for longer, so three to four times daily application is sufficient throughout the treatment course.
Administration	Eye drops (optic) and ear drops (otic) are formulated differently. **Ear drops should not be put into the eye**, where they can cause injury with burning, stinging and blurred vision.
Communication	For eye drops or ointment, advise that **transient blurred vision** may occur and that they should not drive until vision is clear. Soft contact lenses may be damaged by eye drop preservatives and all contact lenses should be avoided during ocular infections. Emphasise the importance of ensuring that eye drops/ointments are kept sterile. They should check the preparation is sealed when they receive it, wash hands before use, take care not to touch the tip, and discard any remaining drug at the end of the course. If they purchase chloramphenicol over the counter for a self-diagnosed eye infection, they should seek medical advice if there is no improvement after 2 days or if symptoms worsen, as this may indicate an incorrect diagnosis or superinfection with resistant organisms.
Monitoring and stopping	**Efficacy** of topical treatment for eye infections is monitored by improvement in symptoms and signs (e.g. grittiness, redness, pus). **Safety** monitoring is only required during systemic therapy, when it should be guided by a specialist. Full blood count should be monitored closely and the drug stopped if there are any signs of myelosuppression. The duration of antibiotic therapy is a balance between ensuring effective treatment of infection, and reducing adverse reactions and emergence of antimicrobial resistance. For **eye infections**, treatment should be continued for 48 hours after healing, avoiding prolonged topical treatment (>5–7 days) to limit toxicity.
Cost	Chloramphenicol eye drops are inexpensive and can be purchased from pharmacies without prescription.

Clinical tip—Systemic chloramphenicol is not currently first-line treatment for any indication in the UK. However, as multidrug resistance to antibiotics evolves, 'older', more toxic, antibiotics may increasingly be needed. You will need to demonstrate continued professional development to adapt to changes in antimicrobial prescribing.

Clindamycin

CLINICAL PHARMACOLOGY

Common indications	❶ As topical treatment to the skin for **acne vulgaris** and by vaginal administration for **bacterial vaginosis.** ❷ Orally or parenterally for the treatment of moderate-to-severe infections including **cellulitis**, **osteomyelitis**, **septic arthritis**, and **intraabdominal infection**. Usually second- or third-line treatment, given in combination with other antibiotics. ❸ For treatment of *Plasmodium falciparum* **malaria**, with **quinine**.
Spectrum of activity	Clindamycin is active against **Gram-positive aerobes** (staphylococcus and streptococcus), explaining its clinical utility in skin, bone, and joint infections; and against a wide range of **anaerobes**, explaining its utility in intraabdominal sepsis and bacterial vaginosis.
Mechanisms of action	Clindamycin has a similar mechanism of action to **macrolides** and **chloramphenicol**, in that it binds to bacterial **ribosomes** and inhibits the early stages of bacterial **protein synthesis**. It is mainly **bacteriostatic**—inhibiting bacterial growth—thus facilitating clearance of microorganisms by the immune system. Bacteria resist the actions of clindamycin by modifying target proteins, reducing binding affinity.
Important adverse effects	Clindamycin is generally well tolerated, but side effects, including **diarrhoea**, **abdominal pain**, **skin rash,** and **abnormal liver enzyme levels** occur in between 1-in-10 and 1-in-100 people. **Antibiotic-associated colitis** (see **Penicillins, broad-spectrum**) occurs more frequently with clindamycin than other antibiotics. You should have a high index of suspicion for *Clostridioides difficile* colitis if diarrhoea occurs. Consider sending a stool sample to test for *C. difficile* toxin and change or stop the antibiotic if appropriate. GI side effects are much rarer with topical application but may still occur. Other rare, but severe, adverse reactions to clindamycin include **blood dyscrasias** (e.g. neutropenia) and **severe cutaneous adverse reactions**, such as Stevens–Johnson syndrome (SJS) and drug reaction with eosinophilia and systemic symptoms (DRESS).
Warnings	Clindamycin should not be prescribed if there is a history of ✖ **clindamycin hypersensitivity.** It is a useful option where penicillin is contraindicated by allergy, as there is no cross-sensitivity between these drug classes. It should be used with caution in ▲ **inflammatory bowel disease**. Clindamycin should be avoided in ✖ **acute porphyria** unless needed for a serious or life-threatening infection.
Important interactions	Clindamycin can enhance the effect of neuromuscular blocking drugs such as suxamethonium chloride, atracurium besilate, and pancuronium bromide, delaying postoperative recovery.

PRACTICAL PRESCRIBING

Prescription	The dose and route of clindamycin depend on the nature and severity of the indication, and whether oral administration is feasible. You should refer to the BNF and local protocols for guidance. The strength of topical clindamycin is expressed as a percentage (1%), which indicates the number of grams of drug (1 g) in 100 g of cream. For **acne,** topical clindamycin 1%–2% should be applied thinly one to two times daily. For **bacterial vaginosis,** 5 g of 2% cream (the full contents of one disposable applicator) is applied intravaginally at night.
Administration	Topical clindamycin is available as a cream for skin or vaginal (PV) application, or as a gel for the skin only. Oral clindamycin is formulated as capsules. Parenteral clindamycin can be given IM or IV. As there have been rare reports of cardiorespiratory arrest with rapid IV administration, clindamycin must be diluted in 5% glucose or 0.9% sodium chloride and infused over 10–60 minutes.
Communication	Explain that the aim of treatment is to get rid of infection and improve symptoms. Before prescribing, always check for **allergies** to clindamycin. Advise patients (especially those taking *systemic* clindamycin) to let you know immediately if they develop **severe, persistent or bloody diarrhoea**, as this could be a sign of a rare but serious side effect (*C. difficile* colitis) that may require them to stop treatment. Advise those using clindamycin for vaginal treatment that sexual intercourse and use of other vaginal products such as tampons during treatment are not recommended. Advise that clindamycin cream may weaken condoms and diaphragms, reducing contraceptive efficacy.
Monitoring and stopping	Monitor **efficacy** by looking for improvement in symptoms, signs and markers of inflammation (CRP, white cell count). Monitor **safety** by asking about bowel habit and by measuring liver enzymes and renal function in those requiring systemic treatment for more than 10 days. The duration of antibiotic therapy is a balance between ensuring effective treatment of infection and reducing adverse reactions and emergence of antimicrobial resistance. Always set a stop or review date when prescribing antibiotics, referring to local protocols for guidance. Prolonged systemic treatment is required for **deep-seated infection,** e.g. osteomyelitis. For **acne,** topical treatment should be continued for at least 6 months, stopping as soon after this as is possible.
Cost	Relatively inexpensive orally and topically, but more costly when prescribed for injection or where a prolonged course is required.

Clinical tip—Clindamycin is reserved for serious infections because the risk of side effects, particularly *C. difficile* infection, is greater than with other antibiotics. Limiting its use also reduces emergence of bacterial resistance, preserving its efficacy for when more commonly used antibiotics are ineffective. Always follow local antibiotic guidelines to play your part in preserving antibiotics for the future.

Corticosteroids, inhaled

CLINICAL PHARMACOLOGY

Common indications	❶ **Asthma:** to treat airway inflammation and control symptoms where occasional use of a short-acting β$_2$-**agonist** is insufficient. ❷ **Chronic obstructive pulmonary disease (COPD):** to control symptoms and prevent exacerbations. Place in therapy depends on whether there are features suggesting the disease is likely to be responsive to steroids (e.g. atopy, higher blood eosinophils, variable airflow obstruction). In COPD *with features of asthma or steroid responsiveness*, an inhaled corticosteroid (ICS), with a long-acting β$_2$-**agonist** (LABA), is recommended for first-line regular therapy (i.e. if a short-acting bronchodilator is insufficient). In COPD *without* features of asthma or steroid responsiveness, an ICS is recommended for second-line regular therapy (i.e. if regular treatment with a long-acting β$_2$-**agonist** and long-acting **antimuscarinic** (LAMA) is insufficient).
Mechanisms of action	Corticosteroids pass through the plasma membrane and interact with receptors in the cytoplasm. The activated receptor then passes into the nucleus to modify transcription of a large number of genes. Pro-inflammatory interleukins, cytokines, and chemokines are downregulated, while antiinflammatory proteins are upregulated. In the airways, this reduces mucosal inflammation, widens the airways, and reduces mucus secretion. This improves symptoms and reduces exacerbations in asthma and COPD.
Important adverse effects	The main adverse effects of inhaled corticosteroids are in the respiratory tract, including **changes in taste sensation** and **voice**, and **oral candidiasis** (thrush infection). In people with COPD, inhaled corticosteroids cause a dose-dependent increase in the risk of **pneumonia.** Systemic absorption can occur, particularly at high doses and with prolonged administration, causing adverse effects seen with **systemic corticosteroids**, including **adrenal suppression, osteoporosis,** and, in children, **growth retardation.** Inhalation of corticosteroids uncommonly triggers **paradoxical bronchospasm**, with an immediate increase in wheezing after taking treatment. This can often be prevented by taking a short-acting bronchodilator before the inhaled corticosteroid.
Warnings	High-dose inhaled corticosteroids, particularly fluticasone, should be used with caution in people with COPD who have a ▲ **history of pneumonia,** and in ▲ **children** due to the risk of growth retardation.
Important interactions	Clinically significant drug interactions are uncommon with inhaled corticosteroids as systemic exposure is generally low. However, **cytochrome P450 inhibitors**, particularly protease inhibitors (e.g. ritonavir, saquinavir; see **Antiviral drugs, other**) and triazole **antifungal drugs** (e.g. itraconazole), increase systemic exposure to inhaled corticosteroids by inhibiting their metabolism. This interaction can result in adverse effects similar to those seen with **systemic corticosteroids**.

PRACTICAL PRESCRIBING

Prescription	As the drugs within this class have similar efficacy, choice is determined by delivery system, dosage, need for combination therapy, and cost. Delivery is by aerosol (metered-dose inhaler (MDI)) or dry powder inhaler (DPI). MDIs require dexterity and coordination, whereas DPIs require good inspiratory effort. The **total daily dose** is categorised as low (≤400 micrograms/day of beclomethasone or equivalent), moderate (>400 to 800) or high (>800). Dosage equivalence depends on the characteristics of the drug and the delivery system. For example, the 'extrafine' formulation of beclomethasone is 2.5 times more potent than a standard inhaler (an equivalent low dose is ≤160 micrograms/day). Fluticasone proprionate is twice as potent as standard budesonide (low dose ≤200 micrograms/day), and fluticasone furoate is five times as potent (low dose ≤80 micrograms/day). Inhaler prescriptions should include the brand name so that the same device is dispensed each time, optimising adherence and inhaler technique.
Administration	Using a spacer with MDIs can improve airway deposition and treatment efficacy and reduce oral adverse effects.
Communication	Explain that you are offering a steroid inhaler to 'dampen down' inflammation in the lung. Advise that, although they won't feel immediate benefits after inhalation, treatment should gradually improve their symptoms and reduce flare ups, if taken regularly. Demonstrate how to use the device and check inhaler technique at every review. Explain that the common side effects of a sore mouth or hoarse voice can be prevented by rinsing and gargling with water after treatment. In COPD, advise about the increased risk of pneumonia. For those on high-dose treatment, explain the small risk of suppression of their natural steroid production and provide a Steroid Emergency Card.
Monitoring and stopping	Monitor efficacy by symptoms, exacerbation frequency, and lung function. For **asthma**, once disease has been controlled on a stable dose for at least 3 months, reduce this slowly with regular review to the lowest dose that maintains control. For **COPD**, inhaled steroids should be continued if there is evidence of improvement, or stopped if not.
Cost	The NHS spends almost £1 billion per year on inhalers. Where clinical factors are equal, the lowest cost inhaler should be prescribed.

Clinical tip—Inhaled corticosteroids are formulated as inhalers containing inhaled corticosteroid (ICS) alone or as dual (ICS/LABA) or triple (ICS/LABA/LAMA) combination inhalers. Benefits of combination inhalers include increased treatment adherence, convenience, and cost-effectiveness. Disadvantages include less flexibility in adjusting dosing and stopping treatment that is ineffective or no longer required.

Corticosteroids, nasal

CLINICAL PHARMACOLOGY

Common indications	❶ Prevention and treatment of seasonal or perennial **allergic rhinitis** where symptoms are moderate to severe, or treatment with **antihistamines** is insufficient. ❷ As first-line treatment to shrink **nasal polyps.**
Mechanisms of action	Corticosteroids have **antiinflammatory effects** and cause **vasoconstriction**. In rhinitis, this reduces mucosal inflammation, oedema, and secretions and improves symptoms. The diverse actions of corticosteroids are also responsible for their adverse effects, with immunosuppressive effects increasing the risk of infection and anti-mitotic effects reducing healing after nasal surgery. Where systemic absorption occurs, metabolic effects and adrenal suppression may be evident (see ADVERSE EFFECTS and **Corticosteroids, systemic**).
Important adverse effects	Nasal corticosteroids commonly (1%–10%) cause **local adverse effects** such as nasal irritation, epistaxis, pharyngitis and change in sense of taste and smell. Headache is also common. **Ocular adverse effects,** which are rare, include glaucoma, cataracts, and central serous retinopathy. People who report blurred or abnormal vision may require ophthalmological review. Around 70% of the dose administered in the nose is swallowed, and some of this may be absorbed. In high-dose treatment for prolonged periods, this may rarely lead to **adrenal suppression** and, in children, **growth retardation**. Systemic adverse effects are less common with mometasone and fluticasone than with beclometasone. This is because the proportion of the dose that enters the circulation in an active form *(bioavailability)* is less than 1% for mometasone and fluticasone, due to extensive first-pass metabolism in the liver by cytochrome P450 (CYP) 3A4 enzymes. The bioavailability of beclomethasone is much higher (about 40%).
Warnings	Nasal corticosteroids should be used with caution if there is ▲ **co-existing nasal infection**, which should be treated first. People with ▲ **nasal trauma or surgery** should not use nasal corticosteroids until healing has occurred. Nasal corticosteroids should be avoided in ▲ **pulmonary tuberculosis**.
Important interactions	Clinically significant drug interactions are uncommon with nasal corticosteroids as systemic exposure is usually low. However, **CYP 3A4 inhibitors**, particularly protease inhibitors (e.g. ritonavir, saquinavir; see **Antiviral drugs, other**) and the triazole **antifungal drugs** (e.g. itraconazole), increase systemic exposure to nasal corticosteroids by inhibiting first-pass metabolism. This interaction can result in adverse effects similar to those seen with **systemic corticosteroids**.

PRACTICAL PRESCRIBING

Prescription	To limit adverse effects, the objective is to control disease with the minimum effective dose and duration of treatment. Nasal corticosteroids are formulated as sprays, which release a fixed amount of drug per actuation (e.g. for mometasone, beclometasone, and fluticasone this is 50 micrograms per actuation). An indicative starting dose is 100 micrograms (2 sprays) to each nostril, once daily for mometasone and fluticasone, or 12-hrly for beclometasone. The dose can be increased for uncontrolled symptoms and reduced to maintenance levels when control is achieved. Fluticasone is also formulated as nasal drops, which may be prescribed where there is poor nasal airflow, e.g. due to polyps. Drops are more likely than sprays to be administered incorrectly, and hence swallowed and absorbed, so they are generally reserved for specialist use.
Administration	Before administration, they should gently blow their nose, shake the spray well, and remove the cap. They should sit upright and tilt their head forwards slightly. They should take the spray in the opposite hand to the nostril they intend to treat and insert the nozzle into the nostril, pointing away from the nasal septum back towards their ear. As they press the button to release the spray they should breathe in gently through their nose, then take the nozzle out and breathe through their mouth. This is repeated for a second spray in the same nostril if required and, after swapping hands, in the other nostril.
Communication	Explain that the steroid spray will reduce inflammation in the lining of the nose. This will improve symptoms such as nasal blockage and discharge, but the benefit will come on slowly over days or weeks, and only if they take treatment regularly. Demonstrate how to use the nasal spray and reinforce the importance of doing this correctly. Explain that common side effects include nasal irritation or bleeding, and that they should take a short break from treatment if these occur.
Monitoring and stopping	Efficacy is monitored by symptoms. Treatment controls inflammation but does not cure the underlying condition so symptoms can recur on stopping therapy. Aim to reduce dose and stop treatment in those with intermittent symptoms or where the trigger is removed (see CLINICAL TIP). Longer-term treatment may be needed for chronic inflammation or nasal polyps, with occasional interruption to check for resolution.
Cost	Nasal corticosteroid sprays are inexpensive. Beclometasone and fluticasone sprays can be purchased from a pharmacy.

Clinical tip—Nasal corticosteroids work best for seasonal rhinitis (hay fever) if started early in the season, before symptoms start. In the UK, this is around March for tree pollen allergy, May for grass pollen allergy, and September for mould spore allergy. Treatment may be stopped when the allergy season is over.

Corticosteroids, systemic

CLINICAL PHARMACOLOGY

Common indications

❶ Allergic or inflammatory disorders, e.g. **anaphylaxis;** exacerbations of **asthma** or **chronic obstructive pulmonary disease (COPD).**
❷ Suppression of autoimmune disease, e.g. inflammatory bowel disease, inflammatory arthritis.
❸ To reduce tissue damage due to excessive inflammation in response to infection, e.g. in severe **bacterial meningitis, COVID-19, and croup.**
❹ In the treatment of some **cancers** as part of chemotherapy or to reduce tumour-associated swelling.
❺ Hormone replacement in **adrenal insufficiency** or **hypopituitarism.**

Mechanisms of action

Corticosteroids bind to cytosolic glucocorticoid receptors, which translocate to the nucleus and bind to glucocorticoid-response elements, which regulate gene expression. Corticosteroids are used to **modify the immune response.** They **upregulate antiinflammatory genes** and **downregulate pro-inflammatory genes** (e.g. cytokines, tumour necrosis factor α). Direct actions on inflammatory cells include suppression of circulating monocytes and eosinophils. Their metabolic effects include increased gluconeogenesis from circulating amino and fatty acids, released by catabolism (breakdown) of muscle and fat. Corticosteroids also have mineralocorticoid activity, stimulating Na^+ and water retention and K^+ excretion by the kidneys. This effect is greatest with hydrocortisone and negligible with dexamethasone.

Important adverse effects

Immunosuppression increases the risk and severity of infection. **Metabolic** effects include diabetes mellitus and osteoporosis. Increased catabolism causes proximal muscle weakness and skin thinning with easy bruising and gastritis. **Mood** and **behavioural changes** include insomnia, confusion, psychosis, and suicidal ideas. Hypertension, hypokalaemia, and oedema can result from **mineralocorticoid** actions. Corticosteroid treatment suppresses pituitary adrenocorticotropic hormone (ACTH) secretion, switching off the stimulus for adrenal cortisol production. In *prolonged treatment*, this can cause **adrenal atrophy,** reducing endogenous cortisol secretion. If the exogenous steroid is then withdrawn suddenly, an **adrenal crisis** with cardiovascular collapse may occur. Slow withdrawal is required to allow recovery of adrenal function. **Chronic glucocorticoid deficiency** (e.g. during treatment withdrawal) can cause fatigue, weight loss and arthralgia.

Warnings

Corticosteroids should be prescribed with caution in people with ▲ **infection** and in ▲ **children** (in whom they can suppress growth).

Important interactions

Corticosteroids increase the risk of peptic ulceration and GI bleeding when used with **NSAIDs** and enhance hypokalaemia when used with β₂-**agonists,** theophylline, **loop** or **thiazide diuretics.** Their efficacy may be reduced by ▲ **cytochrome P450 inducers** (e.g. phenytoin, **carbamazepine,** rifampicin). Corticosteroids reduce the beneficial immune response to **vaccines.**

PRACTICAL PRESCRIBING

Prescription	Corticosteroids vary in potency. For example, the antiinflammatory activity of hydrocortisone 100 mg is approximately equivalent to prednisolone 25 mg and dexamethasone 4 mg. Systemic corticosteroid treatment can be given orally or by IV or IM injection. In emergencies (e.g. for vasogenic oedema associated with **brain tumours**), dexamethasone is prescribed at a high dose (e.g. 8 mg twice daily orally or IV), then weaned as symptoms improve. In **acute asthma,** prednisolone is usually prescribed at a dose of 40 mg orally daily. Where oral administration is inappropriate (e.g. **inflammatory bowel disease flares, anaphylaxis**), IV hydrocortisone may be used. In long-term treatment, e.g. for **inflammatory arthritis,** to limit adverse effects, use the lowest effective dose. This may be reduced by co-prescription of a steroid-sparing agent (e.g. azathioprine, **methotrexate**). In those at risk of adverse effects, consider offering **bisphosphonates** and **proton pump inhibitors** to mitigate these.
Administration	Once-daily corticosteroid treatment should be taken in the morning, to mimic the natural circadian rhythm and reduce insomnia.
Communication	Explain that treatment should suppress the underlying disease process but it usually takes 1–2 days before they will start to feel better. For those who require prolonged treatment, warn them **not to stop treatment suddenly,** as this could make them very unwell. Provide a Steroid Emergency Card and explain its importance. Discuss the benefits and risks of steroids, including longer-term risks of osteoporosis, bone fractures and diabetes.
Monitoring and stopping	Monitoring of **efficacy** will depend on the condition treated, e.g. peak flow recordings for asthma, blood inflammatory markers for inflammatory arthritis. In prolonged treatment, monitor for **safety** by, for example, measuring glucose and haemoglobin A_{1c} (HbA_{1c}) to identify diabetes mellitus, or performing dual-energy X-ray absorptiometry (DEXA) to measure bone density. The **duration** of systemic corticosteroid treatment should be as short as possible to control disease while minimising adverse effects. There is a risk of adrenal suppression if systemic corticosteroids are taken for more than 3 weeks (or 1 week at high dose), when treatment should be withdrawn gradually to prevent adrenal crisis.
Cost	Prednisolone, hydrocortisone, and dexamethasone are available in non-proprietary forms and are inexpensive.

Clinical tip—People taking long-term corticosteroid therapy have atrophic adrenal glands and may be unable to increase cortisol secretion in response to stress (e.g. acute illness). You may therefore need to provide this artificially by increasing the dose of corticosteroid treatment. Common practice is to double the regular dose during acute illness, reducing back to the maintenance dose on recovery.

Corticosteroids, topical

CLINICAL PHARMACOLOGY

Common indications	Inflammatory skin conditions, e.g. **eczema, psoriasis**, to treat disease flares or control chronic disease where **emollients** alone are ineffective.
Mechanisms of action	Corticosteroids have **antiinflammatory** and **immunosuppressive** effects (see **Corticosteroids, systemic**). In skin disease they suppress inflammation during flares and reduce recurrence during maintenance therapy, but they are not curative. Other actions, including metabolic effects and adrenal suppression, contribute to their adverse effects. Topical corticosteroids are classified depending on their type, concentration, and formulation as mildly potent (e.g. hydrocortisone 0.1%–2.5%), moderately potent (e.g. betamethasone valerate 0.025%) potent (e.g. betamethasone valerate 0.1%) or very potent (e.g. clobetasol propionate 0.05%). Potency determines efficacy and safety, with more potent corticosteroids being used to treat more severe disease, and also more likely to cause adverse events.
Important adverse effects	Where corticosteroids are applied topically, adverse effects are mostly limited to the **site of application**. These include skin thinning, striae, telangiectasia, contact dermatitis, and worsening and spreading of untreated infection. When used on the face, they can cause perioral dermatitis and cause or exacerbate acne. As topical corticosteroids do not cure the underlying skin condition, **withdrawal reactions** can occur on treatment cessation, particularly after prolonged treatment with moderate- to high-potency corticosteroids. These commonly manifest as a flare of skin inflammation occurring days to weeks after treatment cessation, which may be more extensive and uncomfortable than the original condition. **Systemic adverse effects** are rare, but include adrenal suppression, Cushing's syndrome and, in children, growth retardation. They are more likely when systemic absorption is increased, for example in prolonged treatment, larger areas of application, poor skin condition (inflammation or thinner skin at extremes of age), higher potency of corticosteroid, and use of occlusive dressings.
Warnings	You should not use topical corticosteroids where ▲ **untreated bacterial, viral or fungal infection** is present as this can cause it to worsen or spread. Avoid prescribing potent corticosteroids for use on the ▲ **face, genitals, and axillae** where the skin is thin or flexural.
Important interactions	**Emollients** increase the efficacy of topical corticosteroids and may allow a lower-potency drug to be used, reducing adverse effects. The order of application of emollients and topical corticosteroids to the affected area is probably not important. However, application should be separated by 15 minutes between to allow full absorption of one treatment before applying the other. There are generally no significant adverse drug interactions when corticosteroids are used topically.

PRACTICAL PRESCRIBING

Prescription	The goal is to control disease with the lowest potency corticosteroid for the shortest possible duration. When prescribing for an **eczema flare,** steroid potency should match disease severity (e.g. mild for mild flares; potent for severe flares). Prescribe treatment once daily for 7–14 days, or until 48 hours after symptoms resolve, whichever is sooner. Frequent flares or chronic disease may necessitate **maintenance treatment.** This should be with the lowest potency steroid that controls the disease, either daily or intermittently (e.g. 2 days per week). Prescriptions should specify the name, strength, and potency of the topical corticosteroid; its formulation (e.g. lotion, cream, ointment); and the amount to be supplied, e.g. 'hydrocortisone 1% (mild) cream, supply 30 g'. Note the strength is expressed as a percentage, indicating the mass of drug in grams (e.g. 1% = 1 g) in 100 g of cream. Specify where on the body the drug should be applied. The amount supplied depends on the coverage required. For example, 30–60 g of cream is sufficient for an adult to treat both arms for 1 week.
Administration	Corticosteroids should be **applied very thinly** and **only to the area of skin where disease is active.** Formulation is guided by patient preference (see **Emollients**). Most people prefer creams, particularly on visible areas of skin. Ointments have greater emollient effect and may be more effective, but are less well tolerated. Wash hands after application (unless they are being treated!).
Communication	Explain that topical corticosteroids should improve the skin condition by reducing inflammation, but may not take full effect for 1–2 weeks. Advise application at the time of day best for them, but at least 15 minutes before or after emollients. Explain that treatment should be applied thinly and indicate the approximate amount they should use (see CLINICAL TIP). Reassure them that side effects are uncommon if treatment is used as advised, but skin damage and withdrawal reactions can occur if it is applied to the wrong areas or for too long.
Monitoring and stopping	Monitor skin inflammation visually and by enquiring about symptoms. For disease flares, advise continuing treatment for 48 hours after eczema has cleared or return for review in 14 days if this has not occurred. Maintenance therapy should be continued indefinitely, with occasional treatment interruptions to see if it is still required.
Cost	Most topical corticosteroids are relatively inexpensive. Mild topical corticosteroids can be purchased from a pharmacy.

Clinical tip—A practical, albeit very approximate, method for specifying the amount of topical corticosteroid cream required is the 'finger-tip unit' (FTU). One FTU is the amount of ointment or cream squeezed from a tube with a standard 5-mm diameter nozzle from the tip of an adult index finger to the first (distal) crease. This amount should cover an area equivalent to the palms and fingers of both hands.

Digoxin

CLINICAL PHARMACOLOGY

Common indications	❶ In **atrial fibrillation (AF)** and **atrial flutter,** digoxin is used to reduce the ventricular rate. However, a β-blocker or non-dihydropyridine **calcium channel blocker** is usually more effective. ❷ In **severe heart failure,** digoxin may be added if treatment with an **ACE inhibitor,** β-blocker and either an **aldosterone antagonist** or **angiotensin receptor blocker** is insufficient, or at an earlier stage if there is co-existing AF.
Mechanisms of action	Digoxin is negatively chronotropic (it reduces the heart rate) and positively inotropic (it increases the force of contraction). In **AF and flutter,** its therapeutic effect arises mainly via an indirect pathway involving **increased vagal (parasympathetic) tone.** This reduces conduction at the atrioventricular (AV) node, preventing some impulses from being transmitted to the ventricles, thereby reducing the ventricular rate. In **heart failure,** it has a direct effect on myocytes through **inhibition** of **Na$^+$/K$^+$-ATPase pumps,** causing Na$^+$ to accumulate in the cell. As cellular extrusion of Ca^{2+} requires low intracellular Na$^+$ concentrations, elevation of intracellular Na$^+$ causes Ca^{2+} to accumulate in the cell, increasing contractile force.
Important adverse effects	Adverse effects of digoxin include **bradycardia, GI upset, rash, dizziness,** and **visual disturbance** (blurred or yellow vision). Digoxin is proarrhythmic and has a low therapeutic index: that is, the safety margin between the therapeutic and toxic doses is narrow. A wide range of arrhythmias can occur in **digoxin toxicity** and these may be life threatening.
Warnings	Digoxin may worsen conduction abnormalities, so is contraindicated in ✖ **second-degree heart block** and ✖ **intermittent complete heart block.** It should not be used in those with or at risk of ✖ **ventricular arrhythmias.** The dose should be reduced in ▲ **renal failure,** as digoxin is eliminated by the kidneys. Certain electrolyte abnormalities increase the risk of digoxin toxicity, including ▲ **hypokalaemia, ▲ hypomagnesaemia,** and ▲ **hypercalcaemia.** Potassium disturbance is probably the most important of these, as digoxin competes with potassium to bind the Na$^+$/K$^+$-ATPase pump. When serum potassium levels are low, competition is reduced and the effects of digoxin are enhanced.
Important interactions	**Loop** and **thiazide diuretics** can increase the risk of digoxin toxicity by causing hypokalaemia. **Amiodarone, calcium channel blockers, spironolactone,** and **quinine** can all increase the plasma concentration of digoxin and therefore the risk of toxicity.

PRACTICAL PRESCRIBING

Prescription	Digoxin is available as an oral or IV preparation. The effect of IV digoxin is seen at about 30 minutes, compared with about 2 hours following an oral dose. Intravenous administration is therefore usually unnecessary. By either route, a **loading dose** is required if a rapid effect is needed. A common approach is to give 500 micrograms of digoxin, followed by 250–500 micrograms 6 hours later, depending on response. Thereafter, the usual **maintenance dose** is 125–250 micrograms daily. Take care to ensure the loading dose(s) are prescribed for once-only administration, and not confused with regular maintenance doses. If prescribing by hand, be sure to write 'micrograms' in full.
Administration	Oral digoxin can be taken with or without food. Intravenous doses must be given slowly.
Communication	Depending on the indication, explain that you are offering a treatment which should slow down their abnormally fast heart rate and/or help their heart beat more efficiently. Outline common side effects such as sickness, diarrhoea, and headache. Ask them to seek advice if side effects are particularly bad or seem to get progressively worse, as this may suggest the dose is too high.
Monitoring and stopping	The best guides to the efficacy of digoxin are symptoms and heart rate. Check the electrocardiogram (ECG), electrolytes, and renal function periodically, particularly if there is a reason to suspect a change in the way the body handles drugs (e.g. during acute illnesses). Note that therapeutic doses of digoxin can cause ST-segment depression (the 'reverse tick' sign) on the ECG. This is an expected effect and does not signify toxicity. In acute therapy, continuous cardiac monitoring is advisable. Digoxin level monitoring is not helpful routinely, but may add value if toxicity or non-adherence is suspected. To guide dosage adjustment, levels should be checked at least 6 hours after the last dose. Although there is an approximate relationship between plasma concentrations and risk of toxicity, high concentrations do not always indicate toxicity, and 'therapeutic' concentration do not exclude it. Digoxin should be stopped if adverse effects outweigh its benefits, or if the indication for treatment is definitively treated (e.g. electrophysiological treatment of the arrhythmia).
Cost	Digoxin is available in inexpensive non-proprietary forms.

Clinical tip—Because digoxin's effect on ventricular rate in AF relies on parasympathetic ('rest and digest') tone, it tends to be lost during stress and exercise. Digoxin is therefore now rarely used on its own for AF, although it may be an option in people who are sedentary.

Dipeptidylpeptidase-4 inhibitors

CLINICAL PHARMACOLOGY

Common indications	In **type 2 diabetes,** dipeptidylpeptidase-4 (DPP-4) inhibitors are options for *combination therapy* with **metformin** (and/or other antihyperglycaemic agents) if blood glucose is not adequately controlled, or as *monotherapy* if **metformin** is contraindicated or not tolerated.
Mechanisms of action	The incretins (glucagon-like peptide-1 (GLP-1) and glucose-dependent insulinotropic peptide (GIP)) are released by the intestine throughout the day, but particularly in response to food. They promote insulin secretion and suppress glucagon release, lowering blood glucose. Incretins are rapidly inactivated by hydrolysis by the enzyme **DPP-4.** DPP-4 inhibitors ('gliptins') therefore lower blood glucose by **preventing incretin degradation** and increasing plasma concentrations of their active forms. The actions of the incretins are *glucose dependent,* occurring when blood glucose is elevated, so they do not stimulate insulin secretion at normal blood glucose concentrations or suppress glucagon release in response to hypoglycaemia. This means that DPP-4 inhibitors are less likely to cause hypoglycaemia than **sulphonylureas,** which stimulate insulin secretion irrespective of blood glucose.
Important adverse effects	DPP-4 inhibitors are generally well tolerated. Common side effects are GI upset, headache, nasopharyngitis, and peripheral oedema. **Hypoglycaemia** can occur, particularly where DPP-4 inhibitors are prescribed in combination with other drugs that cause hypoglycaemia, such as **sulphonylureas** or **insulin.** All the DPP-4 inhibitors are associated with a small risk of **acute pancreatitis,** affecting 0.1%–1% of people taking the drugs. This should be suspected if there is persistent abdominal pain and usually resolves on stopping the drug.
Warnings	DPP-4 inhibitors are contraindicated in people with a history of ✖ **hypersensitivity** to the drug class and should not be used in the treatment of ✖ **type 1 diabetes** or ✖ **ketoacidosis.** As there is animal evidence of reproductive toxicity and insufficient human data to ascertain safety, they should not be used during ✖ **pregnancy** or ✖ **breastfeeding.** They should be used with caution in ▲ **older people** (>80 years) and those with a ▲ **history of pancreatitis.** Many of the DPP-4 inhibitors are renally excreted, so a dose reduction may be required in ▲ **moderate-to-severe renal impairment** and some (e.g. saxagliptin) should be avoided in ▲ **hepatic impairment.**
Important interactions	Risk of hypoglycaemia is increased by co-prescription with other antihyperglycaemic drugs, including **sulphonylureas** and **insulin,** and by alcohol. **β-blockers** may mask symptoms of hypoglycaemia. The efficacy of DPP-4 inhibitors is reduced by drugs that elevate blood glucose, e.g. **prednisolone, thiazide,** and **loop diuretics.**

PRACTICAL PRESCRIBING

Prescription	DPP-4 inhibitors are taken orally, usually once daily: e.g. sitagliptin 100 mg daily. They are also available in fixed-dose combinations with **metformin**. As metformin needs to be taken two to three times daily, these compound products contain half the daily dose of the DPP-4 inhibitor (e.g. sitagliptin 50 mg with metformin 1 g) and are taken twice daily. Advantages of compound preparations include reduced tablet burden and improved treatment adherence. Disadvantages include inflexible dosage options, and difficulty identifying the culprit drug if adverse effects occur.
Administration	DPP-4 inhibitors are formulated as tablets. They may be taken with or without food.
Communication	Advise that you recommend a 'gliptin' tablet to help control the blood sugar level and reduce the risk of diabetic complications, such as kidney disease. Explain that tablets are not a replacement for lifestyle measures and should be taken in addition to a healthy, balanced diet and regular exercise. Advise them to stop taking the drug and seek urgent medical attention if they develop symptoms that could indicate acute pancreatitis (e.g. severe and persistent stomach and/or back pain) or allergy (e.g. rash, swelling of face, lips, tongue or throat).
Monitoring and stopping	Assess blood glucose control by measuring **HbA$_{1c}$**. When a DPP-4 inhibitor is used as monotherapy, the target HbA$_{1c}$ is usually <48 mmol/mol; when used as part of combination therapy the target is <53 mmol/mol. An HbA$_{1c}$ >58 mmol/mol is generally a trigger to intensify therapy with another agent. Home capillary blood glucose monitoring is not routinely required. Measurement of renal function before treatment can determine need for dose adjustment for sitagliptin and saxagliptin. Drug treatment for type 2 diabetes may be required indefinitely. However, as the treatment options expand, it is increasingly common for individual agents to be stopped and switched, or others added in, depending on efficacy and tolerance.
Cost	Monotherapy with a DPP-4 inhibitor is around 10-fold more expensive than monotherapy with **metformin**. The cost of a DPP-4 inhibitor alone is the same as its cost in a fixed-dose combination with metformin. However, in the long term, as generic products emerge and their cost falls, using fixed-dose combinations (which are less amenable to generic substitution) generally costs more.

Clinical tip—Although DPP-4 inhibitors improve glycaemic control, there is no evidence that they reduce the risk of vascular complications. This contrasts with **metformin**, **sodium–glucose co-transporter 2 (SGLT-2) inhibitors**, and **GLP-1 agonists**. They also do not have the weight loss benefits of these alternative options.

Direct oral anticoagulants

CLINICAL PHARMACOLOGY

Common indications	**❶ Venous thromboembolism** (VTE, the collective term for deep vein thrombosis and pulmonary embolism): Direct oral anticoagulants (DOACs) are an option for treatment and prevention of recurrence (secondary prevention) of VTE. **Heparin** and **warfarin** are alternatives. DOACs are also indicated for primary prevention of VTE in elective hip or knee replacement surgery. **❷ Atrial fibrillation (AF):** DOACs are indicated to prevent stroke and systemic embolism in non-valvular AF associated with at least one risk factor (including previous stroke, symptomatic heart failure, diabetes mellitus, or hypertension). **Warfarin** is an alternative.
Mechanisms of action	The coagulation cascade is a series of reactions triggered by vascular injury that generates a fibrin clot. The DOACs act on the final common pathway of the coagulation cascade, comprising factor X, thrombin, and fibrin. Api**xa**ban, edo**xa**ban, and rivaro**xa**ban directly **inhibit activated factor X (Xa),** preventing conversion of prothrombin to thrombin. Dabigatran directly **inhibits thrombin,** preventing the conversion of fibrinogen to fibrin. All DOACs therefore **inhibit fibrin formation,** preventing clot formation or extension in the veins and heart. They are less effective in the arterial circulation where clots are largely platelet driven, and are better prevented by **antiplatelet** agents.
Important adverse effects	**Bleeding** is an important adverse effect, most commonly epistaxis, GI, and genitourinary haemorrhage. The risk of intracranial haemorrhage and major bleeding is less with DOACs than with **warfarin**. However, the risk of **GI bleeding** is greater, possibly due to intraluminal drug accumulation causing local anticoagulant effects. Other adverse effects include **anaemia**, **GI upset**, **dizziness,** and **elevated liver enzymes**.
Warnings	DOACs should be avoided in people with ✖ **active, clinically significant bleeding** and in those with ✖ **risk factors for major bleeding**, such as peptic ulceration, cancer, and recent surgery or trauma, particularly of the brain, spine or eye. As DOACs are excreted by multiple routes, including cytochrome P450 (CYP) enzyme metabolism and elimination in faeces and urine, dose reduction or an alternative agent may be required in ▲ **hepatic** or ▲ **renal disease**. DOACs are contraindicated in ✖ **pregnancy** and ✖ **breastfeeding**, where the risk of harm to the baby is unknown, but has been seen in animal studies.
Important interactions	Risk of bleeding with DOACs is increased by concurrent therapy with **other antithrombotic agents** (e.g. ▲ **heparin**, ▲ **antiplatelets,** and ▲ **NSAIDs**). Other interactions can arise with drugs that affect DOAC **metabolism** (e.g. CYP inducers/inhibitors) or **excretion** (through induction/inhibition of transport proteins). For example, the anticoagulant effect is *increased* by ▲ **macrolides**, ▲ protease inhibitors, and ▲ **fluconazole** and *decreased* by ✖ rifampicin and ✖ phenytoin.

PRACTICAL PRESCRIBING

Prescription	The **dosage regimens** of DOACs vary by indication. For example, rivaroxaban is prescribed at 20 mg orally daily for prevention of stroke in AF, and 10 mg daily to prevent VTE following hip or knee replacement. For the treatment of VTE, 15 mg 12-hrly is prescribed for the first 3 weeks, reducing to 20 mg daily thereafter. **Duration of treatment** also varies by indication: e.g. 14 days following knee replacement; lifelong for AF. DOACs are usually started without need for initial **heparin** treatment, as onset of action is rapid. However, where dabigatran or edoxaban are used to treat VTE, 5 days of prior anticoagulation with heparin is recommended to align with the clinical trial evidence base.
Administration	DOACs are taken orally. In the outpatient setting, this is advantageous over **heparin**, which requires injection. Rivaroxaban, but not other DOACs, must be taken with food as this affects its absorption. Factor Xa inhibitors can be crushed to aid administration and are suitable for use with compliance aids (e.g. 'dosette boxes'). However, dabigatran must be stored in its original packaging and swallowed whole.
Communication	Advise that DOACs work by reducing the ability of blood to clot and thus that the main side effect is an increased risk of bleeding. Provide an alert card and advise that this should be shown at all healthcare contacts, particularly if they have an accident, need surgery or start a new medication. They should contact a healthcare professional immediately if they have prolonged or serious bleeding; or weakness, tiredness or breathlessness, which could be signs of anaemia. Otherwise they should take the DOAC at the same time each day until advised to stop.
Monitoring and stopping	Clinical monitoring for signs of bleeding is important, but laboratory monitoring of anticoagulant effect is not required. Duration of treatment depends on the indication (e.g. VTE: at least 3 months, AF: indefinite). Due to their short half-life, DOACs are stopped 24–72 hours prior to surgery (depending on the procedure's bleeding risk).
Cost	One month's supply of a DOAC to treat VTE costs around £50, whereas a warfarin tablets costs <£1. However, this difference is offset by lower monitoring costs with DOACs than warfarin.

Clinical tip—In emergencies, dabigatran can be reversed with idarucizumab (a humanised monoclonal antibody fragment that binds to dabigatran and its metabolites). Apixaban and rivaroxaban can be reversed with ande**xa**net alfa (a recombinant, modified form of human factor Xa that acts as a 'decoy receptor' for factor Xa inhibitors). Always seek advice from a haematology specialist in such cases.

Diuretics, loop

CLINICAL PHARMACOLOGY

Common indications	❶ For relief of breathlessness in **acute pulmonary oedema** in conjunction with **oxygen** and **nitrates**. ❷ For symptomatic treatment of fluid overload in **chronic heart failure.** ❸ For symptomatic treatment of fluid overload in **other oedematous states,** e.g. due to renal disease or liver failure, where they may be given in combination with other diuretics.
Mechanisms of action	As their name suggests, loop diuretics act principally on the ascending limb of the loop of Henle, where they **inhibit** the **Na⁺/ K⁺/2Cl⁻ co-transporter.** This protein is responsible for transporting sodium, potassium, and chloride ions from the tubular lumen into the epithelial cell. Water then follows by osmosis. Inhibiting this process has a potent diuretic effect. In addition, loop diuretics have a direct effect on blood vessels, causing dilation of capacitance veins. In acute heart failure, this reduces preload and improves contractile function of the 'overstretched' heart muscle. Indeed, this is probably the main benefit of loop diuretics in acute heart failure, as illustrated by the fact that a clinical response usually occurs before diuresis is evident.
Important adverse effects	Water losses due to diuresis can lead to **dehydration** and **hypotension.** Inhibiting the Na⁺/K⁺/2Cl⁻ co-transporter increases urinary losses of sodium, potassium, and chloride ions. Indirectly, this also increases excretion of magnesium, calcium, and hydrogen ions. You can therefore associate loop diuretics with almost any **low electrolyte state** (i.e. hyponatraemia, hypokalaemia, hypochloraemia, hypocalcaemia, hypomagnesaemia, and metabolic alkalosis). Hypernatraemia may also occur, due to loss of water in excess of sodium. A similar Na⁺/K⁺/2Cl⁻ co-transporter is responsible for regulating endolymph composition in the inner ear. At high doses, loop diuretics can affect this too, leading to **hearing loss** and **tinnitus.**
Warnings	Loop diuretics are contraindicated in severe ✖ **hypovolemia** and ✖ **dehydration**. They should be used with caution in ▲ **hypokalaemia,** ▲ **hyponatraemia** and in people at risk of ▲ **hepatic encephalopathy** (where hypokalaemia can cause or worsen coma). In chronic use, loop diuretics inhibit uric acid excretion, which can worsen ▲ **gout.**
Important interactions	Loop diuretics have the potential to affect **drugs that are excreted by the kidneys.** For example, ▲ lithium levels are increased due to reduced excretion. The risk of ▲ **digoxin** toxicity may also be increased, because of diuretic-associated hypokalaemia. Loop diuretics can increase the ototoxicity and nephrotoxicity of ▲ **aminoglycosides**.

PRACTICAL PRESCRIBING

Prescription	In the management of acute pulmonary oedema, you usually prescribe the initial dose of the loop diuretic intravenously, due to its more rapid and reliable effect. A typical choice is furosemide 40 mg IV, initially as a once-only dose. Then, depending on clinical response (see MONITORING), additional IV bolus doses, regular oral maintenance doses or, in resistant cases, an IV infusion may be required.
Administration	IV doses of furosemide should be administered slowly, at a rate no greater than 4 mg/min. Oral maintenance doses should be taken in the morning (with a second dose in the early afternoon in the case of twice-daily administration) to avoid causing nocturia.
Communication	Explain that you are offering a treatment for their water retention, in an effort to improve their symptoms of puffiness or breathlessness (as applicable). The medicine will inevitably cause them to need to pass urine more often. Provided they do not take doses late in the day, it should not affect them at night. Advise them to seek advice if they develop an acute illness that may put them at risk of dehydration.
Monitoring and stopping	For **efficacy** in the acute management of pulmonary oedema, evidence for a good response will include improvements in symptoms (e.g. breathlessness) and signs (e.g. tachycardia, hypertension, oxygen requirement). Urine output typically increases later, indicating onset of the diuretic effect. Over a period of several days, body weight monitoring (aiming for losses of no more than 1 kg/day) may be a useful measure of effect. For **safety,** periodic monitoring of serum sodium, potassium, and renal function is also advisable, particularly in the first few weeks of therapy. Deteriorating renal function should prompt a review of fluid status and consideration of dose reduction (or cessation of therapy). In the acute setting, once a target weight/ fluid status is achieved, doses may need to be reduced to a dose that maintains a target weight. If prescribed for simple gravitational oedema, stop after a few days and encourage movement, raising the legs, and support stockings as longer-term alternatives.
Cost	Tablet and injectable forms of furosemide and bumetanide are cheap. Oral solutions are considerably more expensive (about 20 times more in the case of furosemide; over 100 times for bumetanide).

Clinical tip—The proportion of furosemide absorbed from the gut (its *bioavailability*) is highly variable, both between and within individuals. It tends to be particularly low in severe fluid overload, due to gut wall oedema. This problem can be circumvented by administering furosemide IV, but this will not always be possible or desirable. In such cases, bumetanide may be a better choice, as there is some evidence that its bioavailability is more predictable. Bumetanide 1 mg is equivalent to about 40 mg of furosemide.

Diuretics, thiazide, and thiazide-like

CLINICAL PHARMACOLOGY

Common indications	❶ As an alternative first-line treatment for **hypertension** where a **calcium channel blocker** would otherwise be used, but is either unsuitable (e.g. due to oedema) or there are features of heart failure. ❷ Add-on treatment for **hypertension** if blood pressure (BP) is not adequately controlled by a **calcium channel blocker** plus an **angiotensin-converting enzyme (ACE) inhibitor** or **angiotensin receptor blocker (ARB)**.
Mechanisms of action	Thiazide diuretics (e.g. bendroflumethiazide) and thiazide-like diuretics (e.g. indapamide, chlortalidone) differ chemically but have similar effects and clinical uses. We refer to them here collectively as 'thiazides'. Thiazides **inhibit** the **Na$^+$/Cl$^-$ co-transporter** in the distal convoluted tubule of the nephron. This prevents reabsorption of sodium and its osmotically associated water. The resulting diuresis causes an initial fall in extracellular fluid volume. Over time, compensatory changes (e.g. activation of the renin–angiotensin system) tend to reverse this, at least in part. The longer-term antihypertensive effect may be mediated by vasodilation, the mechanism of which is incompletely understood.
Important adverse effects	Preventing sodium ion reabsorption from the nephron can cause **hyponatraemia,** although this is not usually problematic. The increased delivery of sodium to the distal tubule, where it can be exchanged for potassium, increases urinary potassium losses and may therefore cause **hypokalaemia.** This, in turn, may cause **cardiac arrhythmias.** Thiazides may increase plasma concentrations of glucose (which may unmask type 2 diabetes), low-density lipoprotein (LDL)-cholesterol, and triglycerides. However, their net effect on cardiovascular risk is protective. They may cause **impotence** in men.
Warnings	Thiazides should be avoided in ✖ **hypokalaemia** and ▲ **hyponatraemia.** As they reduce uric acid excretion, they may precipitate acute attacks of ▲ **gout.**
Important interactions	The effectiveness of thiazides may be reduced by **NSAIDs** (although low-dose **aspirin** is not a concern). The combination of thiazides with other drugs that lower the serum potassium concentration (e.g. ▲ **loop diuretics**) is best avoided. If combination treatment is essential, it should prompt more intensive electrolyte monitoring.

PRACTICAL PRESCRIBING

Prescription	Indapamide (e.g. 2.5 mg orally daily) and chlortalidone (12.5–25 mg orally daily) are the recommended options for hypertension. Historically in UK practice, bendroflumethiazide 2.5 mg daily has been widely used, but this is not recommended because there is limited evidence to support it. There is little to be gained from higher-dose treatment, as this tends just to increase side effects without significantly improving antihypertensive effect.
Administration	It is generally best to take the tablet in the morning, so that the diuretic effect is maximal during the day rather than at night and does not therefore interfere with sleep.
Communication	Explain that you are offering treatment with a 'water tablet' for their high blood pressure. If they have leg swelling, it may also help with this. Enquire whether they have any difficulty getting to the toilet in time (either because of mobility issues or sensations of urgency), since the water tablet is likely to make them pass water more often. Advise them to seek advice if they develop an acute illness that may put them at risk of dehydration. Also advise that 'antiinflammatory drugs' (**NSAIDs**) like ibuprofen, which can be bought without prescription, may reduce the effectiveness of diuretics. At review, ask men directly about the possible side effect of impotence, as this may not be volunteered without prompting.
Monitoring and stopping	The best measure of efficacy is BP control. Measure serum electrolyte concentrations before starting the drug, at 2–4 weeks into therapy, and after any change in therapy that might alter electrolyte balance. Electrolyte abnormalities should prompt consideration of an alternative agent. Antihypertensives may be required indefinitely, but treatment aims should be reviewed regularly. For example, easing of blood pressure targets in those aged over 80 years or who develop frailty or multimorbidity may allow dose reduction or discontinuation.
Cost	Indapamide, chlortalidone, and bendroflumethiazide are available in non-proprietary forms and are inexpensive. Indapamide is also available in branded modified-release (MR) forms. These are more expensive but there is no convincing evidence that they are clinically superior.

Clinical tip—One of the main adverse effects of thiazides is *hypokalaemia,* while one of the main adverse effects of **ACE inhibitors** and **ARBs** is *hyperkalaemia*. Moreover, these drug classes have a synergistic BP-lowering effect: thiazides tend to activate the renin–angiotensin system, while ACE inhibitors/ARBs block it. Consequently, the combination of a thiazide and an ACE inhibitor/ARB is very useful in practice, both to improve BP control and to maintain neutral potassium balance.

Dopaminergic drugs for Parkinson's disease

CLINICAL PHARMACOLOGY

Common indications	**❶** To improve motor symptoms in **Parkinson's disease.** Levodopa is preferred if motor symptoms are impacting quality of life. Dopamine agonists (e.g. ropinirole, pramipexol) are options for milder symptoms, or as add-on treatment in advanced disease. **❷** Levodopa and dopamine agonists are options for **secondary parkinsonism** (parkinsonian symptoms due to a cause other than idiopathic Parkinson's disease), but addressing the underlying cause (e.g. discontinuation of an offending drug) generally takes precedence.
Mechanisms of action	In Parkinson's disease, there is a deficiency of dopamine in the nigrostriatal pathway that links the substantia nigra in the midbrain to the corpus striatum in the basal ganglia. Via direct and indirect circuits, this causes the basal ganglia to exert greater inhibitory effects on the thalamus which, in turn, reduces excitatory input to the motor cortex. This generates the features of Parkinson's disease, such as bradykinesia and rigidity. Treatment seeks to increase dopaminergic stimulation to the striatum. It is not possible to give dopamine itself because it does not cross the blood–brain barrier. By contrast, levodopa (L-dopa) is a **precursor of dopamine** that can enter the brain via a membrane transporter. Ropinirole and pramipexol are relatively selective **agonists** for the D_2 **receptor,** which predominates in the striatum.
Important adverse effects	All dopaminergic drugs can cause **nausea** and **hypotension.** They can also cause **sleepiness, confusion,** and **hallucinations**, which are more common with dopamine agonists than levodopa. Conversely, excessive and involuntary movements (**dyskinesias**) are more problematic with levodopa. A particular problem with levodopa is the **wearing-off effect,** where symptoms worsen towards the end of the dosage interval. This tends to worsen in more advanced disease. It can be overcome to an extent by increasing the dose or frequency, but this can exacerbate dyskinesias early in the dosage interval. When these occur together, this is called the **on–off effect.** Modified-release formulations may improve control by providing a more continuous supply of dopamine.
Warnings	Dopaminergic drugs should be used cautiously in ▲ **older people** and in those with existing ▲ **cognitive or psychiatric disease,** due to the risk of causing confusion and hallucinations. Caution is also required in ▲ **cardiovascular disease,** because of the risk of hypotension.
Important interactions	Peripheral dopa-decarboxylase inhibitor (e.g. carbidopa) have a desirable interaction with levodopa, as they reduce its conversion to dopamine outside the brain. This lowers the dose needed for therapeutic effect. Dopaminergic agents should not usually be combined with ▲ **first-generation antipsychotics** (and, to a lesser extent, **second-generation**) or ▲ **metoclopramide** because of their opposing effects on dopamine receptors.

PRACTICAL PRESCRIBING

Prescription	Treatment decisions in Parkinson's disease, including drug choices and dosages, should be made by a specialist multidisciplinary team. In early disease, if symptoms are not impacting quality of life, dopamine agonists may provide sufficient control without causing dyskinesias. If quality of life is impacted, levodopa is preferred. Levodopa is always co-formulated with a peripheral dopa-decarboxylase inhibitor: either benserazide (co-beneldopa) or carbidopa (co-careldopa). A modified-release formulation may be tried if there are significant on–off effects.
Administration	It is very important with levodopa that doses are taken at times that produce the best symptom control. This is especially important to note in people admitted to hospital (see Clinical tip).
Communication	Close communication with specialists in Parkinson's disease is essential. Often a clinical nurse specialist will form the vital link in this partnership. Engage as necessary with the specialist team to support this.
Monitoring and stopping	The best form of monitoring for efficacy and side effects is an assessment by a specialist multidisciplinary team. Blood pressure (BP) should be monitored, particularly in those with existing cardiovascular disease. Dopaminergic therapy should never be stopped abruptly, as this can precipitate neuroleptic malignant syndrome. This is a particularly important issue in people admitted to hospital with an acute illness (see Clinical tip).
Cost	The drugs mentioned here are available in non-proprietary forms. There may be good reasons to use a more expensive branded product in some cases (e.g. when the on–off effect is prominent, switching to an MR form may mitigate this). A gel formulation, administered continuously via a percutaneous jejunostomy tube, is substantially more expensive. It is initiated in specialist practice only.

Clinical tip—Non-specialists are unlikely to play a major role in active prescribing decisions regarding antiparkinsonian therapy. However, you may be integral in *ensuring that therapy is maintained* during hospital admissions. Adhering to the correct timing of doses is essential: ask exactly what time they take each dose and prescribe accordingly. Where appropriate, consider implementing a self-medication approach. Avoid switching between products if possible. However, if the oral route becomes unavailable (e.g. peri-operatively), a transdermal dopamine-agonist preparation may be useful.

Emollients

CLINICAL PHARMACOLOGY

Common indications	As a topical treatment for all **dry** or **scaling skin disorders.** Specifically, emollients are used alone or in combination with **topical corticosteroids** in the treatment of **eczema.** They can reduce skin dryness and cracking in **psoriasis,** where, depending on severity, they are used alone or in combination with other therapies.
Mechanisms of action	Emollients help to **replace water** content in dry skin. They contain oils or paraffin-based products that help to soften the skin and can **reduce water loss** by protecting against evaporation from the skin surface. Many preparations can be used as a soap substitute, as soap is drying to the skin. Bath or shower emollient preparations are also available.
Important adverse effects	Emollients have few adverse effects. The main tolerability issue is that they cause **greasiness** of the skin, but this is integral to their therapeutic effect. Emollient ointments can **exacerbate acne vulgaris** and **folliculitis** by blocking pores and hair follicles.
Warnings	While these drugs are usually very safe to use, paraffin-based emollients are a significant **fire hazard.** The risk is proportional to the paraffin content (highest if >50%), but exists for all emollient products. Emollients also make the skin slippery, which may be a particular hazard when bathing children.
Important interactions	There are no significant interactions with other medications. However, when using more than one topical product, applications should be separated in time. This ensures that small volumes of topical drugs (e.g. topical corticosteroids) are not prevented from reaching the affected skin by large quantities of emollient.

PRACTICAL PRESCRIBING

Prescription	Emollients are emulsions of oil and water formulated as semi-solid **creams** (50% oil, 50% water), semi-liquid **lotions** (less oil, more water) or **ointments** (80% oil, 20% water). The choice of preparation depends on preference; the amount of skin to cover (lotions and creams spread further); and the severity of the condition (ointments are more occlusive and potent and last longer). Prescribe emollients to be applied at least two or three times a day in active disease as their effect is quite short lasting. Supply a sufficient quantity, e.g. 500 g, to provide adequate supply for frequent and widespread application. Continue treatment after improvement of symptoms to prevent recurrence.
Administration	Apply emollients in the direction of hair growth to reduce the risk of folliculitis.
Communication	Explain that you are offering a therapy to improve skin dryness, but that it may take several days or weeks to see the full effect. Encourage them to apply emollients as often as possible. Advise them to use emollients instead of soap for hand-washing as well as when washing in a bath or shower. Warn them that **emollients can make skin and bathroom fittings slippery.** When treating **eczema,** advise application emollient to the whole body, rather than just the affected skin, and to keep using emollients even when the disease is controlled, to stop it returning. If other topical agents are being used, advise them to apply these first and leave 5 minutes before applying an emollient.
Monitoring and stopping	When treating conditions like **eczema** or **psoriasis,** review of symptoms and signs is the best guide to efficacy. If emollients are ineffective, consider a second agent such as a topical corticosteroid. After resolution of acute flare of a skin condition like eczema, emollients are generally continued, although the frequency of application may be decreased.
Cost	Non-proprietary emollients are cheap, around £2–£5 for 500 g. Proprietary preparations are often double this.

Clinical tip—Most people who find emollients ineffective are not applying them frequently enough. Sometimes this is because they find them greasy and unpleasant. In this case, suggest trying cream or a lotion instead of an ointment, but apply it more often.

Gabapentinoids

CLINICAL PHARMACOLOGY

Common indications	❶ Gabapentin and pregabalin are first-line options in **neuropathic pain,** including painful diabetic neuropathy (**carbamazepine** is preferred in trigeminal neuralgia). ❷ Gabapentin and pregabalin are licensed for the prevention of focal seizures (with or without secondary generalisation) in **epilepsy,** although other options, such as **lamotrigine** and **levetiracetam** are preferred. ❸ Pregabalin is an option for **generalised anxiety disorder.**
Mechanisms of action	From a structural point of view, gabapentin and pregabalin (collectively 'gabapentinoids') are related to γ-aminobutyric acid (GABA), the major inhibitory neurotransmitter in the brain. However, they do not bind with GABA receptors and their mechanism of action, although not completely understood, seems to be mediated through **inhibition** of pre-synaptic **voltage-gated calcium (Ca^{2+}) channels** in the neocortex and hippocampus. This reduces Ca^{2+} entry into neurons, and thereby inhibits release of excitatory neurotransmitters such as glutamate. The resulting reduction of neuronal excitability in the brain probably explains the drugs' anticonvulsant effects. These central effects, along with similar effects in peripheral nerves, may also explain the mechanism by which they reduce neuropathic pain.
Important adverse effects	Gabapentinoids are generally better tolerated than older antiepileptic drugs. However, side effects can still be problematic, particularly during treatment initiation. These include **drowsiness, impaired concentration, dizziness,** and **ataxia.** Weight gain is also reported with both drugs. Increasingly, they are recognised as **drugs of misuse and dependency,** presumably for their dissociative effects and relaxation.
Warnings	Both drugs depend on the kidneys for their elimination, so their doses should be reduced in ▲ **renal impairment.** Careful assessment is required to identify risk factors for ▲ **substance misuse**.
Important interactions	The sedative effects of gabapentinoids may be enhanced when combined with other ▲ **sedating drugs** (e.g. **benzodiazepines**). Other than this, gabapentin and pregabalin are notable in having relatively few drug interactions—in contrast to many other antiepileptic drugs, including **carbamazepine, lamotrigine,** and **valproate.** This makes them particularly useful where combination regimens are necessary.

PRACTICAL PRESCRIBING

Prescription	Gabapentin and pregabalin are taken orally. To improve tolerability, they should be started at a low dose. The dose is then increased over subsequent days and weeks to reach a dose that strikes the optimal balance between benefits and side effects. Appropriate escalating-dose regimens are listed in the BNF. In many countries, both drugs are classified as controlled drugs. In the UK, this means that prescriptions must specify the total quantity or dosage units to be dispensed in both words and figures (this does not apply to inpatient prescriptions). It is recommended that no more than a 30-day supply be prescribed at a time.
Administration	There are no special considerations with regard to the oral administration of gabapentin and pregabalin.
Communication	As appropriate for the indication, explain that you are offering a medicine to reduce the severity of their symptoms (e.g. seizure frequency or pain severity). Explain that it commonly causes some drowsiness or dizziness, so you will prescribe a low dose initially, then increase this gradually (make sure they are clear on the dosing instructions). Explain that side effects should improve over the first few weeks. They should avoid driving or operating machines until they are confident that the symptoms have settled. In people with epilepsy, advise that driving is prohibited unless they have been seizure-free for 12 months, and for 6 months after changing or stopping treatment.
Monitoring and stopping	The best guide to clinical effectiveness is enquiry about symptoms (e.g. seizure frequency, pain score) and side effects. Plasma concentration measurement is not required. The drug should be stopped if it is not having a useful effect, or if this is outweighed by adverse effects. In neuropathic pain, use of a validated pain scale, such as the Neuropathic Pain Scale, is advisable to quantify benefit and inform decisions to continue or stop treatment. When stopping, the drug should be tapered gradually to avoid withdrawal reactions and to identify symptoms that may be unmasked by treatment discontinuation.
Cost	Gabapentin and pregabalin are available in both branded and non-proprietary forms. The brand name products are more expensive; there is no reason to prefer them.

Clinical tip—Gabapentin may cause false-positive results for detection of protein on urine dipstick testing. Therefore positive results should be verified by sending a sample to the laboratory for quantitative analysis (e.g. a spot sample for protein:creatinine ratio), which is not affected by gabapentin.

Glycopeptide antibiotics

CLINICAL PHARMACOLOGY

Common indications	❶ Treatment of **complicated skin and soft tissue, bone and joint infections; infective endocarditis;** and other infections caused by Gram-positive organisms where infection is severe and/or penicillins cannot be used due to allergy or resistance (e.g. methicillin-resistant *Staphylococcus aureus* (MRSA)). ❷ Vancomycin is a first-line treatment for ***Clostridioides difficile* colitis.**
Spectrum of activity	Glycopeptide antibiotics have a **relatively narrow spectrum** of activity against Gram-positive bacteria, notably *Staphylococcus* spp. (including MRSA), *Streptococcus* spp., and *C. difficile*. They are inactive against Gram-negative organisms.
Mechanisms of action	Glycopeptide antibiotics **inhibit growth and cross-linking of peptidoglycan chains**. This inhibits synthesis of the cell wall in Gram-positive bacteria, causing cell lysis (**bactericidal**). They are inactive against most Gram-negative bacteria, which have a different (lipopolysaccharide) cell wall structure. Acquired resistance to glycopeptide antibiotics is increasingly reported. One mechanism is bacterial modification of cell wall structure to prevent antibiotic binding.
Important adverse effects	**Pain and thrombophlebitis** from vancomycin infusion are common. Rapid infusion of vancomycin (and, less often, teicoplanin) may cause **vancomycin flushing syndrome** ('red man syndrome') due to direct, non-immune release of histamine. This presents with a pruritic erythematous rash over the upper body, occasionally with hypotension. True **immune-mediated allergy** to glycopeptide antibiotics, including immediate and delayed hypersensitivity (see **Penicillins, broad-spectrum**), may also occur. Glycopeptide antibiotics cause **nephrotoxicity** and **ototoxicity**, which is more common at higher doses. Rarely, idiosyncratic reactions may occur, including **blood dyscrasias** (neutropenia, thrombocytopenia) and **severe cutaneous adverse reactions**.
Warnings	Glycopeptide antibiotics should be used with caution in people with ▲ **immune-mediated hypersensitivity** (there is cross-sensitivity between vancomycin and teicoplanin) and those with ▲ **hearing impairment**, who are at increased risk of ototoxicity. People with ▲ **reduced renal function,** including ▲ **neonates** and ▲ **older adults**, are at increased risk of nephrotoxicity. Glycopeptide antibiotics are renally excreted and may accumulate in renal impairment. Dose adjustment based on plasma drug concentration monitoring is important to reduce toxicity.
Important interactions	Glycopeptide antibiotics increase the risk of ototoxicity and/or nephrotoxicity when prescribed with other drugs that cause these effects, particularly ▲ **loop diuretics**, ▲ **aminoglycosides**, ▲ **NSAIDs**, and ▲ ciclosporin (an immunosuppressant drug).

PRACTICAL PRESCRIBING

Prescription	Glycopeptide antibiotics are not absorbed from the GI tract, so in systemic infection, they must be given parenterally. *Initial* doses are calculated by weight (e.g. for adults vancomycin 15–20 mg/kg; teicoplanin 6–12 mg/kg), taking account of renal function. Vancomycin (half-life 4–6 hours) is given 8–12 hrly, whereas teicoplanin (half-life 100–170 hours) is given daily after initial 12-hrly loading doses. Subsequent doses are adjusted according to serum antibiotic concentrations (see MONITORING). For *C. difficile* colitis, where the intended site of action is the gut itself, vancomycin must be given orally, typically 125 mg 6-hrly for 10 days.
Administration	When given by intermittent or continuous IV infusion, glycopeptide antibiotics should be diluted to ≤5 mg/mL in glucose 5% or sodium chloride 0.9%. This is particularly important for vancomycin, which should be given no faster than 10 mg/min, and over at least 60 minutes, to reduce the risk of flushing syndrome. Vancomycin should not be given IM because of the risk of muscle necrosis, though teicoplanin can be given by this route. Oral vancomycin is formulated as capsules.
Communication	Explain that the aim of treatment is to get rid of infection and improve symptoms. Ask them to report any ringing in the ears or change in hearing during treatment, as ototoxicity is reversible if treatment is stopped promptly. As always with antibiotics, check for a history of allergy before prescribing.
Monitoring and stopping	In parenteral therapy, pre-dose (trough) plasma drug concentrations should be measured. The dosage should be adjusted to keep trough concentrations high enough for therapeutic effect, while avoiding toxicity. An indicative therapeutic range for vancomycin is 10–20 mg/L but this may vary depending on local assays and bacterial susceptibility. **Efficacy** is assessed by monitoring symptoms, signs, and inflammatory markers. **Safety** is monitored by enquiry about hearing changes and daily measurement of renal function. Platelet and leukocyte counts should be monitored in prolonged courses. The duration of therapy needs to strike a balance between ensuring effective treatment and minimising adverse reactions and resistance. Always set a stop or review date when prescribing antibiotics.
Cost	The cost of medicines is a consideration when developing treatment pathways. For example, NICE considered cost-effectiveness when recommending vancomycin (~£190 per course) as first-line treatment for *C. difficile* colitis, with fidaxomicin (~£1350 per course) as a second-line option if vancomycin is ineffective.

Clinical tip—Prescription of glycopeptides and subsequent dosage adjustment is complex and done relatively infrequently, making it difficult for a novice prescriber to gain expertise in this field. Always consult local guidelines and microbiology or pharmacy colleagues to ensure glycopeptide antibiotic prescription is done safely and effectively.

H₂-receptor antagonists

CLINICAL PHARMACOLOGY

Common indications

❶ **Peptic ulcer disease:** as a second-line option for treatment and prevention of gastric and duodenal ulcers (including **NSAID**-associated ulcers), where **proton pump inhibitor** (PPI) therapy alone is inadequate or not tolerated.

❷ **Gastro-oesophageal reflux disease (GORD)** and **dyspepsia:** as a second-line option for relief of symptoms, where **proton pump inhibitor** (PPI) therapy alone is inadequate or not tolerated.

Mechanisms of action

Histamine H₂-receptor antagonists ('H₂-blockers') **reduce gastric acid secretion.** Acid is normally produced by the proton pump of the gastric parietal cell, which secretes H⁺ into the stomach lumen in exchange for drawing K⁺ into the cell. The proton pump is regulated by, among other things, histamine. Histamine is released by local paracrine cells and binds to H₂-receptors on the gastric parietal cell. Via a second-messenger system, this activates the proton pump. **Blocking H₂-receptors** therefore reduces acid secretion. However, as the proton pump can also be stimulated by other pathways, H₂-blockers cannot completely suppress gastric acid production. In this respect they differ from **PPIs**, which tend to have a more complete acid-suppressive effect. Because of this, PPIs are the preferred first-line agents, and H₂-blockers are reserved for cases in which PPIs are not tolerated or symptoms persist despite PPI therapy.

Important adverse effects

H₂-blockers are generally well tolerated. Side effects are usually mild and include bowel disturbance (diarrhoea or, less often, constipation), headache, and dizziness. Ranitidine products have been found to contain low levels of an impurity called *N*-nitrosodimethylamine, a substance that could cause cancer. There is no evidence that ranitidine increases the risk of cancer, and any theoretical risk associated with the contaminant is likely to be very low. However, at the time of writing, all ranitidine formulations have been withdrawn from the market. Whether it returns will depend on the source of the impurity and whether it can be kept below acceptable levels.

Warnings

H₂-blockers are excreted by the kidneys, so their dose should be reduced in renal impairment. Like **PPIs**, they can disguise the symptoms of gastro-oesophageal cancer or significant ulcer disease caused by *H. pylori*. So it is important not just to treat symptoms, but to consider and, as appropriate, investigate their cause.

Important interactions

Cimetidine inhibits cytochrome P450 enzymes, including CYP3A4 and CYP2C19 which is involved in the metabolism of many drugs. It therefore interacts with ▲ **drugs metabolised by cytochrome P450 enzymes,** notably including ▲ aminophylline/theophylline, ▲ **amiodarone,** ▲ **citalopram,** ▲ phenytoin, ▲ **quinine,** and ▲ **warfarin.** Refer to the BNF for a more complete list. Interactions are less problematic for ranitidine and famotidine.

PRACTICAL PRESCRIBING

Prescription	At the time of writing, ranitidine is unavailable due to safety concerns (see ADVERSE EFFECTS). It is not known whether it will return to the market. If available, a typical dosage is 150 mg orally 12-hrly, but this varies by indication. The typical dosage of cimetidine is 400 mg orally 12-hrly, and famotidine 20–40 mg orally 12-hrly. The duration of therapy depends on the indication.
Administration	Oral preparations can be taken before, with or after food.
Communication	Explain that you are offering treatment to reduce stomach acid. This will hopefully improve their symptoms and, if applicable, allow their ulcer to heal. It is reasonable to say that side effects are not usually problematic. Ensure that the intended duration of therapy is clear and emphasise the need to report any 'alarm' symptoms (e.g. weight loss, swallowing difficulty, vomiting blood, altered blood in the stool), should they arise.
Monitoring and stopping	Clinicians should offer testing for *H. pylori* when symptoms of GORD, dyspepsia or peptic ulcer disease are reported (and endoscopy where red-flag symptoms are raised). Where treatment is offered empirically (i.e. without investigation of cause), a maximum 4-week trial of treatment is recommended. Investigations should be carried out if symptoms persist after cessation of this trial, or if any 'alarm' symptoms arise. Acid-suppressive therapy may be stopped following treatment for some indications (e.g. eradication of *H. pylori* or treatment of NSAID-associated ulcer) but may need to be continued for others (e.g. Barrett's oesophagitis with ongoing reflux symptoms). For symptomatic treatment of dyspepsia and GORD, symptoms are the best guide to the effect of therapy and should be reviewed annually. If these have improved, it may be possible to step-down therapy to an **alginate** or **antacid**, taken as required.
Cost	H_2-blockers are available in non-proprietary form and generally inexpensive. Effervescent tablets and oral solutions are about 10 times more expensive than conventional oral formulations.

Clinical tip—H_2-blockers have been superseded by **PPIs** for most indications, due to their more complete acid-suppressing effect. One advantage that H_2-blockers retain, however, is a more rapid onset of effect. This may make them a better choice for suppressing gastric acid production preoperatively. This may be indicated in people with significant GORD due to undergo general anaesthesia, in whom there is a risk that gastric acid may reflux and then be aspirated, causing pneumonitis.

Heparins and fondaparinux

CLINICAL PHARMACOLOGY

Common indications	❶ Heparin, usually low molecular weight heparin (LMWH), is used for prevention of **deep vein thrombosis** and **pulmonary embolism** (collectively **venous thromboembolism (VTE)**) in hospital inpatients. It is also an option for treatment of VTE until oral anticoagulation (e.g. with **warfarin**) is established. Fondaparinux and **DOACs** (e.g. rivaroxaban) are alternatives. ❷ Alongside **antiplatelet drugs**, heparin (usually LMWH) or fondaparinux is given in **acute coronary syndrome (ACS)** to reduce clot progression.
Mechanisms of action	In simple terms, venous and atrial clot formation is driven largely by the coagulation cascade, while arterial thrombosis is more a phenomenon of platelet activation. The coagulation cascade is an amplification reaction between clotting factors that generates a fibrin clot. Antithrombin inactivates clotting factors, particularly factors IIa (thrombin) and Xa, providing a natural break to the clotting process. Heparins and fondaparinux **enhance** the anticoagulant effect of **antithrombin.** The size of heparin molecules determines their molecular specificity: *unfractionated heparin (UFH)* (large and small molecules) promotes inactivation of both factors IIa and Xa, whereas *LMWH* (smaller molecules) is more specific for factor Xa. Fondaparinux is a synthetic pentasaccharide that mimics the sequence of the binding site of heparin to antithrombin and is very specific for factor Xa.
Important adverse effects	The main adverse effect is **haemorrhage.** This risk may be lower with fondaparinux than with LMWH or UFH. **Bruising** may occur, particularly at the injection site. **Hyperkalaemia** occurs occasionally, due to an effect on adrenal aldosterone secretion. Rarely, heparins can cause a dangerous immune reaction characterised by low platelet count and thrombosis **(heparin-induced thrombocytopenia (HIT)).** This is less likely with LMWH than UFH, and far less likely with fondaparinux.
Warnings	Anticoagulants should be used with caution if there are risk factors for bleeding, including ▲ **clotting disorders** and ▲ **severe uncontrolled hypertension**. They should be withheld immediately before and after ▲ **invasive procedures,** particularly lumbar puncture and spinal anaesthesia. In ▲ **renal impairment,** LMWH and fondaparinux accumulate, so a lower dose or UFH should be used instead.
Important interactions	Combining heparins with other antithrombotic drugs (e.g. **antiplatelets**, **warfarin**) has an additive effect. This is sometimes desirable (e.g. in treating ACS), but it is associated with an increased risk of bleeding, so should otherwise be avoided. In major bleeding, protamine is an option to reverse heparin anticoagulation. This is effective for UFH but much less so for LMWH, and ineffective against fondaparinux. Andexanet α is effective, though unlicensed, for reversal of fondaparinux.

PRACTICAL PRESCRIBING

Prescription

Subcutaneous LMWH is preferred in most indications. The dose is specified in units (*never* abbreviate this to 'U', as this can easily be misread as '0') and varies by indication and body weight. Dalteparin 5000 units SC daily is an example for VTE prophylaxis, but refer to local protocols. UFH may be preferred in renal impairment (e.g. heparin 5000 units SC 12-hrly for VTE prophylaxis) or when rapid onset and offset of anticoagulation is required (when it is given as a variable-rate IV infusion).

Administration

Injections are usually given into the subcutaneous tissue of the abdominal wall.

Communication

In VTE prophylaxis, explain that the treatment is intended to reduce the risk of blood clots. Discuss the risks and benefits of anticoagulation, particularly if long-term treatment is envisaged. Advise on the avoidance of activities that may increase bleeding risk and the need to inform healthcare professionals that they are taking anticoagulants. Discuss self-administration (or administration by a caregiver), which is possible with appropriate training. Otherwise administration by a district nurse may be arranged.

Monitoring and stopping

A major advantage of LMWH and fondaparinux over UFH is that their anticoagulant effect is predictable and laboratory monitoring is not routinely required. In selected cases (e.g. renal impairment, pregnancy), plasma anti-Xa activity may be used to guide dosage adjustment. UFH is less predictable, and when used to achieve full ('therapeutic' as opposed to 'prophylactic') anticoagulation, treatment is titrated against the activated partial thromboplastin ratio (APTR) (usual target 1.5–2.5). Full blood count, clotting, and renal profiles should be checked before starting treatment. In prolonged therapy (>4 days), platelet count and serum potassium concentration should be monitored, as the risk of thrombocytopenia and hyperkalaemia increases with duration of therapy. Seek immediate specialist advice if the platelet count drops significantly, as this may signify HIT, which requires urgent management, including the cessation of all heparins. Treatment duration for VTE depends on the indication (e.g. 3 months for provoked DVT), but this should be guided by a specialist.

Cost

When used for VTE prophylaxis, LMWH costs approximately £3 per day, whereas fondaparinux costs ~£6 per day. For UFH infusion, consumables and monitoring increase the costs. Cost is not generally a driver of drug choice for heparins and fondaparinux.

Clinical tip—If warfarin is chosen for VTE treatment, LMWH may initially be given alongside it. This is because there is a delay in the onset of the anticoagulant effect while existing clotting factors are cleared. Due to their short half-lives, the first to be cleared are the natural anticoagulants, proteins C and S, resulting in a transient prothrombotic effect.

Hormone antagonists and agonists used in breast and prostate cancer

CLINICAL PHARMACOLOGY

Common indications	❶ Tamoxifen, anastrozole, and letrozole are used in estrogen (oestrogen)-receptor positive (ER-positive) **breast cancer,** as an adjuvant (after surgery) treatment option to reduce the risk of recurrent disease or to slow progression in advanced disease. ❷ Leuprorelin, bicalutamide, and goserelin are used in **prostate cancer,** as systemic antiandrogen therapy for hormone sensitive tissue subtypes that cannot be resected.
Mechanisms of action	Approximately two-thirds of **breast cancers** express oestrogen receptors (ER-positive), which stimulate cell proliferation. Antagonising oestrogen therefore suppresses tumour growth in ER-positive cancers. Tamoxifen is a **selective oestrogen receptor modulator,** which acts to prevent oestrogen binding to its receptor. Anastrozole and letrozole are **aromatase inhibitors.** They interfere with synthesis of oestrogens outside the ovary (e.g. in fat and muscle) by inhibiting the conversion of androgens to oestrogens by aromatase. They are superior to tamoxifen in post-menopausal women, but ineffective in women with functioning ovaries because they have relatively little effect on *ovarian* oestrogen synthesis. By a similar mechanism, around 90-percent of **prostate cancers** will respond to hormone therapies that suppress androgens. Gonadotrophin-releasing hormone (GnRH, gonadorelin) analogues (e.g. goserelin, leuprorelin) initially over-stimulate production of luteinising hormone (LH) in the anterior pituitary, but **GnRH receptors** are then rapidly **downregulated** causing LH, and consequently androgens, to decrease to 'medical castration' levels. **Androgen receptor inhibitors** like bicalutamide directly block androgen receptors to prevent testosterone driven cancer cell growth.
Important adverse effects	The most common adverse effects of tamoxifen and aromatase inhibitors are symptoms of **oestrogen depletion** (e.g. vaginal dryness, hot flushes, loss of bone density). Tamoxifen increases the risk of **venous thromboembolism** and **endometrial cancer.** Rarely, tamoxifen and aromatase inhibitors can cause **agranulocytosis** and **liver failure.** Antiandrogen therapy may lead to **hair loss, gynaecomastia,** and **mood disturbance.** Bicalutamide may cause **photosensitivity.**
Warnings	Tamoxifen is contraindicated in ✖ **pregnancy** and ✖ **breastfeeding.** Aromatase inhibitors should not be used in ✖ **pre-menopausal women** unless ovarian function is suppressed or ablated (e.g. by oophorectomy). Initial overstimulation of LH production by goserelin and leuprorelin may stimulate tumour growth. This risks causing cord compression if there are **spinal metastases.**
Important interactions	Tamoxifen inhibits a cytochrome P450 enzyme (CYP2C9) responsible for metabolising ✖ **warfarin**, increasing the risk of bleeding. The **selective serotonin reuptake inhibitors (SSRIs)** ✖ fluoxetine, and ✖ paroxetine inhibit hepatic activation of tamoxifen.

letrozole, tamoxifen, anastrozole (breast cancer)
bicalutamide, goserelin (prostate cancer)

PRACTICAL PRESCRIBING

Prescription	These drugs are prescribed by specialists, following decisions made by a multidisciplinary team.
Administration	Tamoxifen, bicalutamide, and aromatase inhibitors are formulated as tablets to be taken with water. It does not matter if they are taken with or without food. GnRH analogues may be formulated as implants or suspension for injection, to be administered from a pre-filled syringe by SC or IM injection.
Communication	Depending on the clinical context, explain the treatment is intended to reduce the risk of recurrence or slow the growth of the tumour. Explain that it works by blocking the effects of hormones in the body on tumour cells. Describe the important adverse effects. For example, for tamoxifen, explain that it can increase the risk of cancer of the lining of the womb, so they should report symptoms such as vaginal bleeding promptly. Explain that it can also increase the risk of blood clots in the leg and lungs (deep vein thrombosis and pulmonary embolism), so it is advisable to seek medical advice immediately if symptoms such as leg swelling or breathlessness occur. As appropriate, advise that tamoxifen affects the development of unborn babies. Therefore women taking tamoxifen should avoid becoming pregnant. They should use barrier protection or non-hormonal contraceptives. For bicalutamide, advise on the use of sunscreen to prevent photo-sensitivity/sunburn.
Monitoring and stopping	Monitoring for disease recurrence or progression should be guided by the multidisciplinary oncology team. All of these drugs can cause changes in liver enzymes and/or bone marrow suppression, so liver function and full blood count should be monitored. Duration of therapy is highly individualised. Tamoxifen, for example, may be taken for 5 years *or* switched to an aromatase inhibitor if menopause intercedes. This is directed by the an oncology specialist.
Cost	These drugs are inexpensive.

Clinical tip—The combination of warfarin and tamoxifen should be avoided due to a significant drug interaction that increases the risk of bleeding. Interactions are common in cancer therapy, and this is one of the reasons that when anticoagulation is required in a person with cancer, a **low molecular weight heparin** is preferable, and perhaps superior, to **warfarin**.

Insulin

CLINICAL PHARMACOLOGY

Common indications	❶ For insulin replacement in **type 1 diabetes,** and control of blood glucose in **type 2 diabetes** if oral antihyperglycaemic treatment is insufficient or poorly tolerated. ❷ Given intravenously, in the treatment of diabetic emergencies such as **diabetic ketoacidosis** and **hyperosmolar hyperglycaemic state,** and for **peri-operative glycaemic control** in selected cases. ❸ To treat **hyperkalaemia,** while other measures (such as treatment of the underlying cause) are initiated. For this indication, it *must* be given with IV glucose.
Mechanisms of action	Exogenous insulin functions similarly to endogenous insulin. It **stimulates glucose uptake and utilisation** from the circulation into tissues, including skeletal muscle and fat. Insulin stimulates glycogen, lipid, and protein synthesis and inhibits gluconeogenesis and ketogenesis. The overall effect is to lower blood glucose concentration, and this is the primary measure of its therapeutic effect. Insulin also **activates Na$^+$/K$^+$-ATPase,** driving K$^+$ into cells, and reducing serum K$^+$ concentrations. However, once insulin treatment is stopped, K$^+$ leaks back out of the cells into the circulation, so this is only a short-term measure while other treatment is commenced. The wide choice of insulin preparations for treatment of diabetes mellitus can be classified as **rapid acting** (immediate onset, short duration)—e.g. NovoRapid® (insulin aspart); **short acting** (early onset, short duration)—e.g. Actrapid® (soluble insulin); **intermediate acting** (intermediate onset and duration)—e.g. Humulin I® (isophane or NPH insulin); and **long acting** (flat profile with regular administration)—e.g. Lantus® (insulin glargine), Levemir® (insulin detemir), Tresiba® (insulin degludec). **Biphasic insulin** preparations contain a mixture of rapid- and intermediate-acting insulins, e.g. NovoMix® 30 (30% insulin aspart, 70% insulin aspart protamine). Where IV insulin is required (hyperkalaemia, diabetic emergencies, peri-operative glucose control), soluble insulin (Actrapid®) is used. To account for the different potencies of insulin preparations, they are dosed in *units*, which correspond to the glucose-lowering activity of a defined mass of an internationally approved 'standard insulin'.
Important adverse effects	The main adverse effect of insulin is **hypoglycaemia,** which can be severe enough to cause coma and death. When administered by repeated SC injection at the same site, insulin can cause fat overgrowth **(lipohypertrophy)**, which may be unsightly or uncomfortable.
Warnings	In ▲ **renal impairment,** insulin clearance is reduced, so there is an increased risk of hypoglycaemia.
Important interactions	Although often necessary, combining insulin with other hypoglycaemic agents increases the risk of hypoglycaemia. Concurrent therapy with **systemic corticosteroids** increases insulin requirements.

PRACTICAL PRESCRIBING

Prescription	For **diabetes mellitus,** insulin regimens need to provide 'peaks' of insulin to deal with the glucose absorbed at mealtimes, and lower 'basal' levels in between. A *'basal–bolus' regimen* comprises a daily long-acting insulin injection, and rapid-acting insulin taken with breakfast, lunch, and evening meals. The advantage of this regimen is flexibility. A *'twice-daily' regimen* uses intermediate-acting or biphasic insulin, taken before breakfast and evening meals; this is less onerous, but also less flexible. Insulin requirements vary widely, so initial dosage selection should be guided by a specialist. In **diabetic emergencies** and **peri-operative glycaemic control,** a 1-unit/mL IV solution is made by diluting soluble human insulin 50 units in 0.9% sodium chloride 50 mL. The infusion rate is adjusted as necessary; consult a local protocol for details. An IV infusion of glucose with sodium chloride and potassium chloride is run in parallel to provide an insulin substrate. In **hyperkalaemia,** glucose must be given with insulin to avoid hypoglycaemia. A reasonable option is Actrapid® 10 units with 20% glucose 125 mL, infused over 15 min.
Administration	SC insulin is usually administered using 'pens', on which the required dose can simply be 'dialled up'. Alternatively, smart pumps monitor glucose continuously and automatically adjust insulin delivery.
Communication	For **diabetes mellitus,** explain that insulin will help to control sugar levels and prevent complications. Highlight the symptoms that indicate hypoglycaemia (e.g. dizziness, agitation, nausea, sweating, and confusion) and explain how to treat it (e.g. a sugary drink then a sandwich). Alongside this, advise on lifestyle measures, including a healthy, balanced diet and regular exercise.
Monitoring and stopping	Capillary blood glucose measurements are the mainstay of monitoring to guide insulin dosing. Haemoglobin A_{1c} should be measured at least annually to assess long-term glycaemic control. Insulin therapy for diabetes mellitus is usually indefinite. Where insulin is given as an IV infusion, serum K^+ should be monitored and replaced as needed.
Cost	The NHS spends over >£300 million/year on insulin, its fourth biggest drug cost.

Clinical tip—Insulin dosage adjustment in hospital is a daunting task for new prescribers. Note the acceptable blood glucose range in acute illness (e.g. 4–12 mmol/L) is broader than the range targeted for long-term diabetes management. If the concentration strays outside the acceptable range, you need to adjust the dose that *precedes* the problem. Generally, increase the dose by about 10% for hyperglycaemia; reduce it by 20% for hypoglycaemia. By definition, you can only do this from the next day—i.e. to improve *future* rather than current glycaemic control. If 'correction' of acute hyperglycaemia is required, it is better to use a rapid-acting insulin (e.g. NovoRapid®) than a short-acting insulin (e.g. Actrapid®).

Iron

CLINICAL PHARMACOLOGY

Common indications	❶ **Treatment of iron-deficiency anaemia.** ❷ **Prophylaxis of iron-deficiency anaemia** in people with risk factors such as a low-iron diet, malabsorption, menorrhagia, gastrectomy, haemodialysis, and infants with low birth weight.
Mechanisms of action	The aim of iron therapy is to replenish iron stores. Iron is essential for erythropoiesis (the formation of new red blood cells). It is required for the synthesis of the haem component of haemoglobin, which gives red blood cells the ability to carry oxygen. Iron is best absorbed in its ferrous state (Fe^{2+}) in the duodenum and jejunum. Its absorption is increased by stomach acid and dietary acids such as ascorbic acid (vitamin C). Once absorbed into the blood stream, iron is bound by transferrin. Transferrin transports it either to be used in the bone marrow for erythropoiesis or to be stored as ferritin in the liver, reticuloendothelial system, bone marrow, spleen, and skeletal muscle.
Important adverse effects	The most common adverse effect of oral iron salts is **GI upset,** including nausea, epigastric pain, constipation, and diarrhoea. The stool may turn black. IV iron administration can cause injection site irritation and hypersensitivity reactions, including anaphylaxis.
Warnings	*Oral* iron therapy may exacerbate bowel symptoms in ▲ **intestinal disease,** including inflammatory bowel disease, diverticular disease, and intestinal strictures. *IV* iron should be used with caution in people with an ▲ **atopic predisposition** due to the risk of anaphylactic reaction.
Important interactions	Oral iron salts can reduce the absorption of other drugs, including **levothyroxine** and **bisphosphonates**. These medications should therefore be taken at least 2 hours before oral iron.

PRACTICAL PRESCRIBING

Prescription	Iron is available for oral or IV administration. IV iron should be reserved for people unable to tolerate sufficient oral iron to correct or prevent deficiency. It is also used in end-stage renal disease, when it may be given with erythropoietin. IV iron replacement does not lead to a more rapid increase in haemoglobin than oral iron (provided oral preparations are tolerated and absorbed). For **treatment of iron-deficiency anaemia,** prescribe 100–200 mg of elemental iron per day. Different oral iron preparations contain different amounts of elemental iron. For example, ferrous sulfate 200 mg contains 65 mg elemental iron. A prescription for ferrous sulfate 200 mg two to three times daily will therefore provide 130–195 mg elemental iron a day. For **prophylaxis of iron-deficiency anaemia,** ferrous sulfate 200 mg daily should be sufficient. GI adverse effects may limit the dosage tolerated; reducing this or switching to an alternative iron salt may improve tolerability.
Administration	Although oral iron salts are better absorbed on an empty stomach, they can be taken with food to reduce GI side effects. IV iron can be given as an injection over 10 minutes or as an infusion. Facilities for the management of anaphylaxis should be available.
Communication	Explain that treatment should top up their iron stores and improve symptoms of anaemia, but that it may take weeks to months before full benefit is seen. Warn them that iron may turn their stools black. Advise them to come back if the iron upsets their stomach, as treatment can be changed to reduce side effects.
Monitoring and stopping	Monitor full blood count until the haemoglobin has returned to normal. You should expect to see the haemoglobin rise by around 20 g/L per month. Once haemoglobin has returned to normal, continue at two to three times daily dosing for a further 3 months to fully replenish iron stores, then drop to once-daily dosing. If the cause of iron deficiency also resolves (e.g. change in diet or successful management of the source of blood loss) consider stopping iron therapy.
Cost	Ferrous sulfate and ferrous fumarate are available in inexpensive non-proprietary forms. Brand name compound preparations with ascorbic acid and modified-release preparations have minimal additional clinical benefit for a considerable increase in cost.

Clinical tip—People with iron deficiency often require colonoscopy to investigate the cause of their anaemia. However, oral iron can turn stools black and sticky. This is problematic for visualising the bowel during lower GI endoscopy as the sticky black stool coats the colon and obscures the endoscopist's view. Iron treatment should therefore be stopped for 7 days before the procedure.

Lamotrigine

CLINICAL PHARMACOLOGY

Common indications	❶ Seizure prophylaxis in **epilepsy.** Specifically, lamotrigine is an option for first-line monotherapy or add-on therapy in focal seizures (with or without secondary generalisation) and generalised tonic–clonic seizures. ❷ **Bipolar depression**, but not mania or hypomania.
Mechanisms of action	The mechanism of action of lamotrigine is incompletely understood. Like **carbamazepine** and phenytoin, it binds to **voltage-sensitive neuronal Na⁺ channels,** producing use-dependent inhibition of Na⁺ influx into the neuron. This impedes repetitive neuronal firing, which is a characteristic of seizure activity. Additionally, lamotrigine reduces release of the excitatory neurotransmitter, glutamate. These effects, and others, likely explain its antiepileptic action. The mechanism by which it reduces depressive symptoms in bipolar disorder is uncertain.
Important adverse effects	The most common adverse effects are **headache, drowsiness, irritability, blurred vision, dizziness,** and **GI upset**. A minority develop a **skin rash** within a few weeks of starting lamotrigine. This is usually mild, but requires urgent review and possibly discontinuation of the drug. This is because it may be the first sign of a **severe hypersensitivity reaction.** Although rare, this may be life threatening, and early discontinuation of the drug is essential (see **Carbamazepine**).
Warnings	Lamotrigine should be avoided if possible in people with a prior history of ▲ **hypersensitivity to other antiepileptic drugs**, due to the risk of cross-reactivity. Lamotrigine is metabolised by hepatic glucuronidation, so dosage reduction may be necessary in moderate or severe ▲ **hepatic impairment**. In general, there is no evidence that lamotrigine exposure in **pregnancy** increases the overall risk of congenital malformations, so it is a reasonable choice in women of childbearing age. During pregnancy, due to changes in lamotrigine metabolism, plasma concentration measurement should be considered to guide dosage adjustment.
Important interactions	Lamotrigine has many interactions arising from its metabolism by glucuronidation. These are of sufficient importance to necessitate pre-emptive dosage modification (see Prescription). Drugs that induce glucuronidation include ▲ **carbamazepine**, ▲ phenytoin, ▲ **oestrogens**, ▲ rifampicin, and ▲ protease inhibitors (see **Antiviral drugs, other**). These can cause lamotrigine concentration to fall, potentially leading to treatment failure. Glucuronidation is inhibited by ▲ **valproate**, causing lamotrigine concentration to rise, increasing the risk of toxicity. Severe hypersensitivity reactions are also more common when lamotrigine is co-administered with valproate.

PRACTICAL PRESCRIBING

Prescription	The dosage of lamotrigine is influence by concurrent drug treatment. When used as monotherapy with no interacting drugs, the starting dosage in adults is 25 mg daily, increased at 2-weekly intervals to a usual maintenance dosage of 200 mg daily. If it is taken with **valproate**, the dosage should be halved (start at 25 mg on alternate days). If it is taken with a drug that induces glucuronidation (see INTERACTIONS), the dosage is doubled (start at 50 mg daily).
Administration	Standard lamotrigine tablets should be swallowed whole with water. Chewable/dispersible tablets can be taken whole, chewed with a little water or dispersed with water.
Communication	Explain that the aim of treatment is to reduce seizure frequency, not to 'cure' epilepsy. Finding the right dosage may take a few weeks, so its effects may not be evident immediately. It is important for good seizure control to avoid missing doses. If a dose is missed, they should take it as soon as they remember. They should not stop treatment abruptly, as this can cause rebound seizures. Most people tolerate lamotrigine well, but side effects such as headache, drowsiness, and irritability can occur. In the first few months of treatment there is a risk of rare but serious allergic reactions. During this time particularly, they should seek immediate medical attention if they develop a rash, ulcers, fever, swollen glands, bleeding/bruising or a sore throat. Advise that driving is prohibited unless they have been seizure-free for 12 months, and for 6 months after changing or stopping treatment.
Monitoring and stopping	Treatment **efficacy** is monitored by comparing seizure frequency before and after starting treatment or dose adjustment. **Safety** and **tolerability** are monitored by enquiring about adverse effects. This is particularly important in the initial few months of treatment, when advice should be given to seek immediate medical attention for any symptoms that could suggest a hypersensitivity reaction (see COMMUNICATION). Plasma lamotrigine concentration measurement is not routinely required, but may be useful if there is an unexplained lack of efficacy, suspected poor adherence, suspected drug interactions or pregnancy. Withdrawal of antiseizure therapy is a specialist area that requires careful consideration of individual risks and benefits. Generally, it is considered after the person has been seizure-free for at least 2 years. The dosage should be tapered over 2–3 months.
Cost	Lamotrigine is available in generic forms which are relatively inexpensive. The tablet formulations are generally cheaper than the dispersible formulations.

Clinical tip—Lamotrigine appears to be unique among agents used in bipolar disorder, in that it effectively treats depressive symptoms but does not increase the risk of a switch to mania.

Laxatives, oral

CLINICAL PHARMACOLOGY

Common indications	❶ **Constipation** ❷ **Bowel preparation** prior to surgery or endoscopy (usually osmotic laxatives only). ❸ **Hepatic encephalopathy** (lactulose only, to reduce ammonia absorption). Suppositoris and enemas (see **Laxatives, rectal**) are alternatives in most indications, and may be used in conjunction with orally administered drugs.
Mechanisms of action	Laxatives may be classified by their mechanism of action as either osmotic or stimulant laxatives. **Osmotic laxatives** are based on **osmotically active substances** (sugars or alcohols) that are not digested or absorbed, and which therefore remain in the gut lumen. For example, macrogol 3350 is a non-absorbable polymer of ethylene glycol; it may be formulated alone, or with electrolytes to counteract water, sodium, and potassium shifts. Osmotic laxatives hold water in the stool, maintaining its volume and stimulating peristalsis. Lactulose has a useful additional effect of reducing ammonia absorption by increasing gut transit rate and acidifying the stool. This latter effect inhibits the proliferation of ammonia-producing bacteria. This is helpful in liver failure, where ammonia plays a major role in encephalopathy) **Stimulant laxatives** (also known as irritant or contact laxatives) increase water and electrolyte secretion from the colonic mucosa, thereby increasing the volume of colonic content and stimulating peristalsis. They also have a direct pro-peristaltic action, although the exact mechanism differs between agents. For example, bacterial metabolism of senna in the intestine produces metabolites that have a direct action on the enteric nervous system, stimulating peristalsis.
Important adverse effects	**Flatulence, abdominal cramps, diarrhoea,** and **nausea** are common adverse effects. With prolonged use, some stimulant laxatives cause **melanosis coli** (reversible pigmentation of the intestinal wall).
Warnings	Laxatives are contraindicated in ✖ **intestinal obstruction** as there is a risk of perforation.
Important interactions	Laxatives have no significant adverse interactions with other drugs. However, there is an important interaction between macrogols (polyethylene glycol) and **starch-based thickeners,** which are used to aid safe swallowing in some people with dysphagia. Allowing the thickened feed to mix with macrogol will make it watery. This increases the risk of aspiration.

macrogol 3350, lactulose (osmotic laxatives)
senna, docusate sodium (stimulant laxatives)

PRACTICAL PRESCRIBING

Prescription	For **constipation,** laxatives are usually taken regularly and the dose titrated to effect. For example, a typical starting dose of senna is 15 mg (2 tablets) orally every evening. Be aware that it may take a few days for an effect to be seen, as the drug needs to pass through the small intestine to the colon. An additional agent (e.g. docusate sodium) may be added if the response is insufficient. When using lactulose to treat or prevent **hepatic encephalopathy,** you might start with 30–50 mL (doubled in constipation) orally 8-hrly, aiming for three soft/loose stools per day. This is higher than the dose of lactulose used for constipation.
Administration	Laxatives may be taken with or without food. Oral solutions can be taken as they are or diluted in another liquid; powdered forms are dissolved in water. Macrogols must not be administered with feeds that contain a starch-based thickener (see INTERACTIONS).
Communication	Explain that the laxative is intended to help make their stool easier to pass. To work, they need to drink plenty of water, aiming for at least 6–8 glasses of liquid per day. Mention that side effects such as abdominal cramps and flatulence can occur, but these may get better over time. Advise that the dose can be adjusted to maintain comfort. If they are regularly passing more than two or three soft stools per day, the dose should be reduced or the laxative stopped (unless it is being used for hepatic encephalopathy).
Monitoring and stopping	In the hospital setting, a stool chart is useful to monitor the effects of treatment. This is particularly important when treating hepatic encephalopathy, where you should also monitor electrolytes. Where the cause for constipation is treated or resolves (e.g. cessation of opioid therapy), laxatives can often be stopped.
Cost	Laxatives are cheap. People who pay for their prescriptions may save money if they buy them over the counter.

Clinical tip—When prescribing **opioid** analgesics to be taken regularly, consider co-prescribing a laxative to prevent constipation. A stimulant (e.g. senna) is a reasonable choice. Constipation is uncomfortable and can contribute to confusion in older people. Pre-empting opioid-induced constipation can increase adherence to treatment, improve symptoms and reduce complications such as delirium.

Laxatives, rectal

CLINICAL PHARMACOLOGY

Common indications	❶ **Constipation** and **faecal impaction.** ❷ **Bowel preparation** prior to surgery or endoscopy. ❸ **Hepatic encephalopathy** as an adjunct to **lactulose,** where this alone does not provide sufficiently frequent bowel movements. **Oral laxatives** are alternatives in most indications and may be used in conjunction with rectally administered drugs.
Mechanisms of action	Glycerol is an **osmotic laxative.** Administered as a suppository (a medicine in solid form, inserted through the anus), it creates a significant osmotic gradient that draws water and electrolytes into the faeces. This increases its volume and stimulates peristalsis that leads to bowel opening. It also has **lubricant** and **faecal softening** effects, and a mild **irritant** effect on the rectal mucosa. The latter augments the stimulus for peristalsis. Sodium acid phosphate with sodium phosphate (more commonly referred to as 'phosphates enema') and sodium citrate are also osmotic laxatives that are administered rectally as enemas (a medicine in liquid form, injected through the anus). By virtue of the volume and liquid form of enemas, their effect is generally more pronounced than suppositories. Arachis oil is a peanut derivative that directly **softens and lubricates** the stool.
Important adverse effects	**Flatulence and abdominal cramps** are common adverse effects. As with other laxatives, **diarrhoea** is a possible complication. Enemas in particular can be uncomfortable because of the relatively large volume that must be instilled into the rectum (>100 mL). Phosphates enemas can cause **pain, volume depletion** (leading to hypotension), and **electrolyte disturbances,** including hyperphosphataemia and hyper- or hypokalaemia.
Warnings	Phosphates enemas can cause significant fluid shifts, so should be used with caution in ▲ **heart failure,** ▲ **ascites** and when ▲ **electrolyte disturbances** are present. Arachis oil should not be used when there is a history of ✖ **peanut or** ▲ **soya allergy.**
Important interactions	There are no significant adverse drug interactions, although the administration of other rectal drugs should be timed to avoid being expelled by the enema or suppository.

PRACTICAL PRESCRIBING

Prescription	Enemas and suppositories are generally used when there is **constipation** complicated by **faecal impaction** that is not resolved with oral **laxatives**. When treating **faecal impaction,** suppositories and enemas are usually prescribed once only or as required with a maximum dose frequency of once in a 24-hour period. For **bowel preparation** (e.g. prior to colonoscopy), you should refer to a local protocol for prescribing advice. When using enemas to treat **hepatic encephalopathy,** phosphates enemas are usually preferred and are generally prescribed if lactulose has failed to yield sufficient response or encephalopathy is severe. Therapy should be guided by an expert but a typical prescription is one phosphates enema rectally daily.
Administration	Suppositories may be self-administered if the person is able to. They should be advised to lie on their non-dominant side and, using their dominant hand, insert the bullet-shaped suppository (pointed end first) through their anus, pushing it as far in as possible. Wetting the suppository first with cold water can aid insertion. Ideally, it should be pushed against the wall of the bowel. They should then try to retain the drug for the first 15–30 minutes, if possible (i.e. initially resisting the urge to go to the toilet), to maximise the effect. The procedure is similar for enemas, but involves squeezing a liquid from a bottle or syringe. The precise details vary by preparation.
Communication	Explain that you are offering treatment with a tablet or liquid (a suppository or enema, respectively) administered into the rectum. The aim is to make their stool softer and easier to pass. Explain how the drug is administered and, as appropriate, that they may be able do this themselves. With enemas, warn that the urge to open their bowels may come rapidly (within minutes) and suddenly after administration. Mention that side effects such as abdominal cramps and flatulence can occur. Explain that these medicines are intended for occasional rather than regular use.
Monitoring and stopping	In the hospital setting, a stool chart is useful to monitor the effects of treatment. This is particularly important when treating hepatic encephalopathy, where you should also monitor electrolytes. Suppositories and enemas should be taken only when needed, generally for short-term or occasional use.
Cost	Enemas and suppositories are cheap. People who pay for their prescriptions may save money if they buy them over the counter.

Clinical tip—In the inpatient setting, when performing a direct rectal examination, it is a good idea to think ahead and bring a glycerol suppository with you. Then, if you find hard/impacted stool, you can treat it immediately, rather than having to come back later or ask someone else to do it.

Leukotriene receptor antagonists

CLINICAL PHARMACOLOGY

Common indications	❶ Initial add-on therapy for chronic **asthma**, where symptoms are not adequately controlled by a short-acting β_2 **agonist** and a low-dose **inhaled corticosteroids** (see Clinical tip). ❷ A treatment option for **allergic rhinitis** in those who also have asthma, where nasal symptoms have not responded to usual treatments such as **antihistamines** and/or **intranasal corticosteroids**
Mechanisms of action	In asthma, leukotrienes produced by mast cells and eosinophils (among other sources) activate the G protein-coupled leukotriene receptor CysLT1. This activates a cascade of pathways that result in inflammation and bronchoconstriction, which contribute to the pathophysiology of asthma. Leukotriene receptor agonists reduce inflammation and bronchoconstriction in asthma by **blocking the CysLT1 receptor** and damping down the inflammatory cascade.
Important adverse effects	Leukotriene receptor antagonists are generally well tolerated. **Headache, abdominal pain,** and **GI upset** are the most common adverse effects, but they are usually mild. They also increase the risk of upper respiratory tract infections. **Neuropsychiatric reactions**, including sleep disturbance, depression, and agitation occur in up to 1 in 100 of those taking montelukast. Rarely, disturbances of attention or memory and, very rarely, hallucinations and suicidal behaviour may occur. **Churg–Strauss syndrome**, an eosinophilic autoimmune disorder, has been seen in association with leukotriene receptor antagonists. However, there is no conclusive evidence that it is an adverse effect of the drug.
Warnings	The safety of leukotriene receptor antagonists in ▲ **pregnancy** is uncertain because of a lack of evidence, although no harmful effects have been demonstrated. However, as poorly controlled asthma is also a risk during pregnancy, it is considered reasonable to continue leukotriene receptor antagonists where they have led to significant improvement in asthma symptoms not achieved with other therapies.
Important interactions	Drugs that induce the cytochrome P450 enzymes that metabolise montelukast (including phenytoin and rifampicin) can cause a reduction in plasma levels of montelukast, potentially reducing its efficacy.

PRACTICAL PRESCRIBING

Prescription	For adults and children aged 15 years and older, montelukast is prescribed at a dosage of 10 mg orally daily, to be taken in the evening. A lower dosage is prescribed for younger children.
Administration	Montelukast is available in tablet, chewable tablet, and granule form for oral administration. Standard tablets can be taken with or without food, but the chewable tablets must be taken 1 hour before or 2 hours after food on an empty stomach. Granules may be easier for younger children to manage and can be administered directly or mixed with a spoonful of cold or room temperature soft food.
Communication	Explain that this medicine should reduce swelling and narrowing of their airways, which should improve symptoms and control their disease. Advise that leukotriene receptor antagonists should be taken in addition to inhaled treatment, and that both types of treatment need to be taken regularly to be effective. Warn that these tablets should *not* be used to treat acute asthma attacks. If they become acutely breathless, they should use their reliever inhaler and seek medical advice. Explain that although side effects with leukotriene receptor antagonists are usually mild, they should look out for signs of rare but serious reactions including changes in behaviour and mood (neuropsychiatric reactions) and to seek medical advice if they develop new or unexplained symptoms such as rash or pins and needles (in view of the possible relationship with Churg–Strauss syndrome, see ADVERSE EFFECTS).
Monitoring and stopping	Monitor **efficacy** by symptom diary and serial measurement of peak expiratory flow rate, and **safety** by enquiring about adverse effects. Consider stopping the leukotriene receptor antagonist if a treatment trial for asthma or rhinitis makes no difference to symptoms or objective measures of disease, or if it causes unacceptable side effects. Where asthma has been well controlled for 3 months on stable treatment, consider decreasing maintenance therapy. This may include stopping the leukotriene receptor antagonist.
Cost	Inexpensive non-proprietary preparations are available.

Clinical tip—The place of leukotriene receptor antagonists (LTRAs) in the treatment of asthma remains controversial. At the time of writing, in the UK, NICE advise that LTRAs should be the first escalation of therapy where a low-dose **inhaled corticosteroid** does not control disease. In contrast, the British Thoracic Society (BTS) and Scottish Intercollegiate Guidelines Network (SIGN) recommend LTRAs as add-on treatment, where disease control is inadequate despite both a **long-acting β_2-agonist** and low-dose **inhaled corticosteroid**. To navigate this complexity, check local guidelines and be aware that those most likely to benefit from a leukotriene receptor antagonist include people with aspirin sensitive, highly atopic and exercise-induced asthma.

Levetiracetam and brivaracetam

CLINICAL PHARMACOLOGY

Common indications	❶ Seizure prophylaxis in **epilepsy.** Levetiracetam is recommended for both generalised tonic-clonic seizures and focal seizures. It can be used as first-line monotherapy, or as an add-on treatment. **Lamotrigine** and **sodium valproate** (for generalised seizures in boys/men) are alternatives. ❷ Levetiracetam is increasingly the preferred option for treating established convulsive **status epilepticus,** following inadequate response to a **benzodiazepine**. Alternatives are phenytoin and **sodium valproate**.
Mechanisms of action	The molecular target of levetiracetam is **synaptic vesicle protein 2A (SV2A)**. SV2A is expressed throughout the brain, in both excitatory and inhibitory synapses, as a glycoprotein located within the membranes of synaptic vesicles. Synaptic vesicles are where neurotransmitters are stored in the pre-synaptic nerve terminal. During depolarisation, synaptic vesicles fuse with the pre-synaptic membrane to release neurotransmitters into the synaptic cleft. Through its effects on synaptic vesicle function, levetiracetam modulates release of neurotransmitters. This inhibits synchronised epileptiform burst firing and reduces propagation of seizure activity. Brivaracetam has a similar action, supplemented with additional activity on voltage-gated Na^+ channels.
Important adverse effects	Levetiracetam and brivaracetam have similar adverse effect profiles. In contrast to many other antiepileptic drugs, they are generally well tolerated. Most have only mild adverse effects, or none at all. **Drowsiness** (affecting about 10%), **weakness, dizziness,** and **headache** are the most common adverse effects. **Mood disturbance** and psychiatric adverse effects are less common (about 5% and 2.5%, respectively), but more likely to cause discontinuation. **Suicidal ideation** and serious **hypersensitivity reactions** have been reported rarely.
Warnings	Levetiracetam is eliminated by the kidneys, so dosage reduction may be required in ▲ **renal impairment**. In contrast, brivaracetam is metabolised in the liver, so caution is required in ▲ **hepatic impairment**. There is no evidence that levetiracetam increases the overall risk of birth defects when taken during pregnancy, although it is difficult to exclude effects on specific congenital defects. Little data is available on the safety of brivaracetam in pregnancy.
Important interactions	In contrast to many other antiepileptic drugs, levetiracetam has few clinically significant interactions, and this is one of its major advantages. In particular, it does not have important interactions with other antiepileptic drugs, hormonal contraception or warfarin. Brivaracetam has potential to interact with cytochrome P450 inducers (e.g. phenytoin, rifampicin) and inhibitors (e.g. some **antifungal drugs**).

PRACTICAL PRESCRIBING

Prescription	For seizure prophylaxis in adults with established epilepsy, a typical initial prescription is levetiracetam 500 mg orally 12-hrly. This is usually increased to 1 g orally 12-hrly after 2 weeks and may then be titrated further according to clinical response (efficacy and adverse effects; max 1.5 g orally 12-hrly). When used in convulsive status epilepticus refractory to **benzodiazepine** treatment, the initial loading dose (40–60 mg/kg) is given IV.
Administration	Tablets should ideally be swallowed whole. They should not be chewed. If necessary to facilitate administration (e.g. in children), they may be crushed and taken with food. IV doses are usually given by infusion over 15 minutes.
Communication	Explain that the aim of treatment is to reduce seizure frequency, not to 'cure' epilepsy. Finding the right dosage may take a few weeks, so its effects may not be evident immediately. It is important for good seizure control to avoid missing doses. If a dose is missed, they should take it as soon as they remember. They should not stop treatment abruptly, as this can cause rebound seizures. Side effects, such as drowsiness and headache, are infrequent and usually mild. A small proportion of people experience mood changes, and they should seek attention if they develop any symptoms of depression. Advise that driving is prohibited unless they have been seizure-free for 12 months, and for 6 months after changing or stopping treatment.
Monitoring and stopping	Treatment **efficacy** is monitored by comparing seizure frequency before and after starting treatment or dose adjustment. **Safety** and **tolerability** are monitored by enquiring about adverse effects, particularly in relation to mood disturbance and suicidal thoughts. There are no specific laboratory monitoring requirements, and measurement of plasma levetiracetam concentration is not required. Withdrawal of antiseizure therapy is a specialist area that requires careful consideration of individual risks and benefits. Generally, it is considered after the person has been seizure-free for at least 2 years. The dosage should be tapered over 2–3 months.
Cost	Levetiracetam should be prescribed generically to allow the cheapest product to be dispensed. The IV formulation is considerably more expensive, so should be used only when oral administration is impossible (see CLINICAL TIP). Brivaracetam is available as a branded product only, which is several-fold more expensive than equivalent generic levetiracetam.

Clinical tip—Levetiracetam's bioavailability (i.e. the proportion of the administered dose reaching the circulation in active form) is reliably high, so there is no need for dose modification when switching between oral and IV administration. For the same reason, IV administration should be stopped in favour of oral administration as early as possible.

Macrolides

CLINICAL PHARMACOLOGY

Common indications	❶ Treatment of **respiratory, skin and soft tissue infections** as an alternative to a penicillin if this is contraindicated (e.g. allergy). ❷ In **severe pneumonia,** added to a penicillin to cover atypical organisms including *Legionella pneumophila* and *Mycoplasma pneumoniae.* ❸ Eradication of *Helicobacter pylori* (e.g. causing **peptic ulcer disease**) in combination with a **proton pump inhibitor** and either **amoxicillin** or **metronidazole.**
Spectrum of activity	Erythromycin was isolated from *Streptomyces erythraeus* in the 1950s. It has a relatively **broad spectrum** of activity against Gram-positive and some Gram-negative organisms. Synthetic macrolides (e.g. clarithromycin and azithromycin) have increased activity against Gram-negative bacteria, particularly *Haemophilus influenzae.*
Mechanisms of action	Macrolides **inhibit bacterial protein synthesis.** They bind to the 50S subunit of the **bacterial ribosome** and block translocation, a process required for elongation of the polypeptide chain. Inhibition of protein synthesis is **bacteriostatic** (stops bacterial growth), which assists the immune system in killing and removing bacteria from the body. Bacterial resistance to macrolides is common, mainly due to ribosomal mutations preventing macrolide binding.
Important adverse effects	Adverse effects are most common and severe with erythromycin but can occur with any macrolide. Macrolides are **irritant,** causing nausea, vomiting, abdominal pain, and diarrhoea when taken orally, and thrombophlebitis when given IV. Other important side effects include **allergy, antibiotic-associated colitis** (see **Penicillins, broad-spectrum**), **cholestatic hepatitis, prolongation of the QT interval** (predisposing to **arrhythmias**) and **ototoxicity** at high doses.
Warnings	Macrolides should not be prescribed if there is a history of ✖ **macrolide hypersensitivity,** although they are a useful option where penicillin is contraindicated by allergy, as there is no risk of cross-sensitivity. Macrolide elimination is mostly hepatic, with a small renal contribution. Caution is therefore required in ▲ **severe hepatic impairment,** and doses should be reduced in ▲ **severe renal impairment.**
Important interactions	Erythromycin and clarithromycin (but not azithromycin) inhibit cytochrome P450 (CYP) enzymes. This increases plasma concentrations and the risk of adverse effects with ▲ **drugs metabolised by CYP enzymes.** For example, with **warfarin** there is an increased risk of bleeding, and with **statins** an increased risk of myopathy. Macrolides should be prescribed with caution in people taking other ▲ **drugs that prolong the QT interval** or cause arrhythmias, such as **amiodarone, antipsychotics, quinine, quinolone antibiotics,** and **selective serotonin reuptake inhibitors (SSRIs).**

PRACTICAL PRESCRIBING

Prescription	Erythromycin has a short plasma half-life of around 2 hours and is usually prescribed at a dosage of 250–500 mg 6-hrly. Clarithromycin is concentrated in tissues and has a longer elimination half-life, so is prescribed at a dosage of 250–500 mg 12-hrly or as a modified-release preparation that allows once-daily dosing. Azithromycin is highly concentrated in tissues and has a long half-life, so is prescribed at a dosage of 250–500 mg daily, with the option for single-dose treatment for some infections (e.g. uncomplicated urethritis). Higher doses and longer courses of treatment are used in more severe infections. Macrolides are also available for IV administration if necessary. The indication, review date, and duration of treatment should be documented on all inpatient antibiotic prescriptions to aid antibiotic stewardship.
Administration	Macrolides can be taken as tablets or oral suspension with or without food (although food may improve GI tolerability). IV macrolides are irritant, so should be diluted in a large volume, e.g. 500 mg in 250 mL sodium chloride 0.9%, before infusion into a large proximal vein and must not be given as IV bolus or IM. The duration of infusion should be at least 60 minutes to reduce the risk of arrhythmias.
Communication	Explain that the aim of treatment is to get rid of infection and improve symptoms. Before prescribing, always check for allergy to macrolides. Advise that they seek medical advice if a rash or other unexpected symptom develops. If an allergic reaction occurs, give written advice not to take this antibiotic in the future and make sure that the allergy is clearly recorded in their notes.
Monitoring and stopping	Check that infection resolves by checking for resolution of symptoms, examination (e.g. resolution of pyrexia, lung crackles) and blood tests (e.g. falling CRP and white cell count). Duration of antibiotic therapy is a balance between ensuring effective treatment of infection, and minimising adverse reactions and resistance. Always set a stop or review date when prescribing antibiotics, referring to local protocols for guidance. IV antibiotics should be switched to oral administration after 48 hours if clinically indicated, the patient is improving, and is able to take oral medication.
Cost	Prompt IV-to-oral switch reduces drug and administration costs, treatment complications, and duration of inpatient stay. Oral macrolides cost around 50 times less than IV macrolides.

Clinical tip—Long-term prophylactic azithromycin is a treatment option for people with COPD who have prolonged, frequent (≥4/year) or severe exacerbations despite smoking cessation and optimisation of all other therapies (see **antimuscarinics, bronchodilators**, β_2**-agonists**, and **corticosteroids, inhaled**). People taking long-term azithromycin should be monitored for hearing loss and reviewed every 6 months, with treatment only continuing if benefits outweigh the risks.

Metformin

CLINICAL PHARMACOLOGY

Common indications	**Type 2 diabetes,** as the first-choice medication for control of blood glucose, used alone or in combination with other oral hypoglycaemic drugs (e.g. **sulphonylureas, dipeptidylpeptidase-4 (DPP-4) inhibitors, sodium–glucose co-transporter 2 inhibitors**) or **insulin.**
Mechanisms of action	Metformin (a biguanide) lowers blood glucose primarily by **reducing hepatic glucose output** (glycogenolysis and gluconeogenesis) and, to a lesser extent, increasing glucose uptake and utilisation by skeletal muscle. It does not stimulate insulin secretion and therefore does not cause hypoglycaemia. The cellular mechanisms are complex, involving **activation** of **adenosine monophosphate-activated protein kinase (AMP kinase).** This is a cellular metabolic sensor, activation of which has diverse effects on cell functions. Its effects on glucose metabolism can be accompanied by other metabolic changes, notably modest weight loss, which can be a desirable side effect (see CLINICAL TIP).
Important adverse effects	Metformin commonly causes **GI upset,** including nausea, vomiting, taste disturbance, anorexia, and diarrhoea. **Lactic acidosis** has been associated very rarely with metformin use, although the evidence for this is largely derived from case reports. There is no strong evidence of an increased risk in general, but metformin may be a contributory factor in people who develop an intercurrent illness that causes metformin accumulation (e.g. renal impairment), increased lactate production (e.g. sepsis, hypoxia) or reduced lactate metabolism (e.g. liver failure).
Warnings	Metformin is excreted unchanged by the kidney. It must therefore be used cautiously in ▲ **renal impairment,** with dosage reduction required if the estimated glomerular filtration rate (eGFR) is <45 mL/min per 1.73 m^2 and the drug stopped if eGFR falls below 30 mL/min per 1.73 m^2. Metformin should be withheld in ✖ **acute kidney injury** or states of ✖ **severe tissue hypoxia,** e.g. sepsis, cardiac or respiratory failure or myocardial infarction. Caution is required in ▲ **hepatic impairment** as clearance of excess lactate may be impaired. Metformin should be withheld during ▲ **acute alcohol intoxication,** and be used with caution in ▲ **chronic alcohol abuse,** where there is a risk of hypoglycaemia.
Important interactions	Renal function should be checked in people taking metformin before they undergo radiological studies involving ▲ **IV contrast media** (e.g. for computerised tomography (CT) scans, coronary angiography). It may be temporarily withheld if renal function is abnormal, due to the risk of metformin accumulation and lactic acidosis. This does not apply to gadolinium-based contrast agents used for magnetic resonance imaging (MRI) scans. Other drugs (e.g. **angiotensin-converting enzyme (ACE) inhibitors**, **NSAIDs**, **diuretics**) with potential to impair renal function should be used with caution (e.g. with intensified renal function monitoring) if combined with metformin. **Prednisolone**, **thiazide**, and **loop diuretics** elevate blood glucose, and therefore oppose the actions of metformin.

PRACTICAL PRESCRIBING

Prescription	Immediate-release metformin should be preferred in the first instance. Starting at a low dose and increasing gradually is the best way to minimise transient GI upset. A common dosage regimen is 500 mg orally once daily with breakfast, increasing the dose by 500 mg weekly. The usual maximum dose is 1 g twice daily with meals. A modified-release preparation may be tried if GI adverse effects are problematic.
Administration	Tablets should be swallowed whole with a glass of water, with or after food to minimise GI side effects.
Communication	Advise that metformin is being offered as a long-term treatment to help control blood sugar and reduce the risk of diabetic complications, such as heart attacks. Explain that lifestyle measures are still important, including a healthy, balanced diet, and regular exercise. Advise that they should seek urgent medical advice if they develop any significant illness (e.g. involving breathlessness, fever, chest pain) as, in addition to investigating and treating the illness, metformin may need to be stopped or withheld (due to the possibility of a rare but serious side effect called lactic acidosis). Advise them always to highlight that they are taking metformin before having a scan or operation.
Monitoring and stopping	Assess blood glucose control by measuring haemoglobin A_{1c} (HbA_{1c}). In treating type 2 diabetes with a single agent, the target HbA_{1c} is usually ≤48 mmol/mol. Treatment is intensified by adding a second agent if the HbA_{1c} is ≥58 mmol/mol, and a new target of ≤53 mmol/mol is then set (balancing the risks of hyperglycaemia against the risks of treatment, particularly hypoglycaemia). Home capillary blood glucose monitoring is not routinely required for people with type 2 diabetes taking metformin. For safety, measure renal function before starting treatment, then at least annually during therapy (more often in people at risk of renal function deterioration). Stop metformin if it is not tolerated; not effective; or if the eGFR is <30 mL/min per 1.73 m^2. A **sulphonylurea**, **DPP-4 inhibitor** or **sodium–glucose co-transporter 2 inhibitor** may then be offered as an alternative. Withhold metformin during significant acute illnesses (see WARNINGS).
Cost	Standard non-proprietary metformin tablets are cheap. Modified-release tablets, compound preparations, and oral solutions are more expensive.

Clinical tip—Increasing body weight increases insulin resistance, which can cause or worsen type 2 diabetes. Initial treatment for type 2 diabetes is therefore a healthy diet with increased physical activity, promoting weight loss if applicable, and this should be tried for at least 3 months before commencing drug therapy (offered if HbA_{1c} is >48 mmol/mol). As an anabolic hormone, **insulin,** and drugs which increase insulin secretion (e.g. **sulphonylureas**), cause weight gain, which can have long-term adverse effects. Metformin, which does not cause weight gain, is therefore usually the first-choice treatment unless contraindicated.

Methotrexate

CLINICAL PHARMACOLOGY

Common indications	❶ For **inflammatory disorders:** as a disease-modifying treatment for **rheumatoid** or **psoriatic arthritis;** to treat or maintain remission in severe **Crohn's disease;** and for severe, treatment-resistant **psoriasis.** ❷ For **neoplastic disorders:** in the cytotoxic treatment of some forms of **cancer,** including some leukaemias, lymphomas, and solid tumours.
Mechanisms of action	Methotrexate **inhibits dihydrofolate reductase**, which converts dietary folic acid to tetrahydrofolate (FH4). FH4 is required for DNA and protein synthesis, so lack of FH4 interferes with cellular division (mitosis). Actively dividing cells are particularly sensitive to the effects of methotrexate, accounting for its efficacy in cancer. Methotrexate also has antiinflammatory and immunosuppressive effects which are seen at lower doses than required for its antimitotic effect and may have a different mechanism. Methotrexate appears to increase adenosine release from cells. Adenosine acts on G protein-coupled receptors to inhibit a raft of inflammatory effects, including T-cell proliferation, phagocytosis, and release of inflammatory mediators such as interleukin (IL)-6, IL-8, and tumour necrosis factor (TNF)-α.
Important adverse effects	Dose-related adverse effects include **mucosal damage** (e.g. sore mouth, GI upset) and **bone marrow suppression** (resulting most significantly in neutropenia and an increased risk of infection). Rarely, **hypersensitivity reactions**, including cutaneous reactions, hepatitis or pneumonitis, may occur. **Long-term use** can cause liver cirrhosis and lung fibrosis. As methotrexate is usually administered once a week (see PRESCRIPTION), there is a risk of toxicity from inadvertent daily administration. This may cause **renal impairment** and **hepatotoxicity. Neurological effects** such as headache, seizures, and coma may also occur. Treatment is with folinic acid, which 'rescues' normal cells from methotrexate effects, and with hydration and urinary alkalinisation to enhance methotrexate excretion.
Warnings	Methotrexate is teratogenic and must be avoided in ✖ **pregnancy.** Both men and women taking the drug should use effective contraception during and for 3 months after treatment. As methotrexate is renally excreted, it is contraindicated in ✖ **severe renal impairment.** As it can cause hepatotoxicity, it should be avoided in ▲ **hepatic impairment.**
Important interactions	Methotrexate toxicity is more likely if it is prescribed with drugs that inhibit its renal excretion, e.g. ▲ **aspirin,** ▲ **NSAIDs,** ▲ **penicillins,** and ▲ **proton pump inhibitors**. Co-prescription with **other folate antagonists,** e.g. ▲ **trimethoprim** and phenytoin, increases the risk of haematological abnormalities. The risk of neutropenia is increased if methotrexate is combined with ▲ **clozapine**.

PRACTICAL PRESCRIBING

Prescription	Methotrexate should only be started by a specialist. For **inflammatory disorders,** methotrexate is typically prescribed at a dose of 7.5–20 mg orally *once weekly*. The dose depends on the indication and is adjusted according to response and adverse effects (which are more common at higher doses). **Folic acid** 5 mg weekly (taken on a different day to methotrexate) can be prescribed to limit adverse effects. For **cancer,** methotrexate may be given by IV, IM or intrathecal routes to induce remission, then orally for maintenance treatment.
Administration	IV and intrathecal administration of methotrexate should be done only by healthcare practitioners who have appropriate training and expertise, and only in carefully regulated circumstances.
Communication	Explain that methotrexate should improve the symptoms of inflammatory disease, but that this may take some time to reach maximum effect. **It is crucial to emphasise the once-weekly nature of treatment.** Ask what day of the week they will take their methotrexate and write this clearly on the prescription. Advise them of the potentially fatal risk of accidental overdose if they take the tablets more frequently, and that they must seek urgent medical attention if they suspect this has occurred. Warn them to seek urgent medical advice if they develop sore throat or fever (which may signify infection), bruising or bleeding (low platelet count), nausea, abdominal pain or dark urine (liver poisoning) or breathlessness (lung toxicity). Advise about the importance of effective contraception (see WARNINGS) and not taking over-the-counter antiinflammatories (see INTERACTIONS). Provide a methotrexate treatment booklet and warning card.
Monitoring and stopping	Monitor **efficacy** by symptoms, examination (e.g. of inflamed joints), and blood tests (e.g. inflammatory markers). **Safety** monitoring is essential as life-threatening adverse effects can be reversed if detected and treated early. Any unexpected symptoms should be reported promptly (see above). Measure FBC, liver, and renal function before starting treatment, then every 1–2 weeks until treatment is established and 2–3 times monthly thereafter. Stop treatment immediately if abnormalities arise or if breathlessness develops.
Cost	Non-proprietary oral methotrexate is available and is inexpensive.

Clinical tip—There are significant restrictions on the prescription of methotrexate in order to reduce medication errors and the risk of toxicity. Foundation year 1 doctors should not initiate a methotrexate prescription. However, they (and other prescribers) may need to review and (if permitted under local policies) continue prescriptions, for example at the time of hospital admission. If in any doubt about the appropriateness of a methotrexate prescription, seek senior, expert advice.

Metronidazole

CLINICAL PHARMACOLOGY

Common indications	❶ Infections from oropharyngeal Gram-negative anaerobes, including **dental infections, infected human/animal bites** and **aspiration pneumonia**. ❷ Eradication of *Helicobacter pylori* (e.g. causing **peptic ulcer disease**) in combination with a **proton pump inhibitor** and either **amoxicillin** or **clarithromycin**. ❸ **Intraabdominal infection** and **pelvic inflammatory disease**, which may involve Gram-negative anaerobes. ❹ **Protozoal infections** including trichomonal vaginal infection, amoebic dysentery, and giardiasis. ❺ *Clostridioides difficile* **colitis**, if IV treatment is required (otherwise **vancomycin** or fidaxomicin is preferred).
Spectrum of activity	Anaerobic bacteria and protozoa.
Mechanisms of action	Metronidazole enters bacteria by passive diffusion. In anaerobic bacteria, reduction of metronidazole generates a **nitroso free radical.** This **binds to DNA,** reducing synthesis and causing widespread damage, DNA degradation, and cell death **(bactericidal).** As aerobic bacteria are not able to reduce metronidazole in this manner, they are not susceptible to its effects. Bacterial resistance to metronidazole is generally low, but increasing. Mechanisms include reduced uptake of metronidazole and reduced generation of nitroso free radicals.
Important adverse effects	As with many antibiotics, metronidazole can cause **GI upset** (such as nausea, vomiting, metallic taste) and immediate and delayed **hypersensitivity** reactions (see **Penicillins, broad-spectrum**). When used at high doses or for a prolonged course, metronidazole can cause neurological adverse effects, including **peripheral** and **optic neuropathy, seizures,** and **encephalopathy.**
Warnings	Metronidazole is metabolised by hepatic cytochrome P450 (CYP) enzymes, so the dose should be reduced in ▲ **severe liver disease.** Metronidazole inhibits the enzyme acetaldehyde dehydrogenase, which is responsible for clearing the intermediate alcohol metabolite acetaldehyde from the body. ✖ **Alcohol** should be avoided while taking metronidazole as the combination causes an unpleasant reaction including flushing, headache, nausea, and vomiting.
Important interactions	Metronidazole has some inhibitory effect on CYP enzymes, reducing metabolism of **warfarin** (increasing the risk of bleeding) and phenytoin (increasing the risk of toxicity, including impaired cerebellar function). The reverse interaction can occur with CYP inducers (e.g. phenytoin, rifampicin), which increase metronidazole metabolism resulting in reduced plasma concentrations and impaired antimicrobial efficacy. Metronidazole also increases the risk of toxicity with lithium.

PRACTICAL PRESCRIBING

Prescription	The oral route is generally preferred, where a typical starting dosage is 400 mg 8-hrly. The IV route, usually at a dose of 500 mg IV 8-hrly, is used for **severe infection** or where oral treatment is not possible. Rectal metronidazole is an alternative in selected cases. Metronidazole can be prescribed for topical administration to treat vaginal infection such as **bacterial vaginosis**, skin infections such as **rosacea** or to reduce odour from an **infected skin ulcer**.
Administration	Oral metronidazole may be taken as tablets or oral suspension. IV metronidazole is given as an infusion over 20 minutes. Topical metronidazole is administered PV or to the skin as a cream or gel.
Communication	Explain that the aim of treatment is to get rid of infection and improve symptoms. Before prescribing, always check personally or get collateral history to confirm that they are not allergic to metronidazole. If an allergic reaction occurs, give written and verbal advice not to take this antibiotic in the future and make sure that the reaction (including its nature) is clearly recorded in the notes. Warn them not to take alcohol during or for 48 hours after systemic treatment, explaining that if they do they may feel very unwell with nausea, vomiting, flushing, and headache.
Monitoring and stopping	Monitor **efficacy** by reviewing symptoms, signs and inflammatory markers to make sure infection has resolved. For treatment exceeding 10 days, monitor **safety** by measuring full blood count and liver enzymes to look for adverse effects. The **duration** of antibiotic therapy is a balance between ensuring effective treatment of infection, and minimising adverse reactions and antimicrobial resistance. Always set a stop or review date when prescribing antibiotics, referring to local protocols for guidance.
Cost	A 7-day course of non-proprietary oral metronidazole tablets (one taken every 8 hr) currently costs around £3.50 if 400-mg tablets are prescribed, but around £39 if 500-mg tablets are prescribed. You should therefore select the lower dose unless there are overwhelming clinical reasons for the higher dose.

Clinical tip—People often ask if they can drink alcohol while they are taking antibiotics. While it is sensible to minimise alcohol consumption when feeling unwell, most antibiotics do not interact with alcohol, and do not preclude alcohol intake. Metronidazole is a clear exception to this, as it may cause a severe reaction (the 'disulfiram-like effect') if alcohol is taken during, or for up to 48 hours after, metronidazole treatment. **Co-trimoxazole** can cause a similar effect, though more rarely. Alcohol consumption can reduce the effectiveness of **doxycycline** and **erythromycin**.

Monoclonal antibodies

CLINICAL PHARMACOLOGY

Common indications	❶ **Immune-mediated disorders,** e.g. rheumatoid arthritis, psoriasis, psoriatic arthritis, inflammatory bowel disease. ❷ **Allergic disorders,** e.g. asthma, eczema, rhinitis with polyps. ❸ Precision treatment of **cancers,** including haematological (e.g. leukaemias, lymphomas) and solid tumours (e.g. breast and lung cancer). ❹ Prevention of adverse outcomes in high-risk **COVID-19 disease** or **respiratory syncytial virus** infections. ❺ Treatment of some **long-term conditions** with a target amenable to immune manipulation, e.g. osteoporosis, hypercholesterolaemia, migraine, sickle cell disease, haemophilia A.
Mechanisms of action	Monoclonal antibodies (mAbs) are generated by immunising animals with target proteins. B cells are selected and immortalised to create clones that produce homogenous antibodies against specific regions (epitopes) on the target protein. As animal antibodies are immunogenic in humans, their structure is altered by genetic engineering to make them more similar (humanised) or identical to human antibodies. Binding of mAbs to their target epitope inhibits or activates biological processes that leads to therapeutic effect. In **inflammatory disease**, mAbs suppress excessive immune responses by targeting components of the immune system. In **cancer**, mAbs may target tumour cells directly, enhance anti-tumour immune responses, alter the tumour microenvironment (e.g. inhibiting angiogenesis) or deliver targeted chemotherapy or radioisotopes. In **infection**, mAbs neutralise pathogens. In other conditions, mAbs target key proteins in disease pathology. For example, denosumab inhibits RANKL, an essential osteoclast protein, thereby decreasing bone resorption in the treatment of osteoporosis.
Important adverse effects	All mAbs can cause **immediate and delayed hypersensitivity reactions**, including local injection site reactions (common) and systemic reactions including fever, urticaria, and anaphylaxis (rare). Adverse effects of individual mAbs depend on their biological actions. mAbs that target the immune system can cause **immune imbalance**, e.g. immunosuppression, increasing the risk of severe infection or cancer, or overstimulation, leading to development of a new autoimmune condition. Generally, however, due to their precisely targeted effect, monoclonal antibodies are often better tolerated than conventional cytotoxic and immune suppressing treatments.
Warnings	Cautions for individual mAbs vary, so refer to the BNF and seek local specialist guidance. ▲ **Active and latent infection**, including with tuberculosis and hepatitis B or C, should be treated before starting long-term treatment with a mAb that can cause immune suppression.
Important interactions	The risk of severe generalised infection following ✖ live **vaccines** is increased in people treated with mAbs that cause immune suppression.

PRACTICAL PRESCRIBING

Prescription	Monoclonal antibodies are large, stable protein molecules that are eliminated slowly by intracellular catabolism. Long-term treatment is therefore prescribed at 2–4-week intervals (e.g. adalimumab for immune-mediated disorders 40 mg every 2 weeks, omalizumab for allergic disorders 300 mg every 4 weeks). The dosing interval may be longer where the duration of action is prolonged (e.g. denosumab for osteoporosis 60 mg every 6 months). Monoclonal antibody treatment should be initiated and monitored under specialist guidance.
Administration	mAbs have large size, poor membrane permeability, and are digested by gastric proteases. They are therefore administered parenterally by IV, SC or IM injection. Initial administration is under healthcare supervision (see MONITORING). Once established, subcutaneous mAbs can be self-administered at home.
Communication	Explain that monoclonal antibodies are 'precision engineered' antibodies designed to target and improve their disease. Explain that they are given by injection. Outline potential side effects, including general effects such as soreness at the injection site or allergic reactions with symptoms such as rash, dizziness, and wheezing, and effects specific to the mAb. People who experience side effects after taking mAbs at home should consult with their specialist before taking further doses. For those taking mAbs that cause immune suppression, advise that infections may be more frequent or severe while they are taking treatment, and that they should tell their doctor immediately if these occur.
Monitoring and stopping	Treatment **efficacy** should be monitored by pre-defined parameters (e.g. disease activity score for adalimumab, asthma exacerbation rate for omalizumab). For **safety**, monitoring is required for allergic reactions for 1 hour after the first dose of treatment, and after subsequent doses in those at high risk. Other safety monitoring will depend on the individual drug. Treatment should be stopped if there is insufficient response after a pre-defined period or if serious adverse reactions occur.
Cost	mAbs are expensive (e.g. adalimumab ~£600 per dose). 'Biosimilars' that are clinically equivalent to existing mAbs may be authorised once the original patent has expired. They may be cheaper.

Clinical tip—The WHO sets naming conventions for monoclonal antibodies. The first part of the name (prefix) is unique. This is followed by 'infixes' to designate the target class (e.g. *b/ba,* bacterial; *t/tu/ta,* tumour; *v/vi,* viral), and species (e.g. *o,* mouse; *u,* human; *zu,* humanised). For example, *den-os-u-mab* targets bone *(os)* and is human *(u),* whereas *oma-li-zu-mab* is immunomodulating *(li)* and humanised *(zu).* Until 2021, all had the suffix *'mab'*; but since 2022, additional suffixes have been added (e.g. *-ug,* unmodified immunoglobulin; *-ment,* fragment).

Nitrates

CLINICAL PHARMACOLOGY

Common indications	❶ Short-acting nitrates (glyceryl trinitrate) are used in **acute angina** and chest pain associated with **acute coronary syndrome (ACS).** ❷ Long-acting nitrates (e.g. isosorbide mononitrate) are used for **prophylaxis of angina** where a **β-blocker** and/or a **calcium channel blocker** are insufficient or not tolerated. ❸ IV nitrate infusions are used in the treatment of **ACS** (if there is ongoing ischaemia), **pulmonary oedema** (usually in combination with **furosemide** and **oxygen**), and **hypertensive emergencies** (although other agents, such as **labetalol** or sodium nitroprusside, are preferred).
Mechanisms of action	Nitrates are rapidly converted to **nitric oxide (NO)** following absorption. NO **increases cyclic guanosine monophosphate (cGMP) synthesis** and **reduces intracellular Ca^{2+}** in vascular smooth muscle cells, causing them to relax. This results in venous and, to a lesser extent, arterial vasodilation. Relaxation of the venous capacitance vessels reduces cardiac preload and left ventricular filling. These effects reduce cardiac work and myocardial oxygen demand, relieving angina and cardiac failure. Nitrates can relieve coronary vasospasm and dilate collateral vessels, improving coronary perfusion. They also relax the systemic arteries, reducing peripheral resistance and afterload. However, most of the antianginal effects are mediated by reduction of preload.
Important adverse effects	Due to their vasodilator effects, nitrates commonly cause **flushing, headaches, light-headedness,** and **hypotension.** Regular use of nitrates can lead to **tolerance,** with reduced symptom relief despite continued use. This can be minimised by careful timing of doses to avoid significant nitrate exposure overnight, when it tends not to be needed (see CLINICAL TIP).
Warnings	Nitrates are contraindicated in ✘ **severe aortic stenosis,** where arterial constriction is necessary to maintain blood pressure in the face of relatively fixed cardiac output. Abrupt vasodilation due to nitrate administration may therefore cause cardiovascular collapse. Nitrates should be avoided in ✘ **hypotension.**
Important interactions	Nitrates must not be taken concurrently with ✘ **phosphodiesterase (PDE) inhibitors** (e.g. sildenafil). This is because PDE is responsible for metabolising cGMP, and so PDE inhibitors enhance and prolong the hypotensive effect of nitrates. Nitrates should also be used with caution in people taking antihypertensive medication, in whom they may precipitate hypotension.

PRACTICAL PRESCRIBING

Prescription	In **stable angina,** glyceryl trinitrate (GTN) is prescribed sublingually as tablets or spray for immediate relief of chest pain. GTN has a plasma half-life of <5 minutes, so has a very quick onset and offset of action. In **ACS** and **heart failure,** GTN is prescribed as a continuous IV infusion. Give clear instructions on starting dose (e.g. 1 mg/hr), alongside instructions on dose titration (see Monitoring). Isosorbide mononitrate (ISMN) has a plasma half-life of 4–5 hours and is prescribed two to three times daily as immediate-release tablets for the prevention of recurrent angina. ISMN is also available as modified-release (MR) tablets or transdermal patches, which are prescribed once daily. When prescribing MR preparations, include the brand name, since there are important differences between preparations.
Administration	Intravenous GTN is usually administered as an adjustable infusion, using a solution containing GTN 50 mg in 50 mL (1 mg/mL).
Communication	As appropriate, explain that this is a treatment to relieve chest pain, breathlessness or to treat hypertension. Advise that it may cause headache, but that this is normally short-lived. As nitrates are probably more effective at preventing than terminating angina, advise them to use sublingual GTN *before* tasks that normally bring on their angina. Due to the risks of postural hypotension, it is a good idea to sit down and rest before and for 5 minutes after taking GTN. For regularly administered nitrates, advise on the times that doses should be taken (see Clinical tip).
Monitoring and stopping	**Resolution of symptoms** is the best indicator of efficacy. When administering by IV infusion, monitor **blood pressure** frequently (e.g. every 15 minutes initially). The infusion rate should be adjusted to relieve symptoms while avoiding hypotension (e.g. 'Increase GTN infusion rate by 0.5 mL/hr every 15–30 minutes until chest pain/breathlessness relieved, provided systolic BP is >90 mmHg'). Owing to the development of tolerance, continuous IV infusions of nitrates are usually stopped after 24–48 hours, in favour of oral agents. It may be possible to stop chronic nitrate treatment following successful percutaneous intervention or bypass surgery.
Cost	Non-proprietary GTN and ISMN are inexpensive. GTN tablets must be discarded after 8 weeks, so a spray may be a better choice for people with infrequent symptoms.

Clinical tip—Where nitrates are taken regularly, there is a risk of tolerance (tachyphylaxis), which can reduce efficacy. To prevent this, time doses to ensure there is a 'nitrate-free period' every day during a time of inactivity, usually overnight. For example, take twice-daily ISMN morning and mid-afternoon (rather than evening) to provide an 18-hour gap between doses in the afternoon and the following morning.

Nitrofurantoin

CLINICAL PHARMACOLOGY

Common indications
❶ Nitrofurantoin is a first-line option for acute, uncomplicated **lower urinary tract infection (UTI)** (an alternative is **trimethoprim**).
❷ It can also be used for **prophylaxis of recurrent UTIs**.

Spectrum of activity
Nitrofurantoin is active against most organisms that cause uncomplicated UTIs, including *Escherichia coli* (Gram-negative) and *Staphylococcus saprophyticus* (Gram-positive).

Mechanisms of action
Nitrofurantoin is metabolised (reduced) in bacterial cells by nitrofuran reductase. Its active metabolite **damages bacterial DNA** and causes cell death **(bactericidal).** Bacteria with lower nitrofuran reductase activity are resistant to nitrofurantoin. Some organisms that are less common causes of UTI (such as *Klebsiella* and *Proteus* species) have intrinsic resistance to nitrofurantoin. It is relatively rare for *E. coli* to acquire nitrofurantoin resistance. Nitrofurantoin requires concentration in the urine by renal excretion for therapeutic effect against UTIs; for the same reason, it is not useful for infections elsewhere in the body.

Important adverse effects
As with many antibiotics, nitrofurantoin can cause **GI upset** and immediate and delayed **hypersensitivity** reactions (see **Penicillins, broad-spectrum**). Nitrofurantoin, specifically, can turn urine dark yellow or brown. Less commonly, it may cause **chronic pulmonary reactions** (including inflammation (pneumonitis) and fibrosis), **hepatitis,** and **peripheral neuropathy,** which all are more likely with prolonged administration. In neonates, **haemolytic anaemia** may occur because immature red blood cells are unable to mop up nitrofurantoin-stimulated superoxides, which damage red blood cells.

Warnings
Nitrofurantoin should not be prescribed for ✖ **pregnant women towards term**, for ✖ **babies in the first 3 months of life** or for people with ✖ **G6PD deficiency** because of the risk of haemolysis. It is contraindicated in ✖ **renal impairment**, as impaired excretion increases toxicity and reduces efficacy due to lower urinary drug concentrations. Caution is required when using nitrofurantoin for ▲ **long-term prevention of UTIs**, as chronic use increases the risk of pulmonary, hepatic and neurological adverse effects, particularly in older people.

Important interactions
Nitrofurantoin should be used with caution with other drugs that cause ▲ **peripheral neuropathy**, including **amiodarone**, isoniazid, **metronidazole,** and phenytoin.

PRACTICAL PRESCRIBING

Prescription	For **treatment of acute UTI**, a typical dosage is 50 mg orally 6-hrly (immediate-release) or 100 mg orally 12-hrly (modified-release). For **prevention of recurrent UTI**, nitrofurantoin is prescribed at a dosage of 50–100 mg orally nightly, to be taken regularly, or as a single dose of 100 mg to be taken after exposure to a known trigger. Maximum urinary concentrations are usually achieved 2–4 hours after dosing.
Administration	Oral nitrofurantoin is available as tablets, immediate- or modified-release capsules and in suspension. It should be taken with food or milk to minimise GI effects. There is no parenteral formulation.
Communication	Explain that the aim of treatment is to get rid of infection and improve symptoms. Before prescribing, always check for allergy to nitrofurantoin. Advise that urine colour may change to dark yellow or brown during treatment; this is harmless and temporary. Where antibiotics are for prophylaxis, emphasise that this is a long-term medication that should be renewed, rather than a course that should stop. Advise that any unexplained symptoms should be reported promptly, particularly pins and needles or breathlessness, which could be signs of serious side effects.
Monitoring and stopping	Efficacy of **treatment for acute UTI** is determined by resolution of symptoms. For **preventing recurrent UTI**, efficacy is determined by comparing UTI frequency before and during prophylaxis. Safety of long-term treatment is a particular concern, so advice should be given about reporting any new symptoms (see COMMUNICATION) that could indicate neuropathy or pulmonary adverse effects. The duration of therapy is a balance between ensuring effective treatment of infection, and reducing adverse reactions and emergence of resistance. For **treatment of acute UTI**, prescribe nitrofurantoin as a 3-day course for uncomplicated UTIs in women, and as a 7-day course for men and pregnant women. For **prevention of recurrent UTIs**, review long-term treatment every 6 months and stop if ineffective or if features of neuropathy or pneumonitis emerge.
Cost	The drug tariff price (amount paid to pharmacy contractors for dispensing the drug) for a 7-day course of nitrofurantoin is around £10 as tablets or capsules, but around £450 as oral suspension. This formulation should therefore be reserved for people who truly are unable to take tablets or capsules.

Clinical tip—As tissue concentrations of nitrofurantoin are very low, you should not prescribe it for pyelonephritis or other complicated UTIs. Treat these with an IV broad-spectrum antibiotic such as a **penicillin (broad-spectrum)** with a beta lactamase inhibitor, a **cephalosporin** or a **quinolone**, with or without an **aminoglycoside**.

Non-steroidal antiinflammatory drugs (NSAIDs) and COX-2 inhibitors

CLINICAL PHARMACOLOGY

Common indications	❶ 'As-needed' treatment of **mild-to-moderate pain** (e.g. dysmenorrhoea, dental pain, trauma) and **fever. Paracetamol** produces similar analgesic effect, so is preferred in those at risk of adverse effects. ❷ Regular treatment for pain related to inflammation, particularly of the musculoskeletal system, e.g. in **rheumatoid arthritis,** severe **osteoarthritis,** and acute **gout.**
Mechanisms of action	Non-steroidal antiinflammatory drugs (NSAIDs) inhibit prostaglandin synthesis from arachidonic acid by **inhibiting cyclo-oxygenase (COX).** COX exists as two main isoforms. COX-1 is the *constitutive* form. It stimulates prostaglandin synthesis that preserves integrity of the gastric mucosa, maintains renal perfusion (by dilating afferent glomerular arterioles), and inhibits thrombus formation at the vascular endothelium. COX-2 is the *inducible* form, expressed in response to inflammatory stimuli. It stimulates production of prostaglandins that cause inflammation and pain. The therapeutic benefits of NSAIDs are principally mediated by COX-2 inhibition, and adverse effects by COX-1 inhibition, although there is some overlap. Selective COX-2 inhibitors (e.g. etoricoxib) were developed in an effort to reduce the adverse GI effects of NSAIDs.
Important adverse effects	The main adverse effects of NSAIDs are **GI toxicity, renal impairment,** and **major adverse cardiovascular events** (MACE, e.g. myocardial infarction and stroke). The adverse effect profile differs between NSAIDs. Selective COX-2 inhibitors and low-dose ibuprofen are least likely to cause GI toxicity. Cardiovascular events are most likely with COX-2 inhibitors, high-dose ibuprofen and diclofenac, and less likely with naproxen. All NSAIDs, including selective COX-2 inhibitors, can cause renal impairment. Other adverse effects include **hypersensitivity reactions,** e.g. bronchospasm and angioedema, and **fluid retention,** which can worsen hypertension and heart failure.
Warnings	NSAIDs are contraindicated in ✖ **severe renal impairment,** ✖ **heart failure,** ✖ **liver failure** and known ✖ **NSAID hypersensitivity.** They should be avoided in ▲ **peptic ulcer disease** (especially if there are additional risk factors, see CLINICAL TIP), ▲ **cardiovascular disease** and milder forms of ▲ **renal impairment.** If unavoidable, use the safest NSAID for the relevant risk, at the lowest effective dose, for the shortest possible time.
Important interactions	Many drugs increase the risk of NSAID-related adverse effects. For example, **corticosteroids** increase risk of peptic ulceration; ▲ anticoagulants (e.g. **warfarin, direct oral anticoagulants**) and ▲ **selective serotonin reuptake inhibitors (SSRIs)** increase risk of GI bleeding; and ▲ **angiotensin-converting enzyme (ACE) inhibitors, angiotensin receptor blockers** and **diuretics** increase risk of renal impairment. In general, NSAIDs impair the effectiveness of antihypertensives.

ibuprofen, diclofenac, naproxen (NSAIDs)
etoricoxib (COX-2 inhibitor)

PRACTICAL PRESCRIBING

Prescription	NSAIDs have similar antiinflammatory efficacy, so choice depends mostly on adverse effect profile. For example, naproxen is often selected because of its relatively low risk of MACE. However, if cardiovascular risk is low and GI toxicity is a greater concern, low-dose ibuprofen (200–400 mg 8-hrly) may be preferable. Dosage regimens vary with indication. For example, in rheumatoid arthritis, a typical dose of naproxen is 500 mg orally 12-hrly.
Administration	NSAIDs are generally taken orally, but are also available as topical gels, suppositories and injectable preparations. Oral NSAIDs should be taken with food to minimise GI upset.
Communication	Explain that you are recommending an antiinflammatory drug to help improve symptoms of pain, swelling, and/or fever. Warn that the most common side effect is indigestion and advise them to stop treatment and seek medical advice if this occurs. For acute pain, explain that long-term use, e.g. beyond 10 days, is not recommended due to the risk of side effects. If long-term treatment is required, advise that they stop the NSAIDs if they become acutely unwell or dehydrated, to reduce the risk of damage to the kidneys.
Monitoring and stopping	Control of pain and inflammation can be assessed by enquiry about symptoms, examination, and by using scoring systems, e.g. a visual analogue scale for pain. For acute indications, review symptoms after an appropriate interval (e.g. 2 weeks) and stop treatment when pain has become tolerable. When used longer-term for inflammatory conditions, regular treatment for at least 3 weeks is required before the full antiinflammatory effect is seen. Therefore it may be prudent to schedule a review at 4–6 weeks when, depending on response, the treatment may be continued, stopped or an alternative NSAID offered. Routine biochemical monitoring is not required, but renal function should be monitored closely if there is any renal impairment. The NSAID should be stopped if this deteriorates.
Cost	NSAIDs are available in non-proprietary forms, which are inexpensive. For people who pay for their prescriptions, it may be cheaper for them to buy non-proprietary NSAIDs over the counter.

Clinical tip—Protection from NSAID-associated ulcers ('gastroprotection') should be considered for individuals at increased risk of GI complications. Risk factors include age >65 years, previous peptic ulcer disease, co-morbidities (such as cardiovascular disease, diabetes), and concurrent therapy with other drugs with GI side effects, particularly low-dose **aspirin** and **prednisolone**. A PPI (e.g. **lansoprazole** 15–30 mg orally daily) is recommended.

Ocular lubricants (artificial tears)

CLINICAL PHARMACOLOGY

Common indications	For first-line symptomatic treatment of **dry eye conditions,** including **keratoconjunctivitis sicca** and **Sjögren's syndrome,** alongside environmental coping strategies and avoiding precipitants.
Mechanisms of action	In dry eye conditions, ocular lubricants have a **soothing effect** and help **protect the eye surfaces from abrasive damage.** Lubricant *eye drops* typically consist of an electrolyte solution with a viscosity agent, such as a cellulose polymer (e.g. hypromellose). *Gels,* such as carbomer 980 (the active ingredient of Viscotears®), have greater viscosity and are retained in the eye for longer. *Ointments* such as white soft paraffin with liquid paraffin (e.g. Lacri-Lube®) are highly viscous and may provide greater protection, but at a cost of causing blurred vision.
Important adverse effects	Ocular lubricants have few side effects other than mild **stinging** on application and temporary **blurring of vision.** The risk of blurring increases with viscosity and is therefore greatest for ointments. Unless specified as 'preservative-free', it can be assumed that the preparation contains some form of preservative. This may incite a local **inflammatory (allergic) reaction**, particularly in frequent or long-term use.
Warnings	As ocular lubricants are not absorbed, there are no major safety considerations from a systemic illness perspective.
Important interactions	No clinically important interactions arise from the pharmacological effects of ocular lubricants. If more than one type of eye drop is in use, administration should be separated by about 5 minutes. Ocular lubricants should be taken last, otherwise they may be 'washed away' by the other eye drops.

PRACTICAL PRESCRIBING

Prescription	Most ocular lubricants can be purchased from pharmacies without a prescription. Hypromellose 0.3% eye drops are usually tried first at a dose of 1–2 drops three times daily as required. They can be taken more often (up to hourly) if necessary, but if they are required more than four times daily on a regular basis, it may be worth trying a gel (e.g. Viscotears® 1 drop three times daily as required). In severe cases an ointment (e.g. Lacri-Lube®) may be added, although this is generally restricted to bedtime use due to its visual blurring effect. Preservative-free products are preferable for long-term or frequent application (more than four times daily), to avoid adverse reactions to the preservative.
Administration	Ocular lubricants are usually self-administered. After washing their hands, the person tips the head back ('look at the ceiling') and pulls down slightly on the lower eyelid. Then, with the bottle held upside-down just above the eye, they squeeze to release a drop. For drops, they should then close the eye and press gently on the corner nearest the nose for 1 minute. For gels, they should blink a few times to spread it over the eye. They should try not to let the tip of the dispenser touch the eye (or anything else) and should replace the cap directly after use to prevent infection.
Communication	Explain that you are recommending 'artificial tears' in the hope of improving their dry eyes. Explain how to take them and warn that, like most eye drops, they can sting a little when applied. This wears away quickly and they should then experience some relief from their dry eye symptoms. With continued use over days and weeks their symptoms may improve further as previous abrasive damage is repaired. They will probably need to take the treatment indefinitely.
Monitoring and stopping	Symptoms are the best guide to efficacy. Ask the patient to return if their symptoms fail to improve or any problems develop. If the underlying cause of dry eyes can be identified and corrected it may be possible to stop treatment. Otherwise, treatment is continued indefinitely.
Cost	People who pay for their prescriptions will generally save money if they purchase the product over the counter. Preservative-free products are often single-use and expensive, so should be reserved for those requiring frequent or long-term application.

Clinical tip—Critically ill patients in intensive care units may suffer from corneal erosions and microbial keratitis, due to poor eyelid closure and suppression of protective reflexes due to impaired consciousness. Eye care is therefore an essential component of good-quality intensive care. Prescription of an ocular lubricant, e.g. hypromellose 0.3%, 1 drop per eye 4-hrly, should be considered for all patients with impaired consciousness (including due to sedation).

Oestrogens and progestogens

CLINICAL PHARMACOLOGY

Common indications	❶ **Hormonal contraception** in those requiring highly effective, reversible contraception, particularly if its other effects (e.g. improved acne control) are also desirable. ❷ **Hormone replacement therapy (HRT)** to delay **early menopause** and treat distressing **menopausal symptoms** (any age). Systemic formulations (tablets or patches) are used for systemic symptoms (e.g. hot flushes), and vaginal gels for vaginal symptoms (e.g. dryness).
Mechanisms of action	Luteinising hormone (LH) and follicle-stimulating hormone (FSH) control ovulation and ovarian production of oestrogen and progesterone. In turn, oestrogen and progesterone exert predominantly negative feedback on LH and FSH release. In hormonal contraception, oestrogens (e.g. ethinylestradiol) and/or progestogens (e.g. desogestrel) are given to **suppress LH/FSH release** and hence ovulation. Oestrogens and progestogens also have effects outside the ovary. Some, such as in the cervix and endometrium, may contribute to their contraceptive effect (most relevant in progestogen-only contraception). Others offer additional benefits, e.g. reduced menstrual pain and bleeding, and improvements in acne. At the menopause, a fall in oestrogen and progesterone levels may generate symptoms such as vaginal dryness and vasomotor instability ('hot flushes'). Oestrogen replacement (usually combined with a progestogen) alleviates these.
Important adverse effects	Hormonal contraception may cause **irregular bleeding** and **mood changes.** It does not appear to cause weight gain. The oestrogens in combined hormonal contraception (CHC) double the risk of venous thromboembolism (VTE), but the absolute risk is low. They increase the risk of **cardiovascular disease** and **stroke,** most relevant in women with other vascular risk factors. They may be associated with increased risk of **breast and cervical cancer.** In both cases the effect is small, and for breast cancer, it gradually resolves after stopping the pill. Progestogen-only pills do not increase the risk of VTE or cardiovascular disease. The adverse effects of **HRT** are similar to those of CHC but, as baseline rates of disease are higher, the relative risks have more significant effects.
Warnings	Oestrogens and progestogens are contraindicated in women with ✖ **breast cancer.** CHC should be avoided in those with a ✖ personal or ▲ family history of **VTE;** ✖ **thrombogenic mutation**; or risk factors for ▲ **cardiovascular disease** (including age >35 years; migraine with aura; heavy smoking history). Women who have a uterus should not receive oestrogen-only HRT, due to the risk of endometrial benign prostatic enlargement.
Important interactions	▲ **Cytochrome P450 inducers** (e.g. rifampicin, **carbamazepine**) may reduce contraceptive efficacy, particularly of progestogen-only forms. Absorption of ▲ **lamotrigine** may be reduced, impairing seizure control.

ethinylestradiol, estradiol (oestrogens)
levonorgestrel, desogestrel (progestogens)

PRACTICAL PRESCRIBING

Prescription	Hormonal contraception should be prescribed by appropriately trained health professionals only. The **UK Medical Eligibility Criteria for Contraceptive Use** from the Faculty of Sexual and Reproductive Healthcare (FSRH) provide detailed prescribing guidance. CHC is commonly taken as a combined oral contraceptive (COC) pill. A pill containing ethinylestradiol 30 or 35 micrograms is appropriate for most women. Where CHC is contraindicated, a progesterone-only pill (POP) may be suitable. For HRT, combined oestrogen–progestogen therapy (tablet or patch) is prescribed if the woman has a uterus. Women who have had a hysterectomy may receive oestrogen alone. Systemic HRT can either be cyclic (with monthly bleed, usually prescribed for women who are still having periods) or continuous (no bleed, for women who have not had a period for >1 year). For women with vaginal symptoms only, a vaginal oestrogen preparation is best.
Administration	If a COC pill is started within the first 6 days of the woman's cycle, no additional contraception is needed. Beyond this, a barrier method should be used or sex avoided for the first 7 days. Most combined pills are taken for 21 days followed by a 7-day pill-free interval, during which a withdrawal bleed occurs. Some ('everyday') pills are taken throughout the cycle, but the tablets for days 22–28 are inactive. Detailed guidance on how to deal with missed pills is provided by the FSRH and summarised in the BNF. In general, missing one COC pill does not significantly reduce contraceptive efficacy, but missing two or more necessitates additional contraceptive precautions for 7 days.
Communication	Hormonal contraception and HRT should be prescribed only after careful discussion of risks and benefits, which is beyond the scope of this book. Information should be provided on how to take the product (e.g. whether in a cyclic or continuous pattern) and what to expect (e.g. withdrawal bleeding, symptom control). Explain how to deal with missed pills and support this with written guidance.
Monitoring and stopping	Baseline assessment should include relevant history, blood pressure (BP) check and body mass index (BMI). A review should be scheduled at 3 months to check BP check and discuss any issues. Thereafter, annual checks for health changes, BP, and BMI are sufficient. Hormonal contraception can be stopped abruptly if no longer required, whereas for HRT it may be preferable to taper the dose to avoid sudden relapse.
Cost	Hormonal contraception accounts for significant health expenditure. Follow local policies, which are likely to take cost into account.

Clinical tip—Continuous or extended use of the COC pill (i.e. without pill-free intervals) is unlicensed for most brands, but is safe and effective. It eliminates or reduces withdrawal bleeding, which may be a desirable effect for some.

Opioids

CLINICAL PHARMACOLOGY

Common indications	❶ **Acute pain,** e.g. in trauma, surgery or acute coronary syndrome. ❷ **Chronic pain,** as part of a multimodal approach, if non-pharmacological treatments, **paracetamol**, **NSAIDs,** and adjuvant analgesics (e.g. **pregabalin**) are insufficient. ❸ Breathlessness in **palliative care.** ❹ **Acute pulmonary oedema,** alongside **oxygen, furosemide,** and **nitrates**.
Mechanisms of action	*Opioids* include naturally occurring *opiates* (e.g. morphine) and their *synthetic analogues* (e.g. oxycodone). The therapeutic effects of opioids are mediated by **agonism** of **opioid μ (mu) receptors** in the central nervous system (CNS). Activation of these G protein-coupled receptors has several effects that, overall, reduce neuronal excitability and pain transmission. In the medulla, they blunt the response to hypoxia and hypercapnoea, reducing respiratory drive and breathlessness. By relieving pain, breathlessness, and associated anxiety, opioids reduce sympathetic nervous system (fight or flight) activity. In acute coronary syndrome and pulmonary oedema, this reduces cardiac work and oxygen demand. In practical use, opioids are classified by strength. This refers to the intensity of effect that can be elicited with typical therapeutic doses. For example, morphine and oxycodone are *strong opioids,* while codeine and dihydrocodeine are *weak.* The latter examples are prodrugs—they are metabolised in the liver to more active metabolites (including morphine and dihydromorphine, respectively). Tramadol is a synthetic analogue of codeine. It is perhaps best classified as having *moderate* strength. In addition to agonism of the μ receptor, it inhibits neuronal noradrenaline and serotonin uptake. This contributes to analgesia by potentiating descending inhibitory pain pathways.
Important adverse effects	Opioids may cause **respiratory depression**, euphoria, detachment, and in higher doses, **neurological depression.** They can activate the chemoreceptor trigger zone, causing **nausea and vomiting**. **Pupillary constriction** occurs due to stimulation of the Edinger–Westphal nucleus. Activation of μ receptors increases intestinal smooth muscle tone and reduces motility, leading to **constipation.** Opioids may cause histamine release, leading to **itching,** urticaria, vasodilation, and sweating. Prolonged use can lead to **dependence** and **hyperalgesia.**
Warnings	Most opioids rely on the liver and the kidneys for elimination, so doses should be reduced in ▲ **hepatic failure** and ▲ **renal impairment** and in ▲ **older people.** Do not give opioids in ▲ **respiratory failure** except under senior guidance (e.g. in palliative care).
Important interactions	Avoid co-prescription with ▲ **other sedating drugs** (e.g. **antipsychotics, benzodiazepines,** and **tricyclic antidepressants**). Where their combination is unavoidable, close monitoring is necessary.

PRACTICAL PRESCRIBING

Prescription
When treating **acute severe pain** in high-dependency areas (e.g. the emergency or operating department), a strong opioid is given IV for rapid effect. A typical initial prescription is morphine 2–10 mg IV, tailored to pain, age, and other individual factors. In low-dependency areas, oral administration is preferred. A common choice for mild pain is codeine (e.g. 30 mg orally 4-hrly), or for more severe pain, immediate-release oral morphine (e.g. Oramorph® 5 mg orally 4-hrly). When a stable dose of immediate-release morphine is found, it may be converted to a modified-release (MR) form (e.g. MST Continus® 15 mg 12-hrly). Alongside regular treatment, 'breakthrough analgesia' should be prescribed. The breakthrough dose should be about one-sixth of the total daily regular dose (e.g. Oramorph® 5 mg 2-hrly as required). We recommend that the brand name is included in strong oral opioid prescriptions, although local practices may vary. **Chronic pain** often responds poorly to analgesics, so management should focus on non-pharmacological treatments in the first instance.

Administration
IV morphine is given incrementally (1–2 mg every few minutes) to achieve the desired response. IV opioids are usually restricted to high-dependency areas, to monitor for adverse effects.

Communication
Explain that opioid painkillers are most effective for severe, short-term pain, and prolonged use should be avoided due to the risk of dependence and addiction. As applicable, explain the difference between 'slow-release' tablets (taken regularly for 'background' pain control) and 'fast-action' forms (which may be taken regularly or as required). Explain that nausea is a common side effect, but it usually settles after a few days. Constipation is very common; advise good hydration and offer a **laxative** (e.g. senna). Advise that they should not drive if they feel drowsy or confused, and to store opioids safely.

Monitoring and stopping
For acute severe pain, initial parenteral doses are titrated against therapeutic effect (pain severity) and adverse effects (e.g. level of consciousness, respiratory rate). The same general considerations apply for oral treatment. The opioid should be reduced and withdrawn as the acute process resolves. Prolonged treatment is not advisable, but if unavoidable, it should be supported by regular review and an agreed plan for how and when to end treatment. The dose may then need to be tapered slowly to avoid a withdrawal reaction.

Cost
Morphine, codeine, and dihydrocodeine are relatively inexpensive. Synthetic opioids may be more expensive.

Clinical tip—The features of opioid withdrawal are the opposite of the clinical effects of opioids: anxiety, pain, and breathlessness increase; the pupils dilate; and the skin is cool and dry with piloerection ('cold turkey').

Paracetamol

CLINICAL PHARMACOLOGY

Common indications	❶ Paracetamol is a first-line analgesic for most forms of **acute and chronic pain.** It may be used alone for mild pain, or combined with other analgesics (e.g. **opioids, non-steroidal antiinflammatory drugs**). ❷ Paracetamol is an antipyretic that can reduce **fever** and its associated symptoms (e.g. shivering).
Mechanisms of action	The mechanisms of action of paracetamol are poorly understood. In the central nervous system, it acts as a reducing co-substrate of **cyclo-oxygenase 2 (COX-2).** This reduces the availability of oxidised COX-2, necessary for conversion of arachidonic acid to an intermediate metabolite in the prostaglandin synthesis pathway. This interferes with transmission of pain signals between the spinal cord and higher centres, reducing pain sensitivity. It also reduces prostaglandin E_2 (PGE_2) concentrations in the thermoregulatory region of the hypothalamus, reducing fever. However, it has little antiinflammatory action in peripheral tissues. This may be because its effects are inhibited by peroxides, the concentration of which is low in the central nervous system, but high in inflamed tissue. It is likely that other actions of paracetamol and its metabolites contribute to the therapeutic effect. These may include activation of descending serotonergic pathways, and inhibition of neuronal reuptake of endogenous cannabinoids.
Important adverse effects	At treatment doses, paracetamol is very safe with few side effects. Lack of COX-1 inhibition means that it does not cause peptic ulceration or renal impairment or increase the risk of major adverse cardiovascular events (unlike **NSAIDs**). Its safety makes it a popular choice as a first-line analgesic. In **overdose,** paracetamol causes **liver failure.** It is, in part, metabolised by cytochrome P450 (CYP) enzymes to a toxic metabolite (N-acetyl-p-benzoquinone imine (NAPQI)), which is conjugated with glutathione before elimination. In overdose, this elimination pathway is saturated, and NAPQI accumulation causes hepatocellular necrosis. Hepatotoxicity can be prevented by treatment with the glutathione precursor **acetylcysteine**.
Warnings	Paracetamol dose should be reduced in people at increased risk of liver toxicity, either because of *increased NAPQI production* (e.g. in ▲ **chronic excessive alcohol use,** inducing metabolising enzymes) or *reduced glutathione stores* (e.g. in ▲ **malnutrition,** ▲ **low body weight** (<50 kg) and ▲ **severe hepatic impairment**). This is particularly important where paracetamol is given by IV infusion.
Important interactions	There are few clinically significant interactions between paracetamol and other drugs. ▲ **CYP inducers,** e.g. phenytoin and **carbamazepine,** increase the rate of NAPQI production and therefore the risk of liver damage in paracetamol toxicity.

PRACTICAL PRESCRIBING

Prescription	Oral paracetamol is on the 'general sales list', which means that it can be purchased from any retail outlet, although it is also available on prescription. For people unable to take drugs by mouth, paracetamol can be prescribed for IV infusion or rectal administration. By all routes, the usual adult dose is 0.5–1 g every 4–6 hours, maximum 4 g daily (see WARNINGS). Paracetamol can be prescribed for regular administration or to be taken as required, depending on the nature of the pain. When prescribed 'as required', the maximum daily dose must always be stated.
Administration	Oral paracetamol is available as tablets, caplets, capsules, soluble tablets, and oral suspension. IV paracetamol solution may be infused neat over 15 minutes or diluted in 0.9% sodium chloride or 5% glucose solution before administration, depending on the product.
Communication	Explain that you are recommending paracetamol to relieve pain or fever. Effects should be felt around half an hour after taking it. Where regular paracetamol is prescribed, explain the importance of taking it every 6 hours. Warn them not to exceed the recommended maximum daily dose because of the potential risk of liver poisoning. Advise that many medicines purchased from the chemist (e.g. cold and flu preparations) contain paracetamol. Warn them to check the label or ask the pharmacist before taking these with paracetamol.
Monitoring and stopping	Efficacy of paracetamol in pain control can be established by enquiry about symptoms or by using a pain score, e.g. a visual analogue scale. For acute pain, review response to analgesia 1–2 hours after an oral dose. Stop paracetamol when the cause of the pain resolves. In **paracetamol overdose,** blood tests including international normalised ratio (INR), serum alanine aminotransferase, and creatinine concentration should be measured to detect liver and renal injury (see **acetylcysteine and carbocisteine**).
Cost	A single dose of **oral paracetamol** 1 g can cost as little as 2p. The added value of the additional ingredients in expensive branded products is doubtful. As **IV paracetamol** is around 30 times more expensive (65p for 1 g plus infusion costs) than oral formulations, it should be reserved for those unable to take medicines by mouth. Switch from IV to oral as soon as possible.

Clinical tip—When prescribing paracetamol, always check that you are not inadvertently duplicating an existing prescription. For example, if you are prescribing paracetamol regularly, stop any pre-existing 'as required' prescription. Look out for 'co-' drugs (where two drugs are combined into a single preparation) such as **co-codamol** or **co-dydramol**, which contain paracetamol.

Penicillins, antipseudomonal

CLINICAL PHARMACOLOGY

Common indications	Antipseudomonal penicillins are reserved for severe infections, particularly where there is a broad spectrum of potential pathogens, if antibiotic resistance is likely (e.g. hospital-acquired infection) or in people who have immune suppression (e.g. neutropenia). Specific infections treated with these drugs include: ❶ **Lower respiratory tract infection.** ❷ **Urinary tract infection.** ❸ **Intraabdominal infection.** ❹ **Skin and soft tissue infection.**
Spectrum of activity	Antipseudomonal penicillins (e.g. piperacillin) have a **broad spectrum** of activity against a wide range of Gram-positive and Gram-negative bacteria (notably including *Pseudomonas* spp.) and anaerobes. They are formulated with a β-lactamase inhibitor (e.g. tazobactam), which confers antimicrobial activity against β-lactamase-producing bacteria (e.g. *Staphylococcus aureus*, Gram-negative anaerobes).
Mechanisms of action	Penicillins **inhibit enzymes responsible for cross-linking peptidoglycans**. This weakens bacterial cell walls, reducing their ability to maintain an osmotic gradient and resulting in cell swelling, lysis, and death. Penicillins contain a β-lactam ring, which is responsible for their **bactericidal** activity. Side chains attached to the β-lactam ring can be modified to make semi-synthetic penicillins. Piperacillin is similar to ampicillin, but with a longer side chain. This improves its affinity to penicillin-binding proteins, increasing the spectrum of activity.
Important adverse effects	**GI upset** is common. Less frequently, **antibiotic-associated colitis** occurs. Broad-spectrum antibiotics kill normal GI flora, allowing overgrowth of toxin-producing *Clostridioides difficile*. The resulting colitis can be complicated by colonic perforation and/or death. Delayed or immediate **hypersensitivity** may occur (see **Penicillins, broad-spectrum**).
Warnings	Antipseudomonal penicillins should be used with caution in people at risk of ▲ *C. difficile* **infection,** particularly older people and those in hospital. The main contraindication is ✖ **penicillin allergy.** Note that allergy to one type of penicillin implies allergy to all types, as it is due to a reaction to the basic penicillin structure. People with hypersensitivity to penicillins may also react to **cephalosporins** and **other β-lactam antibiotics**. The dose of antipseudomonal penicillins should be reduced in ▲ **moderate/severe renal impairment.**
Important interactions	Penicillins reduce renal excretion of ▲ **methotrexate**, increasing the risk of toxicity. Antipseudomonal penicillins can enhance the anticoagulant effect of **warfarin** by killing normal GI flora that synthesise vitamin K.

PRACTICAL PRESCRIBING

Prescription	Piperacillin is always given with tazobactam. It can be prescribed using the drugs' generic names (piperacillin–tazobactam) or by brand name (e.g. Tazocin®, although note that non-proprietary compound preparations are now available). Piperacillin–tazobactam is given by IV infusion. The usual dose is 4.5 g, containing 4 g of piperacillin and 500 mg of tazobactam, given every 6–8 hours. Document the indication, review date, and treatment duration on all inpatient antibiotic prescriptions to aid antibiotic stewardship.
Administration	Piperacillin with tazobactam is formulated as a powder to be reconstituted in 10 mL sterile water or 0.9% sodium chloride. This is diluted further in 50–150 mL of 0.9% sodium chloride or 5% glucose for IV infusion. Infusion duration varies according to local protocols.
Communication	Explain that the aim of treatment is to get rid of infection and improve symptoms. Before prescribing, always check for allergies to any form of penicillin or other β-lactam antibiotics. Warn them to seek medical advice if a rash or other unexpected symptom develops. If an allergic reaction occurs, give written and verbal advice not to take this antibiotic class in the future and make sure that the reaction (including its nature) is clearly recorded in the notes.
Monitoring and stopping	Efficacy is monitored by resolution of symptoms, signs (e.g. pyrexia, lung crackles) and blood markers (e.g. falling CRP and white cell count). Duration of antibiotic therapy is a balance between ensuring effective treatment and minimising adverse reactions and resistance. Always set a stop or review date when prescribing antibiotics, referring to local protocols for guidance. For IV antibiotics, oral switch should be considered after 48 hours if the patient is improving and able to take oral medication. However, as piperacillin–tazobactam is only available for IV infusion, oral switch is only possible if an alternative antibiotic is available. If piperacillin–tazobactam is the only effective agent, the whole course (usually 5–14 days) must be given IV.
Cost	Due to the costs of the product and the costs of administration and inpatient stay, IV antibiotic treatment is expensive. Use of an outpatient parenteral antimicrobial therapy (OPAT) service can both improve patient experience and reduce costs.

Clinical tip—Each dose of piperacillin–tazobactam contains about 11 mmol Na$^+$ and is infused in 50–150 mL fluid (which may contain more sodium). Take this into account when determining the need for supplementary fluid and electrolyte therapy, particularly in people with heart failure or oedema.

Penicillins, broad-spectrum

CLINICAL PHARMACOLOGY

Common indications	❶ Amoxicillin is used in many infections, including **sinusitis, otitis media,** community-acquired **pneumonia,** and **urinary tract infection (UTI),** and to eradicate *Helicobacter pylori* in **peptic ulcer disease** (with a **proton pump inhibitor** and **clarithromycin** or **metronidazole**). ❷ Co-amoxiclav is a common choice for severe, resistant, and hospital-acquired infections, including **pneumonia, UTI, intraabdominal infection, cellulitis,** and **bone and joint infection.** Unless supported by microbiological evidence of sensitivity, amoxicillin is not generally used for these indications, as resistance is common.
Spectrum of activity	Amoxicillin has a **broad spectrum** of activity against Gram-positive and Gram-negative cocci and bacilli (rods). However, it is inactivated by bacterial penicillinases, and resistance is increasingly prevalent. Combination with clavulanic acid (a β-lactamase inhibitor) as co-amoxiclav restores activity against many amoxicillin-resistant strains.
Mechanisms of action	Penicillins **inhibit enzymes responsible for cross-linking peptidoglycans**. This weakens the bacterial cell wall, reducing its ability to maintain an osmotic gradient, causing cell swelling, lysis, and death. Penicillins contain a β-lactam ring, which is responsible for their **bactericidal** activity. Broad-spectrum penicillins are synthesised by addition of an amino group to the β-lactam ring side chains, broadening activity against aerobic Gram-negative bacteria.
Important adverse effects	**GI upset** is common. Less often but importantly, **antibiotic-associated colitis** may occur. This is where broad-spectrum antibiotics kill normal gut flora, allowing overgrowth of toxin-producing *Clostridioides difficile.* The resulting colitis can be complicated by colonic perforation and/or death. Penicillin **allergy,** affecting 1%–10% of people exposed, usually presents as a **skin rash** 7–10 days after first, or 1–2 days after repeat exposure (delayed IgG-mediated reaction). IgE-mediated (immediate-type) hypersensitivity, including **anaphylaxis,** is less common but important. **Acute liver injury** (cholestatic jaundice or hepatitis) may develop during or shortly after co-amoxiclav treatment, and generally improves if treatment is stopped.
Warnings	The main contraindication is ✖ **severe allergy** to a β-lactam antibiotic. Broad-spectrum penicillins should be avoided in ▲ **young people with a sore throat,** as they can cause a rash with glandular fever that may be mislabelled as penicillin allergy. They should be used with caution in older or hospitalised people at risk of ▲ **C. difficile infection,** and in those with a history of ▲ **penicillin-associated liver injury**. Dosage should be reduced in ▲ **severe renal impairment** (risk of crystalluria).
Important interactions	Reduced renal excretion of ▲ **methotrexate** increases the risk of toxicity. Broad-spectrum penicillins can enhance the anticoagulant effect of **warfarin** by killing normal gut flora that synthesise vitamin K.

PRACTICAL PRESCRIBING

Prescription	For **severe infection,** broad-spectrum penicillins are prescribed for IV administration at a high dose, e.g. amoxicillin 1 g 8-hrly, co-amoxiclav 1.2 g 8-hrly (contains 1 g amoxicillin, 200 mg clavulanic acid). For **mild-to-moderate infection,** broad-spectrum penicillins are prescribed orally at a lower dose, e.g. amoxicillin 250–500 mg 8-hrly, co-amoxiclav 625 mg 8-hrly (500 mg amoxicillin, 125 mg clavulanic acid). Co-amoxiclav doses can either be stated as the amounts of amoxicillin and clavulanic acid separately or together as shown above. Document the indication, review date, and treatment duration on all inpatient antibiotic prescriptions to aid antibiotic stewardship.
Administration	Amoxicillin and co-amoxiclav are available as capsules, tablets, and oral suspensions. Co-amoxiclav suspension may cause dental staining. IV preparations may be given by slow injection or infusion.
Communication	Explain that the aim of treatment is to get rid of infection and improve symptoms. Before prescribing, always check for allergies to any β-lactam antibiotic (including penicillins, **cephalosporins,** and **carbapenems**). Warn them to seek medical advice if a rash or other unexpected symptom develops. If an allergic reaction occurs, give written and verbal advice not to take this antibiotic class in the future and make sure that the reaction (including its nature) is clearly recorded in the notes.
Monitoring and stopping	Check that infection resolves by resolution of symptoms (e.g. cough, dysuria), signs (e.g. pyrexia, lung crackles), and blood markers (e.g. falling CRP and white cell count), as appropriate. Duration of antibiotic therapy is a balance between ensuring effective treatment of infection and minimising adverse reactions and resistance. Always set a stop or review date when prescribing antibiotics, referring to local protocols for guidance. IV antibiotics should usually be switched to oral administration after 48 hours if the patient is improving and is able to take oral medication.
Cost	An IV dose of amoxicillin/co-amoxiclav costs ∼10 times more than an oral dose. Prompt IV-to-oral switch reduces complications and costs of antibiotic treatment and facilitates early discharge.

Clinical tip—When the cause of infection is unknown, broad-spectrum antibiotics are started 'empirically' to cover a wide range of possible organisms. As broad-spectrum antibiotics drive bacterial resistance and antibiotic-associated infections, such as *C. difficile* colitis, limiting their use is important. Refer to a local antimicrobial protocol for guidance on the appropriate use of broad-spectrum antibiotics in empirical treatment. Change from broader to narrower spectrum antibiotics when microbiological test results allow.

Penicillins, narrow-spectrum

CLINICAL PHARMACOLOGY

Common indications	❶ Benzylpenicillin/phenoxymethylpenicillin (penicillin): streptococcal infections, including **tonsillitis, pneumonia,** and **endocarditis;** and meningococcal disease, including **meningitis** (although **cephalosporins** are usually preferred in hospital settings). ❷ Penicillinase-resistant penicillin (flucloxacillin): staphylococcal infections including **skin, soft tissue, bone and joint infections, otitis externa,** and **endocarditis.**
Spectrum of activity	Narrow-spectrum penicillins are active against **Gram-positive organisms** (penicillin—streptococci, bacillus, and some anaerobes (clostridia); flucloxacillin—staphylococci) and **Gram-negative cocci** (penicillin—meningococcus and gonococcus). Narrow-spectrum antibiotics can reduce emergence of antimicrobial resistance, but often need to be combined with other antibiotics for optimal treatment, particularly where the infecting organism has not been identified or infection is severe.
Mechanisms of action	Penicillins **inhibit enzymes responsible for cross-linking peptidoglycans**. This weakens the bacterial cell wall, reducing its ability to maintain an osmotic gradient, causing cell swelling, lysis, and death. Originally isolated from moulds, penicillins comprise a β-lactam ring, responsible for **bactericidal** activity, and a side chain that modifies their properties and antimicrobial spectrum. Some bacteria produce β-lactamase enzymes, which break the β-lactam ring, conferring resistance. Flucloxacillin contains an acyl side chain that protects the β-lactam ring and is effective against β-lactamase-producing staphylococci. Meticillin-resistant *Staphylococcus aureus* (MRSA) resists flucloxacillin by changes in its target enzyme to reduce penicillin-binding affinity. Bacteria can also acquire efflux pumps to reduce intracellular drug concentrations.
Important adverse effects	Minor **GI upset** is common. Penicillin **allergy** affects 1%–10% of people. This is usually IgG-mediated (delayed-type) hypersensitivity, causing **skin rash.** IgE-mediated (immediate-type) hypersensitivity, including **anaphylaxis,** is less common but important. **Neurological toxicity** (including convulsions and coma) can occur at very high doses or in toxic accumulation due to renal failure. Flucloxacillin rarely causes **liver toxicity,** which can be severe.
Warnings	Dose reduction is required in ▲ **severe renal impairment.** The main contraindication is ✖ **allergy** to any penicillin. Note that allergy to one type of penicillin implies allergy to all types as it is due to a reaction to the basic penicillin structure. Severe hypersensitivity to any β-lactam antibiotic generally precludes use of the others.
Important interactions	All penicillins reduce renal excretion of ▲ **methotrexate,** increasing the risk of toxicity.

flucloxacillin, benzylpenicillin, phenoxymethylpenicillin

PRACTICAL PRESCRIBING

Prescription	For **severe infections**, narrow-spectrum penicillins are prescribed for IV administration at high dose (e.g. benzylpenicillin 1.2 g every 4–6 hours, flucloxacillin 1–2 g 6-hrly). As penicillins are rapidly excreted by the kidney and have a short half-life, they need to be administered frequently to maintain therapeutic plasma levels. A prolonged course (e.g. 6 weeks) of high-dose IV antibiotics may be required for deep-seated infections such as osteomyelitis or endocarditis. Phenoxymethylpenicillin (penicillin V, only available orally) should not be used for severe infections as it is less active than benzylpenicillin and GI absorption is unpredictable. For **less severe infections**, flucloxacillin (e.g. 250–500 mg 6-hrly) or phenoxymethylpenicillin (e.g. 500 mg 6-hrly) are prescribed orally. Document the indication, review date, and treatment duration on all inpatient antibiotic prescriptions to aid antibiotic stewardship.
Administration	IV benzylpenicillin and flucloxacillin can be given either as a slow injection or by infusion. Phenoxymethylpenicillin and flucloxacillin are available orally as tablets or capsules and as oral solutions for infants and those with difficulty swallowing.
Communication	Explain that the aim of treatment is to get rid of infection and improve symptoms. Before prescribing, always check for a history of allergy to any β-lactam antibiotic (including penicillins, **cephalosporins,** and **carbapenems**). Warn them to seek medical advice if a rash or other unexpected symptoms develop. If an allergic reaction occurs, give written and verbal advice not to take this antibiotic class in the future and make sure that the reaction (including its nature) is clearly recorded in the notes.
Monitoring and stopping	The duration of antibiotic therapy is a balance between ensuring effective treatment and minimising adverse reactions and resistance. Always set a stop or review date when prescribing antibiotics, referring to local protocols for guidance. IV antibiotics should be switched to oral administration after 48 hours if clinically indicated and the patient is improving (e.g. resolution of pyrexia, tachycardia) and able to take oral medication.
Cost	Cost does not determine choice between narrow-spectrum penicillins.

Clinical tip—Many people say they are 'allergic' to penicillin. Check this is true hypersensitivity, with features of skin rash, bronchospasm or anaphylaxis, rather than a dose-related side effect such as vomiting. A prior anaphylactic reaction to any β-lactam antibiotic is a contraindication to prescription of any other β-lactam antibiotic, whereas these antibiotics can be used in the context of non-immunological intolerance if there is a compelling indication. Discuss this with the patient and consider whether any pre-emptive treatment (e.g. an antiemetic) may be appropriate.

Phosphodiesterase (type 5) inhibitors

CLINICAL PHARMACOLOGY

Common indications	❶ Erectile dysfunction ❷ Primary pulmonary hypertension
Mechanisms of action	A key local mediator in the initiation and maintenance of an erection is **nitric oxide (NO).** This is synthesised in the penis in response to parasympathetic stimulation induced by physical (sexual) stimulation and psychological arousal. NO activates soluble guanylyl cyclase, which produces the second-messenger cyclic guanosine monophosphate (cGMP). This, in turn, activates protein kinase G, which causes vasodilation in penile arteries. The resulting penile engorgement (and its secondary effects on venous outflow) produces an erection. Phosphodiesterase type 5 (PDE-5) degrades cGMP to GMP, terminating its effect. PDE-5 inhibitors therefore **increase cGMP concentration** in the penis, improving the likelihood of achieving an erection and prolonging its duration. PDE-5 is also expressed in pulmonary vasculature, where it causes pulmonary arterial vasodilation by a similar mechanism. PDE-5 inhibitors are therefore also used to treat primary pulmonary hypertension.
Important adverse effects	Most adverse effects of PDE-5 inhibitors are predictable from their vasodilator action. **Headache** is most common, along with **flushing, dizziness,** and **nasal congestion. Hypotension** and **arrhythmias** occur uncommonly and may rarely be associated with **acute coronary syndrome**. Prolonged, painful erection in the absence of stimulation (**priapism**) is a rare adverse effect which requires urgent medical review. **Visual symptoms,** including **colour distortion,** are due to inhibition of PDE type 6 in the retina, where it is involved in phototransduction.
Warnings	PDE-5 inhibitors should not be taken by people in whom vasodilation could be dangerous, including those with ✖ **recent stroke** or ✖ **recent acute coronary syndrome,** or who have ✖ **significant cardiovascular disease**. PDE-5 inhibitors should be avoided or used at a lower dose in people with severe ▲ **hepatic** or ▲ **renal impairment,** due to reduced metabolism and excretion.
Important interactions	Do not prescribe PDE-5 inhibitors for people taking any drug that increases NO concentration, particularly ✖ **nitrates** or ✖ nicorandil, as their combined effects on cGMP (see Mechanisms of action) can cause marked arterial vasodilation and cardiovascular collapse. Caution is also required in people taking other ▲ **vasodilators,** including **α-blockers** (separate from PDE-5 inhibitor doses by at least 4 hours) and **calcium channel blockers**. Plasma concentrations and adverse effects of PDE-5 inhibitors are increased by ▲ **cytochrome P450 inhibitors,** e.g. **amiodarone, diltiazem,** and **fluconazole.**

PRACTICAL PRESCRIBING

Prescription	For **erectile dysfunction,** a typical prescription is for sildenafil 50 mg orally, taken 1 hour before sex, no more than once per day. Sildenafil is available from pharmacies without prescription. Tadalafil has a much longer duration of action than sildenafil (up to 36 hours, versus 4–6 hours), so the timing of administration is less important. Treatment for **pulmonary hypertension** should be started under the direction of a specialist. The licensed dose for this indication is 20 mg three times daily.
Administration	Absorption of oral sildenafil and onset of effect will be delayed if it is taken with food. This does not apply to tadalafil.
Communication	For the treatment of erectile dysfunction, explain that you are prescribing a drug that will help them to have and maintain an erection, but that the drug will not produce an erection without sexual stimulation or arousal. For sildenafil, advise that sildenafil should be taken an hour before sex to allow sufficient time for absorption. Warn him to seek medical advice if the erection does not subside within 2 hours after sexual activity has finished. He should also report significant visual symptoms.
Monitoring and stopping	Enquire about therapeutic efficacy and side effects and adjust dosing or stop treatment as necessary. People with pulmonary hypertension should have regular monitoring with a specialist.
Cost	PDE-5 inhibitors should be prescribed by non-proprietary (generic) name to allow the cheapest product to be dispensed. Branded products (e.g. Viagra®) are expensive. Formulations of sildenafil licensed for use in pulmonary hypertension (which are dosed in multiples of 20 mg, rather than the 25-mg multiples used in erectile dysfunction) are more expensive: a 20-mg tablet of sildenafil is approximately £5 compared to 25 p for a 25-mg tablet.

Clinical tip—Some people take the recreational drug amyl nitrite ('poppers') as an aphrodisiac. Warn that it is very dangerous to do this while there is any sildenafil, tadalafil or vardenafil in their system, as the combination can cause a sudden and severe drop in blood pressure. This is due to the same interaction as with medicinal nitrates (see INTERACTIONS).

Potassium, oral

CLINICAL PHARMACOLOGY

Common indications	Prevention and treatment of **potassium depletion** and **hypokalaemia.** Addition of a drug with potassium-sparing diuretic effects (e.g. an **aldosterone antagonist** or amiloride) is preferred when potassium losses are due to **loop-** or **thiazide-diuretic** therapy. IV potassium chloride is preferred in the initial treatment of hypokalaemia that is severe (<2.5 mmol/L), symptomatic or causing arrhythmias.
Mechanisms of action	Potassium is the predominant cation (positively charged ion) in the intracellular compartment. However, its concentration is measured in serum, and if low this is termed hypokalaemia. Hypokalaemia may be due to potassium depletion (e.g. GI losses) or redistribution (e.g. high-dose β-**agonist** treatment). It has potentially life-threatening effects, particularly in the heart (arrhythmias) and skeletal muscles (weakness). Clinical effects are usually not apparent until the serum potassium falls below 3 mmol/L (normal range 3.5–5.0 mmol/L), unless there is concomitant therapy with **digoxin**. Oral potassium replacement is an option for treatment of hypokalaemia caused by potassium depletion. This is most commonly administered using a combined preparation of potassium bicarbonate and potassium chloride. If losses are due to **loop** or **thiazide diuretic** therapy, supplementation is largely ineffective. This is because although the serum potassium concentration is low, intake and output are in balance. Potassium supplementation results simply in increased potassium excretion and only minimal effect on serum concentration. This can be overcome by starting a potassium-sparing diuretic or **aldosterone antagonist**. Potassium supplementation lacks rationale if hypokalaemia is a result of redistribution, where treatment is best directed at correction of the underlying cause.
Important adverse effects	Oral potassium is unpalatable, which may reduce tolerability. The most important adverse effect is inadvertent **hyperkalaemia**, and for this reason serum potassium should be monitored during treatment (see MONITORING).
Warnings	Potassium supplementation is contraindicated in ✖ **hyperkalaemia** and care must be taken when prescribing for people with, or at risk of, ▲ **renal impairment.**
Important interactions	Particular care should be taken when co-prescribing potassium with ▲ **drugs that increase serum potassium concentration**. These include **angiotensin-converting enzyme (ACE) inhibitors**, **aldosterone antagonists**, **angiotensin receptor blockers**, **heparins**, **NSAIDs,** and potassium-sparing diuretics.

PRACTICAL PRESCRIBING

Prescription	Different preparations contain different amounts of potassium. For example, Sando-K® (potassium chloride with potassium bicarbonate) contains 12 mmol/tablet. A typical prescription might be 1–2 tablets of Sando-K® taken three times a day (total 36–72 mmol/day) for 2–3 days. It is good practice to indicate a stop date and the need to monitor serum potassium concentration in your prescription, to mitigate the risk of rebound hyperkalaemia. Where there are ongoing losses, continuing treatment may be required. Often this will be at a lower dose than that required to replace the initial deficit. Seek advice, as this prescription will need to be individualised.
Administration	Effervescent tablets (e.g. Sando-K®) are stirred in about half a glassful of water for administration. Some people find it easier to take with food.
Communication	Advise that you are prescribing a treatment to replace the low level of potassium, which can have serious complications if not treated. Explain the need for careful monitoring of their potassium levels during treatment. Advise them to seek medical advice if they develop side effects such as weakness, dizziness or palpitations as these may be a sign of a high potassium level.
Monitoring and stopping	Monitor potassium levels daily when treating hypokalaemia and adjust the dose as necessary. Once the serum potassium concentration is normal and the cause of potassium loss has resolved, treatment can be stopped. In the unusual circumstances of ongoing losses requiring continued treatment, less frequent monitoring is possible once a stable dose is achieved. This should be directed by an expert.
Cost	Potassium replacement is inexpensive, at around 10p per tablet of Sando-K®. Modified-release tablets are more expensive at around 70p a tablet.

Clinical tip—Always check the serum magnesium concentration when treating hypokalaemia. If you find hypomagnesaemia, it is important to treat this (e.g. magnesium sulfate 2 g in 50 mL sodium chloride 0.9% over 4 hours, then check response). This is because in low magnesium states, renal losses of potassium increase, making treatment of hypokalaemia more difficult. The mechanism by which this happens is not well understood.

Prostaglandin analogue and carbonic anhydrase inhibitor eye drops

CLINICAL PHARMACOLOGY

Common indications	Topical prostaglandin analogues are the first-line choice to lower intraocular pressure in **open-angle glaucoma** and **ocular hypertension.** Prostaglandin analogues are generally preferred over topical β-blockers as they cause fewer systemic side effects. Topical carbonic anhydrase inhibitors are second-line options, if topical prostaglandin analogues are not tolerated or insufficient.
Mechanisms of action	Glaucoma is characterised by progressive optic nerve damage associated with visual field loss and eventually blindness. It is usually associated with elevated intraocular pressure (ocular hypertension), and lowering intraocular pressure reduces glaucoma progression. Intraocular pressure is determined by the balance of aqueous humour production from ciliary processes, and outflow via the trabecular ('conventional') and uveoscleral ('non-conventional') pathways. **Prostaglandin F$_{2\alpha}$** analogues act via prostaglandin receptors to increase expression of matrix metalloproteinases, reducing resistance to aqueous humour outflow, primarily in the uveoscleral pathway. In contrast, **carbonic anhydrase inhibitors** reduce aqueous humour production. By inhibiting bicarbonate formation, they interfere with Na^+ transport across the ciliary epithelium and, in turn, the flow of water by osmosis.
Important adverse effects	Topical prostaglandin analogues and carbonic anhydrase inhibitors have few systemic side effects. Locally, they commonly cause **eye discomfort** immediately after administration, and **blurred vision.** Prostaglandin analogues also cause transient **conjunctival reddening (hyperaemia)** and may cause a **permanent change in eye colour** by increasing the amount of melanin in stromal melanocytes of the iris. This affects about a third of people and is most noticeable if treatment is restricted to one eye.
Warnings	Caution is needed when contemplating prostaglandin analogue treatment in eyes in which the lens is absent (▲ **aphakia**) or artificial (▲ **pseudophakia**); and in people with or at risk of ▲ **iritis, uveitis, or macular oedema.** In **severe asthma,** there is a theoretical risk of provoking bronchoconstriction, but in practice this does not seem to be a problem. It is certainly less of a concern than with topical β-blockers.
Important interactions	There are no clinically important adverse drug interactions with topical prostaglandin analogues. Systemic absorption of topical carbonic anhydrase inhibitors generates a risk of interactions, but these are not usually problematic.

latanoprost (prostaglandin analogue)
brinzolamide (carbonic anhydrase inhibitor)

PRACTICAL PRESCRIBING

Prescription	The decision to offer pharmacological treatment in **ocular hypertension** is made by a specialist, taking into account factors such as age, intraocular pressure, and central corneal thickness. Those with confirmed **open-angle glaucoma** should be offered pharmacological treatment, again by a specialist. Usually this is with latanoprost 0.005% eye drop solution, 1 drop administered to the affected eye(s) once daily. The starting dose of brinzolamide is 1 drop twice daily.
Administration	It is best to administer latanoprost eye drops in the evening. Contact lenses should be removed before instilling prostaglandin analogue or carbonic anhydrase inhibitor eye drops. They may be reinserted 15 minutes later.
Communication	Explain that the aim of treatment is to reduce the risk of sight loss. Advise on how to administer the eye drops correctly. When prescribing topical prostaglandins, warn about the possibility of a change in eye colour. This advice may be tailored to the individual, since it is most likely in those with mixed-colour irides (i.e. brown plus another colour), and very rare in those with a homogenous eye colour ('pure' blue, grey, green, or brown). Explain that colour change is usually only slight and is not harmful, but if it occurs it is likely to be permanent.
Monitoring and stopping	Monitoring should be by regular review with a clinician experienced in managing glaucoma. The intensity of follow-up and dose adjustment depends on intraocular pressure and risk of conversion from ocular hypertension to glaucoma.
Cost	The generic forms of latanoprost are substantially less expensive than branded products.

Clinical tip—Advice that may be given for all eye drops is that it is helpful to gently compress the medial canthus (the nasal 'corner') of the eye for about 1 minute, immediately after instilling the drop. This reduces drainage through the lacrimal duct, lowering systemic absorption of the drug.

Prostaglandins and analogues

CLINICAL PHARMACOLOGY

Common indications	❶ **Induction of labour** (dinoprostone); **oxytocin** is a second-line option. ❷ **Erectile dysfunction** (alprostadil), although it is largely superseded by **sildenafil** for this indication. ❸ **Medical termination of pregnancy** (misoprostol). ❹ As a vasodilator in **pulmonary hypertension** and **peripheral vascular disease** causing debilitating pain or ischaemia (iloprost).
Mechanisms of action	Prostaglandins are a family of **lipid autacoids** ('local messengers') synthesised from arachidonic acid. They are produced by all cells, but the relative importance of each one varies between tissues. **Prostaglandin (PG) E$_2$** (dinoprostone) is synthesised by the uterine mucosa (decidua) and cells lining the amniotic sac during pregnancy. It stimulates uterine contraction and acts on collagenase enzymes that thin and soften the cervix, facilitating cervical effacement. It plays a key role in the initiation of labour, and this is exploited therapeutically to induce labour. **PGE$_1$** (alprostadil, and its synthetic analogue misoprostol) is produced in vascular smooth muscle, where it stimulates cAMP production, causing muscle relaxation and vasodilation. Applied locally to the penis, alprostadil induces erection, and so is an option for the treatment of erectile dysfunction. Misoprostol may be administered systemically or vaginally to simulate uterine contraction. It is used in combination with the antiprogestogen mifepristone for medical termination of pregnancy. Iloprost is a synthetic analogue of **prostacyclin (PGI$_2$)** that has vasodilatory effects by relaxing smooth muscle. This is useful in pulmonary hypertension and peripheral vascular disease.
Important adverse effects	Dinoprostone may cause **uterine hyperstimulation** that can be harmful to the fetus and increase the risk of uterine rupture. Alprostadil may cause prolonged painful erections **(priapism)** that can lead to tissue ischaemia. Iloprost may cause problematic **hypotension** when given systemically. Prostaglandins may cause nausea and vomiting from stimulation of gastro-intestinal smooth muscle.
Warnings	Induction of labour with dinoprostone should not be attempted if there are ✖ **risk factors for difficult delivery** (e.g. fetal malposition, placenta praevia, previous difficult delivery) or fetal or maternal complications (e.g. fetal distress, previous caesarean section or major uterine surgery). In general, due to their vasodilating effects, prostaglandins should be used with caution in people with ▲ **severe cardiac disease**. Iloprost should be avoided in people with a significant ▲ **bleeding risk.**
Important interactions	Dinoprostone has a synergistic effect with ▲ **oxytocin** and so appropriate monitoring must be in place to pick up adverse effects (including to the fetus). Iloprost may impair platelet function and so should be used with caution with other drugs that can cause bleeding such as ▲ **direct oral anticoagulants** and ▲ **warfarin.**

PRACTICAL PRESCRIBING

Prescription	Dinoprostone is administered as a gel, pessary or vaginal tablet (dose 1–3 mg). It may be repeated after 6 hours. If a pessary is used, it must be removed after adequate cervical effacement (or prior to starting **oxytocin**). Alprostadil is prescribed for urethral application with a maximum frequency of 7 doses per week and/or 2 doses per day. Misoprostol and iloprost are used in specialist practice only; consult local protocols and seek expert advice for details.
Administration	Dinoprostone is usually administered by a midwife or doctor to ensure correct placement in the posterior fornix. Alprostadil is most conveniently administered into the urethra using cream from a pre-filled syringe, or a urethral stick that delivers a medicated pellet. Misoprostol may be taken at home, usually as a sublingual or buccal preparation. Iloprost administration, as an IV infusion or by nebuliser, is complex, and given under specialist direction only.
Communication	For dinoprostone, explain that the drug will help to soften the cervix and stimulate labour to begin. If the woman is going to go home, explain the symptoms of labour and advise on when to re-attend. For alprostadil, explain that the drug will stimulate an erection and should be administered around 15–30 minutes before sex. Explain how to administer the medicine (which varies according to the product) and signpost the written instructions in the Patient Information Leaflet. Advise that medical attention should be sought if the erection lasts more than 4 hours. For misoprostol, explain that the drug will stimulate uterine contraction, which will cause some abdominal pain (cramps). Bleeding (spotting to clots) will occur and may continue until the next period, which itself may be unpredictable. Advise on the need to report excessive bleeding. If symptoms of pregnancy continue, a pregnancy test can be repeated 3 weeks after therapy is taken (any earlier and residual hormones may cause a false positive).
Monitoring and stopping	Appropriate monitoring of the mother and fetus should be in place to ensure safe onset of labour for dinoprostone. The benefits and side effect of alprostadil are ascertained by symptom enquiry.
Cost	The drug costs for dinoprostone and misoprostol generally represent a small fraction of the cost of the treatment pathway. Alprostadil is available only in proprietary products with an applicator device and is more expensive than generic sildenafil tablets. Iloprost is expensive.

Clinical tip—NSAIDs work by inhibiting cyclooxygenases (and therefore the production of prostaglandins), and gastric ulceration is an important adverse effect. From this, you can deduce that prostaglandins may be used to provide gastroprotection. While **proton pump inhibitors** are preferred, misoprostol is an alternative for people who cannot tolerate PPIs.

Proton pump inhibitors

CLINICAL PHARMACOLOGY

Common indications	❶ Prevention and treatment of **peptic ulcer disease,** including NSAID-associated ulcers. ❷ Treatment of **gastro-oesophageal reflux disease** (GORD) and **dyspepsia,** including in the management of Barrett's oesophagus. ❸ Eradication of *Helicobacter pylori* **infection,** for which they are used in combination with antibiotic therapy.
Mechanisms of action	Proton pump inhibitors (PPIs) reduce gastric acid secretion. They act by **irreversibly inhibiting H⁺/K⁺-ATPase in gastric parietal cells.** This is the 'proton pump' responsible for secreting H⁺ and generating gastric acid. An advantage of targeting the final stage of the process is that they suppress gastric acid production almost completely. They differ in this respect to **H₂-receptor antagonists.** In Barrett's oesophagus, acid-suppressive therapy may prevent progression to cancer as well as treating reflux symptoms.
Important adverse effects	Common side effects of PPIs include **GI upset** and **headache.** By increasing the gastric pH, PPIs may reduce one of the body's defences against infection, and in this respect there is some evidence that they increase the risk of *Clostridioides difficile* colitis. Prolonged treatment with PPIs can cause **hypomagnesaemia** which, if severe, can lead to neuromuscular symptoms (including tetany in extreme cases) and arrhythmias.
Warnings	PPIs may **mask symptoms** of gastric or oesophageal cancer and significant ulcer disease caused by *H. pylori,* so prescribers should enquire about 'alarm symptoms' before and during treatment (see COMMUNICATION). There is epidemiological evidence that PPIs, particularly at high dose for prolonged courses in older people, can increase the risk of fracture. People with or at risk of ▲ **osteoporosis** should therefore be identified and treated as appropriate.
Important interactions	Historically, there has been concern that PPIs, particularly omeprazole, may reduce the antiplatelet effect of ▲ **clopidogrel** by decreasing its activation by cytochrome P450 enzymes. This has not been borne out in large-scale clinical trials or systematic reviews. However, as a precaution, the Medicines and Healthcare Products Regulatory Agency (MHRA) continues to recommend against concomitant use of clopidogrel with omeprazole. Other PPIs may be co-prescribed with clopidogrel if indicated.

PRACTICAL PRESCRIBING

Prescription	The route and dose of PPI depends on the drug and indication. A typical prescription, for example for prevention of NSAID-associated peptic ulcers, would be lansoprazole 30 mg orally daily. Combination treatment for *H. pylori* eradication is more complex, but options are helpfully summarised in the BNF.
Administration	Oral PPIs are best taken in the morning, with or without food. IV preparations are given by slow injection or infusion.
Communication	Explain that you are offering treatment to reduce stomach acid production. This will hopefully improve symptoms and, if applicable, allow their ulcer to heal. Ensure that the intended duration of therapy has been made clear (e.g. a 7-day course to eradicate *H. pylori,* or long-term therapy to protect against ulcers) and how success will be judged (e.g. evidence of healing on endoscopy, or simply by resolution of symptoms). Ask them to report any problems, particularly 'alarm' symptoms (weight loss, swallowing difficulty, vomiting blood, altered blood in the stool).
Monitoring and stopping	Offer testing for *H. pylori* when symptoms of GORD, dyspepsia or peptic ulcer disease are reported (and endoscopy if there are 'alarm' symptoms). Where treatment is offered empirically (without investigation of cause), a maximum 4-week trial of treatment is recommended. Investigations should be carried out if symptoms persist after cessation of this trial, or if any 'alarm' symptoms arise. Acid-suppressive therapy may be stopped following treatment for some indications (e.g. eradication of *H. pylori* or treatment of NSAID-associated ulcer) but may need to be continued in others (e.g. Barrett's oesophagitis with ongoing reflux symptoms). For symptomatic treatment of dyspepsia and GORD, symptoms are the best guide to the effect of therapy and should be reviewed annually. If these have improved, it may be possible to step-down therapy to an **alginate** or **antacid**, taken as required. In prolonged use (>1 year) check serum magnesium levels due to the risk of hypomagnesaemia. When withdrawing prolonged therapy, reduce the dose and/ or frequency over a few weeks to avoid a rebound of symptoms. **Alginates** and **antacids** can be useful to control symptoms during this period.
Cost	Relatively inexpensive non-proprietary formulations are available and should be preferred in most cases.

Clinical tip—When undergoing investigation for *H. pylori* infection, PPIs should preferably be withheld for 2 weeks before testing. This is because they increase the chance of a false-negative result. This applies to all *H. pylori* tests.

Quinine

CLINICAL PHARMACOLOGY

Common indications	❶ Quinine is an option for nocturnal **leg cramps,** but only if these are severe, impacting on quality of life (e.g. regularly disrupt sleep) and refractory to non-pharmacological methods such as passive stretching exercises. It is likely that many quinine prescriptions for this indication are inappropriate. ❷ A first-line treatment option for *Plasmodium falciparum* **malaria.**
Mechanisms of action	**Leg cramps** are caused by sudden, painful involuntary contraction of skeletal muscle. Quinine is thought to act by reducing the excitability of the motor end plate in response to acetylcholine stimulation. This reduces the frequency of muscle contraction. In **malaria,** quinine interferes with detoxification of haem monomers, which are produced from digestion of haemoglobin within the malarial parasite. The monomers accumulate, impairing membrane integrity and killing the parasites in the schizont stage. In contrast to other antimalarials, *P. falciparum* resistance to quinine is uncommon.
Important adverse effects	Although quinine is usually safe at recommended doses, it is potentially very toxic and can be fatal in overdose. It can cause **tinnitus, deafness** and **blindness** (which may be permanent), **GI upset,** and **hypersensitivity** reactions. Quinine **prolongs the QT interval** and may therefore predispose to arrhythmias, particularly after administration of IV loading doses. **Hypoglycaemia,** caused by stimulation of insulin secretion, can occur and is particularly problematic in malaria, since this condition also predisposes to hypoglycaemia.
Warnings	Quinine should be prescribed with caution in people with existing ▲ **hearing or visual loss.** It is teratogenic, so should not be used in the ▲ **first trimester** of pregnancy, although in the case of malaria its benefit may outweigh this risk. Quinine should be avoided in people with ▲ **glucose-6-phosphate dehydrogenase (G6PD) deficiency,** in whom it may precipitate haemolysis.
Important interactions	Quinine should be prescribed with caution in people taking other ▲ **drugs that prolong the QT interval** or cause arrhythmias such as **amiodarone, antipsychotics, quinolones, macrolides,** and **selective serotonin reuptake inhibitors**.

PRACTICAL PRESCRIBING

Prescription	If indicated for nocturnal **leg cramps,** quinine should be prescribed at a dose of 200–300 mg orally nightly, for a 4-week trial (see MONITORING). In the treatment of **malaria,** higher doses of quinine are required and should be initiated under specialist direction. Quinine may be prescribed for oral administration in uncomplicated malaria (alongside another antimalarial medication such as **doxycycline**). Alternatively, in severe cases it may be prescribed for IV administration, although this requires use of a 'special-order' (unlicensed) product. IV doses are based on body weight.
Administration	Oral quinine for **leg cramps** should be taken in the evening. For **malaria**, oral quinine doses should be taken at 8-hrly intervals. IV quinine is given by slow infusion.
Communication	For nocturnal **leg cramps,** explain that you are recommending a 4-week trial of quinine in the hope of reducing the frequency of cramps. Explain that if there is no improvement after 4 weeks, they are unlikely to experience any benefit and should stop taking it. Ask them to report any adverse effects, such as hearing loss, visual disturbance, and palpitations immediately, as quinine is potentially harmful to the ears, eyes and heart.
Monitoring and stopping	In the treatment of **leg cramps,** review symptoms after 4 weeks and stop quinine if there has not been a significant improvement. If continued treatment is indicated, review again at 3 months and consider a trial discontinuation at that stage. Aim to avoid long-term use due to the potential for serious adverse effects. It is likely that many prescriptions for quinine are inappropriate due to its poor risk–benefit balance. If you encounter a patient on long-term quinine therapy, take the opportunity to discuss the value of a trial of discontinuation. Monitoring and duration of therapy for **malaria** should be guided by specialists.
Cost	Oral quinine sulfate is available in non-proprietary formulations and is relatively inexpensive. Other formulations (including solutions for IV infusion) are purchased from special-order manufacturers and may be expensive.

Clinical tip—Although quinine is commonly prescribed for people with nocturnal leg cramps, its benefit is modest, reducing the frequency of cramps only by around 20%, and its toxicity may be significant. Before starting treatment, you should first exclude reversible causes, such as electrolyte disturbances and side effects from other drugs (e.g. **statins**, β_2-**agonists**) and encourage non-pharmacological treatments such as passive stretching exercises. Correction of vitamin and mineral deficiencies, including B vitamins and iron respectively, may also be beneficial.

Quinolones

CLINICAL PHARMACOLOGY

Common indications	Systemically administered quinolones are best reserved for severe bacterial infections in which other treatment options are limited. With these caveats in mind, they are used in: ❶ **Urinary tract infection (UTI)** (mostly Gram-negative organisms). ❷ **Severe gastroenteritis** (e.g. due to *Shigella*, *Campylobacter*). ❸ Lower respiratory tract infections, including **infective exacerbation of COPD** and **pneumonia** (Gram-positive and Gram-negative organisms).
Spectrum of activity	Quinolones have a relatively **broad spectrum** of activity, particularly against Gram-negative bacteria. Ciprofloxacin is unusual among oral antibiotics in having significant activity against *Pseudomonas aeruginosa*. Moxifloxacin and levofloxacin have enhanced activity against Gram-positive organisms (so are preferred over ciprofloxacin for treatment of lower respiratory tract infections.
Mechanisms of action	Quinolones kill bacteria **(bactericidal effect)** by **inhibiting DNA synthesis.** However, resistance is problematic. Some bacteria prevent intracellular accumulation of the drug by reducing permeability and/or increasing efflux. Others develop protective mutations in target enzymes. Quinolone resistance genes are spread horizontally between bacteria by plasmids, accelerating acquisition of resistance.
Important adverse effects	Quinolones are generally well tolerated although they can cause **GI upset** and immediate- and delayed-type **hypersensitivity** reactions (see **Penicillins, broad-spectrum**). Quinolones and **cephalosporins** are the antibiotics most commonly associated with ***Clostridioides difficile* colitis**. Class-specific adverse reactions may be **neurological** (convulsions, peripheral neuropathy), **musculoskeletal** (tendon damage and rupture) or **cardiovascular** (QT interval prolongation, valvular regurgitation, and aortic aneurysm/dissection). Although rare, these may be disabling and long-lasting or irreversible.
Warnings	A careful risk–benefit assessment and consideration of other options are required before prescribing quinolones. They should be used with caution in ▲ **pregnancy** and in ▲ **children and young adults** who are growing (risk of arthropathy); ▲ **adults >60 years** (risk of tendon damage); people with ▲ **renal impairment**; and people with or at risk of ▲ **neurological** or ▲ **cardiovascular** morbidity.
Important interactions	Drugs containing divalent cations (e.g. **calcium**, **iron**, **antacids**) reduce absorption and efficacy of quinolones. Ciprofloxacin inhibits certain cytochrome P450 (CYP) enzymes, increasing risk of toxicity from some drugs, notably ▲ **theophylline**. Co-prescription of ▲ **NSAIDs** increases the risk of **seizures**, and ▲ **prednisolone** increases the risk of **tendon rupture.** Caution is required in people taking other ▲ **drugs that prolong the QT interval** or that cause arrhythmias, such as **amiodarone**, **antipsychotics**, **quinine**, **macrolide antibiotics,** and **SSRIs.**

PRACTICAL PRESCRIBING

Prescription	Quinolones are rapidly and extensively absorbed from the intestine, so high plasma concentrations can be achieved by oral administration. Intravenous prescription should therefore be reserved for people unable to take drugs orally or absorb them from the GI tract (see also COST). They are eliminated by the kidney and have relatively long plasma half-lives, so are administered every 12–24 hours. Typical dosages are ciprofloxacin 250–750 mg orally 12-hrly or 400 mg IV 12-hrly; levofloxacin 500 mg oral/IV daily; and moxifloxacin 400 mg oral/IV daily.
Administration	Oral quinolones are available as tablets, with ciprofloxacin also being formulated as a (more expensive) oral suspension. IV quinolones come pre-prepared in solution for infusion, usually over 60 minutes.
Communication	Explain that these are effective antibiotics. However, they have important potential side effects, affecting the tendons, muscles, joints, and nerves, so they are offered only when other options are limited. Advise them to look out for pain or swelling, changes in sensation (touch, vision, hearing, taste, and smell) or mood. If any of these develop, they should stop taking the antibiotic and contact a doctor immediately for advice. Advise that ciprofloxacin should not be taken with dairy products. It must be separated from calcium/iron supplements and antacids by at least 2 hours, as these interfere with absorption, making the antibiotic less effective.
Monitoring and stopping	Check that infection resolves by resolution of symptoms, signs (e.g. pyrexia, lung crackles) and blood markers (e.g. falling CRP and white cell count) as appropriate. Duration of antibiotic therapy is a balance between ensuring effective treatment and minimising adverse reactions and resistance. Always set a stop or review date when prescribing antibiotics, referring to local protocols for guidance.
Cost	Switch IV quinolone prescriptions to oral as soon as possible. This is good practice as it reduces the cost of the drug (oral quinolone preparations cost around 20 times less than IV quinolone preparations), as well as reducing administration costs, treatment complications and duration of inpatient stay.

Clinical tip—Quinolones can be prescribed for topical administration as eye and ear drops for superficial bacterial infections, and by inhalation of nebulised solution (levofloxacin) to control chronic pulmonary infections due to *Pseudomonas aeruginosa* in cystic fibrosis. As systemic absorption can occur, there is still a risk of adverse reactions and drug interactions with topical quinolones, particularly where high doses are given by nebulisation. Patients starting inhaled therapy should be given the same advice about adverse reactions as those taking systemic treatment.

Serotonin 5-HT₁-receptor agonists (triptans)

CLINICAL PHARMACOLOGY

Common indications	In **acute migraine** with or without aura, serotonin 5-HT$_1$-receptor agonists, often referred to as 'triptans', are used to reduce the duration and severity of symptoms. **Paracetamol** and **NSAIDs** are alternative options and may be combined with triptans.
Mechanisms of action	Serotonin 5-HT$_1$-receptor agonists relieve the symptoms of acute migraine, including headache and nausea. Although the mechanisms underlying migraine are not completely understood, the primary disturbance is thought to be a slowly propagating wave of cortical depolarisation (cortical spreading depression). This is associated with local vasoconstriction and, depending on the area of the brain affected, may cause early focal neurological symptoms (aura). Subsequently, activation of trigeminal nerve afferents that innervate cerebral blood vessels and the meninges (the trigeminovascular pathway) causes release of vasoactive peptides such as calcitonin gene-related peptide (CGRP). This, in turn, simulates neurogenic inflammation and dilation of cranial blood vessels, causing headache and other symptoms of acute migraine. Triptans are thought to act by **inhibiting neurotransmission** in the peripheral trigeminal nerve and in the trigeminocervical complex (via 5-HT$_{1B}$ and 5-HT$_{1D}$ receptors) and **constricting cranial blood vessels** (via 5-HT$_{1B}$ receptors).
Important adverse effects	Common adverse effects of triptans include **chest and throat discomfort**, which can be intense but resolves quickly. Rarely, triptans can cause **angina** and **myocardial infarction** due to coronary vasospasm. Other common adverse effects include nausea and vomiting, tiredness, dizziness, and transient high blood pressure. In general, adverse effects are more common with SC administration of sumatriptan than with other drugs by other routes.
Warnings	Due to their vasoconstrictor properties these drugs should not be used in ✖ **ischaemic heart disease**, ✖ **cerebrovascular disease**, ✖ **peripheral vascular disease**, and ✖ **uncontrolled hypertension**. Triptans should also not be used in ✖ **hemiplegic migraine** or ✖ **migraine with brainstem aura** (e.g. with vertigo or diplopia).
Important interactions	Triptans may increase the risk of **serotonin toxicity** and **serotonin syndrome** when given in combination with other **serotonergic drugs**, such as ✖ monoamine oxidase inhibitors, ▲ **tramadol**, ▲ **selective serotonin reuptake inhibitors,** and ▲ **tricyclic antidepressants**.

PRACTICAL PRESCRIBING

Prescription	The usual dose of sumatriptan for the treatment of migraine is 50–100 mg orally, repeated if the migraine recurs (but not if it failed to respond to the initial dose). Small (2-tablet) packs of sumatriptan can be purchased over the counter from pharmacies by patients with confirmed migraine. Intranasal or SC formulations (which require prescription) may be useful alternatives if vomiting precludes oral treatment.
Administration	Tablets should be swallowed whole with water. To use the nasal spray, they should first blow their nose if it is blocked. Then they should insert the nozzle into a nostril, block the other nostril with their finger, and push the plunger as they breathe in through the nose.
Communication	Explain that you are recommending a treatment they can use to shorten the duration and intensity of migraines. Advise that it is more effective if given early in the attack, so they should take the treatment as soon as they feel the migraine coming on, ideally within 6 hours of onset of a moderate-to-severe headache. Explain that it can be taken in combination with **paracetamol** and/or an **NSAID** such as ibuprofen. Explain the treatment only works when a migraine has started and advise them not to take it to prevent an attack. Explain the main side effects, particularly that they may feel heaviness or pressure in the chest or throat which should pass quickly. If it does not, or if it is severe, they should seek medical help as there is a very small risk of heart attack. Encourage them to seek further advice if they are having frequent migraines—four or more attacks a month—as they may then benefit from preventative treatments (see CLINICAL TIP).
Monitoring and stopping	Schedule a follow-up appointment to check if the treatment is effective. The interval will depend on the frequency of attacks, and therefore the opportunity to test the treatment's effect. Triptans work in around two-thirds of people, and if one triptan is ineffective, it may still be worth trying another. Where triptans are not effective, they should be stopped. Always consider alternative causes of headache (including medication-overuse headache) if treatment is ineffective.
Cost	Triptans are available in inexpensive non-proprietary formulations, but also as expensive branded products. Therefore, unless a particular formulation is needed, prescribe generically to allow the least expensive product to be dispensed.

Clinical tip—Preventative treatment for migraine should be considered for people who have four or more attacks per month, particularly if they are impacting quality of life. The first-line options are propranolol (a β-blocker), amitriptyline (a **tricyclic antidepressant**), and antiepileptic agents topiramate and **valproate**. **Monoclonal antibodies** that target CGRP (e.g. galcanezumab) or its receptor (e.g. erenumab) are alternatives if first-line agents are ineffective or not tolerated, but only under specialist direction.

Sodium–glucose co-transporter 2 inhibitors

CLINICAL PHARMACOLOGY

Common indications	❶ **Type 2 diabetes,** usually in combination with other antidiabetic drugs (e.g. **metformin, insulin**), but also as an option for monotherapy if metformin is not tolerated. ❷ Symptomatic chronic **heart failure with reduced ejection fraction,** inadequately controlled with a **β-blocker, ACE inhibitor/ angiotensin receptor blocker**, and an **aldosterone antagonist**. ❸ **Chronic kidney disease (CKD) with albuminuria,** alongside an **ACE inhibitor/angiotensin receptor blocker**.
Mechanisms of action	These drugs selectively and reversibly **inhibit** the **sodium–glucose co-transporter 2 (SGLT2)** in the proximal convoluted tubule of the nephron. SGLT2 mediates active transport of glucose and sodium from filtrate into blood, controlling sodium content of the filtrate and, under physiological conditions, recovering most of the filtered glucose. SGLT2 inhibition impairs glucose reabsorption in the nephron, increasing renal excretion of glucose (glycosuria) and treating hyperglycaemia. Additionally, by increasing renal sodium excretion (natriuresis) and water excretion (osmotic diuresis), SGLT2 inhibitors reduce extracellular water volume, blood pressure, and cardiac preload. Increased sodium delivery to the macula densa (in the wall of the distal tubule) triggers tubuloglomerular feedback mechanisms that reduce intra-glomerular pressure. Together, these actions have favourable effects on renal and cardiovascular outcomes in type 2 diabetes, heart failure, and CKD.
Important adverse effects	As the effect of SGLT2 inhibitors diminishes at lower serum glucose concentrations, they **rarely cause hypoglycaemia**, although they may exacerbate hypoglycaemia due to other glucose-lowering drugs. Osmotic diuresis can cause **thirst** and, in the context of intercurrent illness, increase the risk of **hypovolaemia** and **electrolyte disturbance**. Glycosuria increases the risk of **genital and urinary tract infections**, and, rarely, **Fournier's gangrene** (acute necrotic infection of the perineum). SGLT2 inhibitors have been associated with ketoacidosis with a near-normal glucose concentration (**euglycaemic diabetic ketoacidosis**). This is rare in type 2 diabetes, but common if the drugs are used in type 1 diabetes (which is not recommended).
Warnings	SGLT2 inhibitors should be withheld during ▲ **intercurrent illness** that causes or presents a risk of ✖ **volume depletion or hypotension.**
Important interactions	SGLT2 inhibitors augment the effects of **other glucose-lowering drugs** (insulin, sulphonylureas, etc), with both therapeutic benefit and increased risk of hypoglycaemia; ▲ **blood pressure-lowering drugs,** with increased risk of hypotension; and ▲ **diuretics,** with increased risk of volume depletion.

PRACTICAL PRESCRIBING

Prescription	For most indications, a typical starting dose for canagliflozin is 100 mg orally once daily, and for dapagliflozin is 10 mg orally daily. If an SGLT2 inhibitor is started for a reason other than glycaemic control (i.e. for heart failure or CKD), their other antihyperglycaemic treatment may need to be adjusted to accommodate its glucose-lowering effect.
Administration	Canagliflozin and dapagliflozin are formulated as tablets which are swallowed with water. They can be taken with or without food, and at any time of day, though this should be the same time each day.
Communication	As appropriate for the indication, explain the reason for starting the medicine. Explain that it acts by increasing the amount of sugar passed in the urine, which in turn increases the amount of water. This is helpful in diabetes, heart failure, and kidney disease, but it does also increase the risk of urine and genital infections. Advise them to look out for symptoms such as vaginal discharge, burning sensation when passing water or fever and to consult a doctor or pharmacist if these occur. Explain that as it will cause them to pass more water than normal, this may make them thirsty. They can manage this simply with increased water intake (*not* sugary drinks!). However, if it is severe, or if they feel faint, dehydrated or develop an illness that makes it more difficult for them to keep hydrated, they should stop taking the medicine and seek urgent medical advice.
Monitoring and stopping	Renal function should be checked before initiation of treatment and then at least once a year. More frequent monitoring is needed in CKD. If an intercurrent illness develops, particularly if severe enough to require hospital admission, you should assess volume status carefully, and temporarily stop treatment if there is dehydration, hypovolaemia or hypotension (or a risk of these developing). Treatment with SGLT2 inhibitors is usually indefinite, if tolerated.
Cost	While they remain under patent protection, SGLT2 inhibitors are costly relative to other medicines used for the same indications. However, health economic evaluation suggests they are cost-effective if used in accordance with national guidelines.

Clinical tip—As SGLT2 inhibitors work by promoting glycosuria, people taking these drugs will almost inevitably have positive urinalysis ('dipstick test') for glucose, even if their serum glucose concentration is normal. This is expected and should not cause alarm. However, if they have urinary ketones, you should be concerned about the risk of euglycaemic diabetic ketoacidosis. Withhold the drug, check acid–base status (e.g. by arterial or venous blood gas analysis) and seek expert advice.

Statins

CLINICAL PHARMACOLOGY

Common indications	**❶ Primary prevention of major adverse cardiovascular events** (e.g. myocardial infarction, stroke) in people over 40 years of age with a 10-year cardiovascular risk >10%, as assessed using a validated tool. **❷ Secondary prevention of major adverse cardiovascular events** in people with ischaemic heart disease (including after acute coronary syndrome), stroke, and peripheral vascular disease. **❸ Dyslipidaemia** (e.g. primary hypercholesterolaemia, mixed dyslipidaemia, familial hypercholesterolaemia).
Mechanisms of action	Statins slow the atherosclerotic process and may even reverse it. They act by competitive **inhibition** of **3-hydroxy-3-methyl-glutaryl coenzyme A (HMG CoA) reductase,** the enzyme that catalyses the rate-limiting step in cholesterol synthesis. This reduces cholesterol production by the liver and stimulates a compensatory increase in low-density lipoprotein (LDL) cholesterol uptake from the blood by hepatocytes. Together, these effects reduce LDL cholesterol levels and also, indirectly, reduce triglycerides and slightly increase high-density lipoprotein (HDL) cholesterol levels. In addition to their lipid-lowering effects, statins may modulate the inflammatory response and improve endothelial function. These effects may be due to reduced production of isoprenoid intermediates in the cholesterol synthesis pathway, which are substrates in the production of various cell-signalling proteins.
Important adverse effects	Statins are generally safe and well tolerated. The most common adverse effects are **headache, GI upset,** and **muscle aches.** Rare but more serious adverse effects are **myopathy** and **rhabdomyolysis.** Statins can cause a **rise in liver enzymes** (e.g. alanine transaminase). Minor biochemical changes are clinically unimportant (see MONITORING), but **drug-induced hepatitis** is a rare but serious adverse effect.
Warnings	Statins should be used with caution in ▲ **hepatic impairment.** With the exception of rosuvastatin, statins are dependent on the kidneys for elimination of their metabolites, so the dose should be reduced in ▲ **renal impairment.** Statins are contraindicated for women who are ▲ **pregnant** (cholesterol is essential for normal fetal development) and should be avoided in ▲ **breastfeeding.**
Important interactions	The metabolism of statins (other than rosuvastatin) is impaired by ▲ **cytochrome P450 (CYP) inhibitors,** such as **amiodarone, diltiazem, itraconazole, macrolides, protease inhibitors,** and grapefruit juice. This leads to accumulation of the statin and/or its metabolites, which may increase the risk of adverse effects. ▲ **Amlodipine** has a similar interaction, although the mechanism is less clear. Dosage reduction of the statin may be necessary. If the CYP inhibitor is being used for a short period only (e.g. clarithromycin for an acute infection), temporarily withhold the statin.

atorvastatin, simvastatin, rosuvastatin, pravastatin

PRACTICAL PRESCRIBING

Prescription	For **primary prevention** of cardiovascular disease, a typical starting prescription is for simvastatin 40 mg orally nightly, or atorvastatin 10 mg orally daily. These dosages are considered 'medium-intensity' therapy. 'High-intensity' therapy (e.g. atorvastatin 80 mg orally daily) is indicated for **secondary prevention** of cardiovascular disease.
Administration	Simvastatin, which has a short half-life, is best taken in the evening, because cholesterol synthesis is greatest in the early-morning hours. This is not necessary for other statins that have a longer half-life.
Communication	Explain that you are offering a medicine to lower cholesterol levels to reduce the risk of a heart attack or stroke. Explain that most people tolerate statins well, but outline the common, mild side effects like headache, stomach upset, and muscle aches. Explain that, rarely, statins can cause muscle inflammation and damage. Therefore, they should seek medical advice if they experience unexplained muscle pain or weakness. Advise them to minimise alcohol consumption. Those taking simvastatin or atorvastatin should avoid grapefruit juice, as this may increase the risk of side effects.
Monitoring and stopping	In the absence of adverse effects, statin therapy is required indefinitely. For **primary prevention** of cardiovascular disease, check a lipid profile before starting treatment and at 3 months, aiming for a 40% reduction in non-HDL cholesterol levels. In **secondary prevention,** a baseline lipid profile is informative but not essential. However, **efficacy** should be monitored by checking target cholesterol levels are achieved, as specified in guidelines. If not, consider increasing the dose, switching to an alternative statin or adding another agent (e.g. ezetimibe). For **safety,** check liver enzymes (e.g. alanine transaminase (ALT)) at baseline and again at 3 and 12 months. A rise in ALT up to three times the upper limit of normal may be acceptable, but the statin should be stopped if this is exceeded. It can be restarted at a lower dose when liver enzymes have returned to normal. Routine monitoring of creatine kinase (CK) is not required, but it should be checked before starting therapy if the person has experienced persistent, generalised, unexplained muscle pains; or during therapy if statin-induced myopathy is suspected.
Cost	Statins that are available in inexpensive non-proprietary forms (e.g. simvastatin, atorvastatin) should be preferred over branded products.

Clinical tip—Do not forget to assess the thyroid status (checking serum thyroid-stimulating hormone (TSH) if there is any clinical uncertainty) before starting a statin. Hypothyroidism is a reversible cause of hyperlipidaemia and should be corrected before reassessing the need for lipid-lowering medications. Furthermore, hypothyroidism increases the risk of myositis.

Sulfonylureas

CLINICAL PHARMACOLOGY

Common indications	In **type 2 diabetes,** sulphonylureas are options for *combination therapy* with **metformin** (and/or other antihyperglycaemic agents) if blood glucose is not adequately controlled, or as *monotherapy* if metformin is contraindicated or not tolerated.
Mechanisms of action	Sulfonylureas lower blood glucose by **stimulating pancreatic insulin secretion.** They **block ATP-dependent K$^+$ channels** in pancreatic β-cell membranes, causing depolarisation of the cell membrane and opening of voltage-gated Ca^{2+} channels. This increases intracellular Ca^{2+} concentrations, stimulating insulin secretion. Sulfonylureas are effective only in people with residual pancreatic function. As insulin is an anabolic hormone, stimulation of insulin secretion by sulfonylureas causes weight gain. Weight gain increases insulin resistance and can worsen diabetes mellitus in the long term.
Important adverse effects	Dose-related side effects such as **GI upset** are usually mild and infrequent. **Hypoglycaemia** is a potentially serious adverse effect, which is more likely with high doses; if drug metabolism is reduced (see WARNINGS); or if other glucose-lowering medications are prescribed (see INTERACTIONS). Depending on the duration of action of the drug, sulfonylurea-induced hypoglycaemia may last for many hours. If severe, it should be managed in hospital. Rare **hypersensitivity reactions** include hepatic toxicity (e.g. cholestatic jaundice), drug hypersensitivity syndrome (rash, fever, internal organ involvement) and haematological abnormalities (e.g. agranulocytosis).
Warnings	Gliclazide is metabolised in the liver and has a plasma half-life of 10–12 hours. Unchanged drug and metabolites are excreted in the urine. A dose reduction may therefore be required in ▲ **hepatic impairment** and blood glucose should be monitored carefully in ▲ **renal impairment.** Sulfonylureas should be prescribed with caution for people at ▲ **increased risk of hypoglycaemia,** including those with hepatic impairment (reduced gluconeogenesis), malnutrition, adrenal or pituitary insufficiency (lack of counter-regulatory hormones), and in older people.
Important interactions	Risk of hypoglycaemia is increased by co-prescription of other ▲ **glucose-lowering drugs,** including **metformin, insulin, DPP-4 inhibitors,** thiazolidinediones (pioglitazone), **sodium–glucose co-transporter 2 inhibitors**, and by alcohol. **β-blockers** may mask symptoms of hypoglycaemia. The efficacy of sulfonylureas is reduced by drugs that elevate blood glucose, e.g. **prednisolone, thiazide,** and **loop diuretics.**

PRACTICAL PRESCRIBING

Prescription	A sulfonylurea with a short duration of action and hepatic metabolism (e.g. gliclazide) is usually preferred, as this reduces complexity and the risk of nocturnal hypoglycaemia. Gliclazide (standard release) is usually started at a dosage of 40–80 mg once daily. The dose is increased gradually until glycaemic targets are achieved, with higher doses (160–320 mg daily) being given in divided doses. Gliclazide is also available as a modified-release (MR) form. It is important to note that these formulations are not therapeutically equivalent: 30 mg MR has a similar effect to that of 80 mg using standard-release tablets.
Administration	Sulfonylureas should be taken with meals (e.g. once daily at breakfast or twice daily at breakfast and evening meal).
Communication	Advise that this medicine is a long-term treatment to control blood sugar and reduce the risk of diabetic complications, such as kidney disease. Tablets are not a replacement for lifestyle measures and should be taken in addition to a healthy diet and regular exercise. Warn about hypoglycaemia, advising them to watch out for symptoms such as dizziness, nausea, sweating, and confusion. If they have a 'hypo', they should take something sugary (e.g. glucose tablets or a sugary drink), then something starchy (e.g. a sandwich), and seek medical advice if symptoms recur.
Monitoring and stopping	Assess blood glucose control by measuring haemoglobin A_{1c} (HbA_{1c}). In treating type 2 diabetes with a single agent, the target HbA_{1c} is usually <48 mmol/mol. Treatment is intensified by addition of a second agent if the HbA_{1c} is >58 mmol/mol, and a new target of <53 mmol/mol is then set (balancing the risks of hyperglycaemia against the risks of treatment, particularly hypoglycaemia). Home capillary blood glucose monitoring is not routinely required, although measurement may be helpful to determine if any unusual symptoms are due to hypoglycaemia. Tests of renal and hepatic function should be considered if there is reason to suspect they may be abnormal. Treatment for diabetes mellitus is indefinite unless, for example, weight loss improves glucose tolerance.
Cost	Non-proprietary gliclazide 80-mg tablets are inexpensive, and considerably cheaper than newer antidiabetic drugs, e.g. **sodium–glucose co-transporter 2 inhibitors**.

Clinical tip—During acute illness, insulin resistance increases and renal and hepatic function may become impaired. All oral glucose-lowering medicines become less effective at controlling blood glucose and side effects are more likely, e.g. hypoglycaemia with sulfonylureas. In hospital inpatients, **insulin** treatment may be required temporarily during severe illness. Insulin has a short half-life and its dosage can be adjusted more easily than can oral medication in response to acute fluctuations in blood glucose.

Tetracyclines and glycylcyclines

CLINICAL PHARMACOLOGY

Common indications	❶ **Acne vulgaris,** particularly where there are inflamed papules, pustules and/or cysts (*Propionibacterium acnes*). ❷ Lower respiratory tract infections, including **infective exacerbation of COPD** (e.g. *Haemophilus influenzae*) and **pneumonia.** ❸ Chlamydial infection, including **pelvic inflammatory disease.** ❹ Other infections such as **typhoid, malaria,** and **Lyme disease.** ❺ Tigecycline is used for **severe skin, soft-tissue, and abdominal infections,** but reserved for cases where other options are limited.
Spectrum of activity	Tetracyclines have a relatively **broad spectrum** of activity against Gram-positive and Gram-negative organisms. Resistance is common, although less problematic for the newer related drug, tigecycline.
Mechanisms of action	Tetracyclines **inhibit bacterial protein synthesis.** They bind to the ribosomal 30S subunit, which is specific to bacteria. This prevents binding of transfer RNA to messenger RNA, interfering with the addition of amino acids to growing polypeptide chains. Inhibition of protein synthesis is **bacteriostatic** (stops bacterial growth), which assists the immune system in killing and removing bacteria. Resistance is widespread, particularly in Gram-positive organisms. A common mechanism is an efflux pump, which allows bacteria to pump out tetracyclines, preventing cytoplasmic accumulation. Tigecycline is a glycylcycline antibiotic which is structurally and mechanistically similar to tetracyclines, but less susceptible to resistance.
Important adverse effects	Like most antibiotics, tetracyclines commonly cause **GI upset,** although with a lower risk of *Clostridioides difficile* infection than other broad-spectrum antibiotics (see **Penicillins, broad-spectrum**). **Hypersensitivity reactions** occur in about 1%, including immediate and delayed reactions. There is no cross-reactivity with β-lactam antibiotics (e.g. penicillins). Tetracycline-specific side effects include **oesophageal** ulceration and dysphagia; **photosensitivity** (an exaggerated sunburn reaction); and **discolouration** and/or hypoplasia of **tooth enamel** in children. Rare but serious adverse effects include **hepatotoxicity** and **intracranial hypertension,** the latter causing headache and visual disturbance.
Warnings	Tetracyclines bind to teeth and bones during childhood development, so should not be prescribed during ✘ **pregnancy,** ✘ **breastfeeding** or for ✘ **children ≤12 years of age.** They should be used with caution in ▲ **renal impairment** as their antianabolic effects can raise serum urea and reduced drug excretion can increase the risk of adverse effects.
Important interactions	Tetracyclines bind to divalent cations. They should therefore not be given within 2 hours of **calcium**, **antacids** or **iron**, which will prevent antibiotic absorption. Tetracyclines can enhance the anticoagulant effect of **warfarin** by killing normal gut bacteria that synthesise vitamin K.

PRACTICAL PRESCRIBING

Prescription	Most tetracyclines are prescribed orally. A loading dose may be required, e.g. doxycycline 200 mg on day 1, then 100–200 mg orally daily. As with other antibiotics, higher doses are prescribed for more severe or difficult-to-treat infections. Tigecycline is prescribed for IV infusion, but only for severe infections with limited treatment options.
Administration	Oral tetracycline products are formulated as capsules or tablets. These should be swallowed whole with plenty of water while sitting or standing to stop them getting stuck in the oesophagus, where they may cause ulceration.
Communication	Explain that the aim of treatment is to get rid of infection and improve symptoms. Before prescribing, always check for history of allergy to tetracyclines. Advise that medical advice should be sought if a rash or other unexpected symptom develops. If an allergic reaction occurs, give written and verbal advice not to take tetracycline antibiotics in the future and make sure that the allergy is clearly recorded in the notes. Advise that treatment should be taken during a meal, with a full glass of water, while sitting or standing. They should avoid indigestion remedies and medicines containing iron or zinc 2 hours before and after taking the antibiotic. During treatment they should protect their skin from sunlight, even on cloudy days.
Monitoring and stopping	Check that infection resolves by resolution of symptoms, signs (e.g. reduction in inflamed papules, pustules, and cysts in acne), and blood markers (e.g. resolution of inflammatory markers in respiratory infection) as appropriate. The duration of antibiotic therapy is a balance between ensuring effective treatment and minimising adverse reactions and resistance. This depends on the indication: for example, 5–7 days in **infective exacerbation of COPD,** 8 weeks in **acne.** Always set a stop or review date when prescribing antibiotics.
Cost	Oral tetracyclines are inexpensive. For example, a 1-week course of doxycycline 100 mg for respiratory infection costs around £1. Tigecycline is expensive (about £300 for 5 days' treatment).

Clinical tip—Demeclocycline is a tetracycline notable for its ability to increase serum sodium concentrations in the syndrome of inappropriate antidiuretic hormone (SIADH). It appears to do this by blocking antidiuretic hormone (ADH) binding to its receptor, although the mechanism is poorly understood. Other non-antibiotic properties of tetracyclines, including antiinflammatory, immune-modulating and neuroprotective effects, are being tested in clinical trials and may lead to new therapeutic applications in the future.

Thyroid hormones

CLINICAL PHARMACOLOGY

Common indications	❶ Primary hypothyroidism. ❷ Hypothyroidism secondary to hypopituitarism.
Mechanisms of action	The thyroid gland produces thyroxine (T_4), which is converted to the more active triiodothyronine (T_3) in target tissues. Thyroid hormones regulate metabolism and growth. Deficiency of these hormones causes hypothyroidism, with clinical features including lethargy, weight gain, constipation and slowing of mental processes. Hypothyroidism is treated by **long-term replacement of thyroid hormones**, usually with levothyroxine (synthetic T_4). Liothyronine (synthetic T_3) has a shorter half-life and quicker onset (a few hours) and offset (24–48 hours) than levothyroxine. It is therefore reserved for emergency treatment of severe or acute hypothyroidism.
Important adverse effects	The adverse effects of levothyroxine are usually due to excessive doses, so are predictably similar to symptoms of hyperthyroidism. These include **GI upset, cardiac** (e.g. palpitations, arrhythmias, angina), and **neurological** (e.g. tremor, restlessness, insomnia) manifestations. **Weight loss** is also an expected and often desirable effect of treatment.
Warnings	Thyroid hormones increase heart rate and metabolism. They can therefore precipitate cardiac ischaemia in people with ▲ **coronary artery disease,** in whom replacement should be started cautiously at a low dose and with careful monitoring. In ▲ **hypopituitarism, corticosteroid** therapy must be initiated before thyroid hormone replacement to avoid precipitating acute adrenal insufficiency (Addisonian crisis).
Important interactions	As GI absorption of levothyroxine is reduced by **antacids, calcium,** and **iron** salts, administration of these drugs needs to be separated from levothyroxine by about 4 hours. An increase in levothyroxine dose may be required in people taking **cytochrome P450 inducers,** e.g. phenytoin, **carbamazepine.** Levothyroxine-induced changes in metabolism can increase requirements for glucose-lowering treatments in diabetes mellitus and may enhance the effects of **warfarin.**

PRACTICAL PRESCRIBING

Prescription	For thyroid hormone replacement, a typical starting dose of levothyroxine is 50–100 micrograms orally daily, except in older people or those with cardiac disease, who should start on 25 micrograms daily. The dose is adjusted monthly in 25–50-microgram increments according to thyroid-stimulating hormone (TSH) level (see MONITORING) to a usual maintenance dose of 50–200 micrograms daily. Liothyronine may be prescribed for IV administration in emergency care. This should be under specialist direction.
Administration	Levothyroxine is available in 25-, 50-, and 100-microgram tablets. A combination may be required for correct dosing (e.g. 175 micrograms will require one tablet of each strength daily).
Communication	Explain that treatment aims to replace a natural hormone that their body has stopped making. This should give them more energy and make them feel better. Advise that it may take some time (months in some cases) to feel 'back to normal'. Emphasise (for most people) that treatment is indefinite, and that they should not stop taking it. Warn of the symptoms of too much treatment (e.g. shakiness, anxiety, insomnia, diarrhoea) and advise them to report these, as their treatment dosage may need to be reduced. If they take calcium or iron replacement, they should separate these from levothyroxine by at least 4 hours.
Monitoring and stopping	The aim of therapy is to relieve symptoms and achieve a euthyroid state. After starting levothyroxine, dose changes should initially be guided by symptoms, which should be reviewed monthly. Thyroid function tests should then be measured at 3 months. In primary hypothyroidism, TSH is the main guide to dosing. It is elevated due to loss of negative feedback of T_4 on the pituitary, but should return to a normal or low-normal level if an adequate replacement dose is given. The dosage should be titrated to achieve this, repeating TSH measurement 3 months after a change. Once stable, an annual clinical review and TSH level is sufficient.
Cost	Non-proprietary levothyroxine treatment costs around £4 per month.

Clinical tip—*Hyper*thyroid symptoms (see ADVERSE EFFECTS) may occur initially when starting levothyroxine. If this happens, continue therapy at a lower dose (rather than stopping it) and monitor symptoms over the next 1–2 weeks to look for the re-emergence of *hypo*thyroid symptoms. Thyroid function tests will be unhelpful in guiding therapy at this stage as it is likely that both TSH and T_4 concentrations will be raised: TSH because it takes weeks for this to fall in response to treatment, and T_4 because the measurement will include exogenous levothyroxine.

Tranexamic acid

CLINICAL PHARMACOLOGY

Common indications	❶ As a second-line treatment for **menorrhagia** (heavy menstrual bleeding) if a levonorgestrel intrauterine system is ineffective, declined or unsuitable, and after the underlying cause has been established (or while awaiting specialist review). An alternative option is **hormonal contraception**. ❷ For **epistaxis** (nose bleeding), as an option if management with first aid, nasal cautery and nasal packing have been unsuccessful. For this indication, it may be applied topically. ❸ In **major trauma**, where early IV administration reduces mortality. ❹ For **post-partum haemorrhage** (PPH) as an option to reduce blood loss in women with established PPH, or those undergoing caesarean section and at high risk of PPH, in addition to **oxytocin, blood products**, and other measures.
Mechanisms of action	Tranexamic acid is an antifibrinolytic drug that can prevent, reduce, and stop bleeding. It is a lysine analogue that acts by competitively binding to **plasminogen**, inhibiting its activation to **plasmin**. Plasmin is a fibrinolytic enzyme, responsible for breaking down (lysing) clots. Inhibiting plasmin production therefore promotes haemostasis.
Important adverse effects	Tranexamic acid tablets are well tolerated. **GI upset** and **rash** are common with IV use. Rare adverse effects include **deep vein thrombosis, pulmonary embolism, seizures,** and **visual disturbance.**
Warnings	Before starting tranexamic acid for abnormal menstrual bleeding, investigations for a cause should be started. Tranexamic acid should be avoided in people with history of ▲ **seizures** and ▲ **thromboembolic disease**, unless the benefits are thought to outweigh these risks (e.g. in major trauma). It should be avoided in overt ✖ **disseminated intravascular coagulation** (DIC), although it is beneficial in trauma-induced coagulopathy, where some features of DIC may be present.
Important interactions	Tranexamic acid can increase the risk of thromboembolism when combined with other drugs which are also ▲ **associated with an increased risk of thromboembolism** (e.g. **combined hormonal contraceptives, tamoxifen**).

PRACTICAL PRESCRIBING

Prescription	Tranexamic acid is available as a tablet or injection. Tablets can be prescribed or bought over the counter for **menorrhagia**, with a typical dose being 1 g orally 8-hrly for up to 4 days, which can be repeated over the long term if needed. For bleeding after **trauma**, a 1 g IV loading dose is given followed by a 1 g IV infusion over 8 hours. For **epistaxis**, tranexamic acid may be used topically (see ADMINISTRATION). This method of administration is 'off-label', as is the use of tranexamic acid in trauma. This means that while it is an approved medicinal product, licensed for use in some indications (such as menorrhagia), it is not licensed for the other uses described. Informed consent should be sought when a drug is used off-label. In an emergency, where it may not be possible to obtain informed consent, it can be prescribed on a best-interests basis.
Administration	Tablets can be taken with or without food and, when given regularly, doses should be spaced evenly throughout the day. For **trauma**, the loading dose is given over 10 minutes followed by a slow IV infusion over 8 hours. For **epistaxis**, it may be administered topically by saturating a nasal pack with the IV formulation before insertion.
Communication	Explain that tranexamic acid is a medicine that helps to control bleeding. It is used to treat heavy periods, nose bleeds, and bleeding after accidents. When taken by mouth, it may take up to 24 hours to see benefit. Usually, it is taken just for a few days when bleeding is most problematic. Explain that most people do not have any side effects. For those who are also taking combined hormonal contraception, explain that there is an increased risk of blood clots in the leg (deep vein thrombosis, DVT) and consider discussing alternative forms of contraception.
Monitoring and stopping	Efficacy should be monitored by reviewing symptoms and signs of bleeding. In long-term treatment for menorrhagia, stop tranexamic acid if it does not improve symptoms or if the underlying cause of the bleeding has been treated (e.g. fibroids removed or established on hormonal contraception).
Cost	Tranexamic acid is available in inexpensive non-proprietary forms.

Clinical tip—Given its proven benefit in reducing deaths from trauma (influential trials include CRASH-2, CRASH-3, and STAAMP), favourable side effect profile and relative ease of administration, tranexamic acid is an appealing treatment for a range of acute bleeding conditions. However, studies in conditions such as intracerebral haemorrhage (e.g. STOP-AUST, TICH-2) and GI bleeding (e.g. HALT-IT) have been unable to replicate this success. Location of bleeding and early treatment appears to be important to prevent adverse outcomes. Therefore a key reason for lack of efficacy in these conditions may be that their presentation can be delayed and the harm from bleeding has already occurred.

Trimethoprim

CLINICAL PHARMACOLOGY

Common indications	Trimethoprim is a first-line antibiotic for ❶ acute lower **urinary tract infection (UTI)** in men and non-pregnant women, provided the risk of trimethoprim resistance is low; and ❷ prevention of **recurrent UTI** if non-antibiotic measures are ineffective. **Nitrofurantoin** is an alternative. Trimethoprim is also an option for ❸ **acne vulgaris** and ❹ **prostatitis**. The main use of co-trimoxazole is ❺ treatment and prevention of **pneumocystis pneumonia** in immune suppression, e.g. HIV infection.
Spectrum of activity	Trimethoprim *ought* to have broad activity against many Gram-positive and Gram-negative bacteria (particularly enterobacteria, e.g. *Escherichia coli*), but this is increasingly **limited by resistance**. Combination with a sulfonamide (e.g. sulfamethoxazole, as co-trimoxazole) **extends the spectrum** to include activity against the fungus *Pneumocystis jirovecii*.
Mechanisms of action	Bacteria are unable to use external sources of folate, so need to make their own for essential functions such as DNA synthesis. Trimethoprim **inhibits bacterial folate synthesis,** slowing bacterial growth (bacteriostasis). Its clinical utility is reduced by widespread bacterial resistance. Mechanisms of resistance include reduced intracellular antibiotic accumulation and reduced sensitivity of target enzymes. Sulfamethoxazole, a sulfonamide, also inhibits bacterial folate synthesis, but at a different step in the pathway. Given together, the drugs cause more complete inhibition of folate synthesis.
Important adverse effects	Trimethoprim most commonly causes **GI upset** and **skin rash** (3%–7%). Severe **hypersensitivity** reactions, including anaphylaxis, drug fever, and erythema multiforme, are rare with trimethoprim, but more common with sulfonamides, limiting their use. As a folate antagonist, trimethoprim can impair haematopoiesis, causing **megaloblastic anaemia, leukopenia,** and **thrombocytopenia.** It can also cause **hyperkalaemia** and elevation of plasma creatinine concentration.
Warnings	Trimethoprim is contraindicated in the ✖ **first trimester of pregnancy** because, as a folate antagonist, it could potentially increase the risk of fetal abnormalities. It should be used cautiously in people with ▲ **folate deficiency,** who are more susceptible to adverse haematological effects. As trimethoprim is mostly excreted unchanged into urine it is less suitable in ▲ **renal impairment;** if it is used, a dose reduction is necessary. ▲ **Neonates,** ▲ **older people,** and individuals with ▲ **HIV infection** are more susceptible to adverse effects.
Important interactions	Use with ▲ **potassium-elevating drugs** (e.g. **aldosterone antagonists**, **ACE inhibitors**, **ARBs**) predisposes to hyperkalaemia. Use with other ▲ **folate antagonists** (e.g. **methotrexate**) and ▲ **drugs that increase folate metabolism** (e.g. phenytoin) increases the risk of adverse haematological effects. Trimethoprim can enhance the anticoagulant effect of warfarin by killing normal gut flora that synthesise vitamin K.

PRACTICAL PRESCRIBING

Prescription	Trimethoprim is prescribed orally. For **acute UTI,** the usual dosage is 200 mg 12-hrly, for a duration appropriate to the severity of infection. As **prophylaxis for recurrent UTI,** it is prescribed at a lower dose (e.g. 100 mg nightly). Co-trimoxazole can be prescribed for oral or IV administration. A weight-based dosage (120 mg/kg per day, oral or IV, in 2–4 divided doses) is given for 14–21 days to treat **pneumocystis infection.** A lower dose (e.g. 960 mg orally three times a week) is used for pneumocystis prophylaxis.
Administration	Oral trimethoprim and co-trimoxazole are available as tablets and suspension. Intravenous co-trimoxazole must be diluted immediately before use (to prevent crystallisation) in 125–500 mL sodium chloride 0.9% or glucose 5%, and infused slowly over 60–90 minutes.
Communication	Explain that the aim of treatment is to get rid of infection and improve symptoms. Where antibiotics are for **prophylaxis**, explain that this is a long-term medication rather than a time-limited course. Before prescribing, always check there is no history of **allergy** to trimethoprim or co-trimoxazole (which they may know by a brand name, Septrin®). As allergic reactions are common with these antibiotics, it is particularly important to warn them to seek medical attention if a rash or other unexpected symptom develops. If an allergic reaction occurs, give them written and verbal advice not to take this antibiotic in the future and make sure the allergy is clearly recorded in the notes.
Monitoring and stopping	Check that **acute infection** resolves by improvement in symptoms (e.g. dysuria), signs (e.g. resolution of pyrexia) and investigations (e.g. fall in inflammatory markers, sterile urine on repeat culture in selected cases), as appropriate. For **long-term treatment,** full blood count monitoring may be useful for early detection and treatment of haematological disorders (e.g. by replacing folate and/or stopping the antibiotic). The duration of antibiotic therapy is a balance between ensuring effective treatment and minimising adverse reactions and resistance. Always set a stop or review date when prescribing antibiotics, following local protocols for guidance.
Cost	Trimethoprim and co-trimoxazole have been on the market for many years and are inexpensive.

Clinical tip—Trimethoprim and creatinine compete for secretion by the renal tubules. Trimethoprim treatment can cause a small reversible rise in serum creatinine concentrations, without reducing the glomerular filtration rate. In renal impairment, increased serum creatinine concentrations compete with trimethoprim for secretion into the urinary tract, potentially reducing efficacy against UTIs.

CLINICAL PHARMACOLOGY

Common indications	**❶ Prevention of post-partum haemorrhage** (PPH), as part of 'active management' of the third stage of labour. Oxytocin and ergometrin are similarly effective, but oxytocin is better tolerated. **❷ Treatment of PPH.** Oxytocin and ergometrin, alone or in combination, are first-line options for treatment of PPH. Oxytocin may also be given by infusion if there is inadequate response. **❸ Induction** and **augmentation of labour.** Oxytocin (but *not* ergometrine) is a second-line option for induction of labour (e.g. after prostaglandin application and artificial rupture of membranes). It is also used in protracted or arrested labour (hypotonic uterine inertia).
Mechanisms of action	Oxytocin is a naturally occurring hormone produced in the hypothalamus and secreted from the posterior pituitary. Oxytocin receptors are expressed on myometrium and endometrium, increasing significantly in density in the latter weeks of pregnancy. At this time, stimulation by oxytocin leads to a rise in intracellular calcium, causing contractions. This is beneficial in the third stage of labour, when it reduces the risk of PPH. It can also be used to stimulate or augment labour, but only after maturation of the cervix and rupture of membranes (naturally or artificially). Ergometrine is an ergot alkaloid that acts on uterine α-adrenergic and 5-HT$_2$ receptors to stimulate contractions. It has a similar effect to oxytocin in PPH.
Important adverse effects	Oxytocin may cause abdominal pain through uterine contraction. When used to stimulate or augment labour, it may cause **uterine hyperstimulation** (more than five contractions in 10 minutes, or lasting more than 2 minutes). This should be managed promptly as it can cause fetal distress, asphyxia, and death and may lead to uterine rupture. Rarely, oxytocin causes **hyponatraemia** and **pulmonary oedema** (SEE CLINICAL TIP). Other adverse effects include nausea and vomiting, headaches, and arrhythmias. Ergometrine has similar adverse effects. In addition, stimulation of extra-uterine α-adrenergic receptors may cause **systemic hypertension, pulmonary oedema, coronary vasospasm,** and **myocardial infarction**.
Warnings	Oxytocin should not be administered for induction or augmentation of labour in atypical fetal presentation (e.g. ✖ **breech**) or ✖ **placenta praevia**. It should be used with caution in those with ▲ **ischaemic heart disease.** Ergometrine should not be given in the ✖ **first or second stage of labour,** or to people with severe ✖ **cardiac disease,** ✖ **hypertension** or ✖ **vascular disease.**
Important interactions	Ergometrine and oxytocin have a synergistic effect on uterine muscle; this may be the therapeutic aim, but it increases pain. Oxytocin may prolong the QT interval and should be used with caution in people with long QT syndrome or taking ▲ **drugs that prolong the QT interval**.

PRACTICAL PRESCRIBING

Prescription	For the **prevention of PPH**, 10 units of oxytocin by IM injection is recommended. For **treatment of PPH,** oxytocin may be prescribed for slow IV injection (which may be repeated) or infusion. For **induction or augmentation of labour,** oxytocin is given as a continuous IV infusion. When prescribing oxytocin, 'units' should be written out in full, rather than abbreviated to 'U', which can be mistaken for '0'.
Administration	For prevention of PPH, oxytocin is administered to the mother by IM injection (usually in the thigh) immediately after the baby is born and before the cord is clamped. If IV administration is required, it should be given by slow injection or infusion, because rapid bolus injection can cause hypotension, tachycardia, and QT interval prolongation.
Communication	Discussion of the benefits and risks of oxytocin to prevent PPH should form part of a broader conversation about active versus physiological ('natural') management of the third stage of labour. In this context, explain that oxytocin (or ergometrine) helps the womb contract and reduces the risk of serious bleeding after birth. For treatment of PPH, explain that the treatment is offered in the hope that by causing contractions it will stop the bleeding. Advise that post-partum contractions may be painful, although not usually more painful than labour itself. For induction or augmentation of labour, an appropriate specialist should discuss the reasons for offering treatment (usually to prevent fetal complication of delayed or prolonged labour) and outline the risks and benefits of treatment, and other treatment and monitoring that may be required.
Monitoring and stopping	Response to treatment in PPH is monitored clinically. For induction of labour, oxytocin infusions are titrated to achieve labour at a maximum of 3–4 contractions every 10 minutes. Where contractions are more frequent or prolonged (see ADVERSE EFFECTS) the infusion should be stopped or dose reduced as appropriate. Oxytocin infusions should be given on a labour ward where monitoring of the mother (blood pressure, heart rate and rhythm, contractions) and fetus can occur. Fluid intake should be monitored during oxytocin infusion (see CLINICAL TIP).
Cost	IM injection of oxytocin is inexpensive.

Clinical tip—Oxytocin has antidiuretic effects and prolonged infusion alongside hypotonic fluids risks causing hyponatraemia and pulmonary oedema. Fluid intake should be carefully monitored and hypotonic solutions (e.g. glucose 5%) avoided.

Vaccines and immunoglobulins

CLINICAL PHARMACOLOGY

Common indications	❶ **Active immunisation** (vaccines), according to a routine immunisation schedule or in specific risk scenarios (e.g. travel) to prevent infection. ❷ **Passive immunisation** (immunoglobulins) to prevent infection in immunodeficiency or as post-exposure treatment of specific infections. ❸ **Prevention of Rh₀ (D) sensitisation** (anti-D immunoglobulin) in rhesus negative women following birth of a rhesus positive infant. ❹ Treatment of immune-mediated conditions (immunoglobulins) such as **Guillain–Barré syndrome.**
Mechanisms of action	Vaccines deliver an **antigen** to induce a protective immune response to a pathogen, without causing disease. The antigen stimulates B cells to produce antibodies (humoral immunity) and activates T cells (cell-mediated immunity). Antibody persistence and memory cells provide long-term protection against infection. To deliver the antigen, vaccines may comprise the **whole pathogen** (live attenuated or killed) or a **subunit** (recombinant protein or inactivated toxin). The latter may be linked **(conjugated)** with another protein to amplify the immune response. Other vaccines contain genetic material encoding the antigen, to be synthesised in vivo by host cells. This may be delivered as **nucleic acid** (e.g. modified messenger RNA (mRNA) in lipid nanoparticles) or in a **viral vector** (e.g. a live, non-replicating adenovirus). Immunoglobulins are human antibodies. **Normal immunoglobulin** is prepared from pooled human plasma and confers passive immunity in immunodeficiency states. It also has complex immunomodulatory effects that are useful in some immune-mediated conditions. **Disease-specific immunoglobulin** is prepared from plasma of donors with high antibody levels against specific diseases (e.g. hepatitis B).
Important adverse effects	**Local reactions** (pain, swelling, redness) and **mild systemic symptoms** (fever, malaise, headache, GI upset, myalgia) are common and short lived. Fever may trigger **febrile convulsions** in susceptible children. Abnormal immune responses to vaccines are rare but can be life threatening (∼1 per million vaccine doses). These include **anaphylaxis** and **delayed immune-mediated reactions** (e.g. vaccine-induced immune thrombotic thrombocytopenia associated with adenoviral-vectored COVID-19 vaccines).
Warnings	Vaccine efficacy is impaired in ▲ **severe immunosuppression,** where there is also a theoretical risk of infection from live attenuated and replicating viral-vector vaccines. Live vaccines should generally be avoided in ▲ **pregnancy** due to a similar theoretical risk of fetal infection. Allergy is not a contraindication unless it was a ✖ **confirmed anaphylactic reaction** to a previous dose or component of the vaccine.
Important interactions	▲ **Drugs with immune suppressing effects** such as **systemic corticosteroids, methotrexate, monoclonal antibodies,** and cytotoxic chemotherapy may reduce the response to vaccination.

vaccines, normal immunoglobulin, tetanus immunoglobulin

PRACTICAL PRESCRIBING

Prescription	In the UK, the routine immunisation schedule is set out in The Green Book. National patient group directions (PGDs) remove the need for individual prescriptions. Vaccines for travel may be prescribed by GPs, pharmacies or private travel clinics. Most prescriptions for immunoglobulins are directed by specialists (but see CLINICAL TIP). Immunoglobulins are dosed in grams or units, usually based on weight. As normal immunoglobulin is a scarce resource, with demand exceeding supply, prior approval from NHS subregional panels is required for all but emergency indications.
Administration	Most vaccines are administered by IM injection. Exceptions are cholera (given orally), Bacillus Calmette–Guérin (BCG; intradermal) and influenza vaccination in children (intranasal). Deep SC injection is preferred over IM injection in those at increased risk of bleeding. Immunoglobulins are given by IM, IV or SC injection. Vaccines and immunoglobulins can be inactivated by heat and light, so must be stored and handled in accordance with the product literature.
Communication	People may be reluctant to come in or bring children for vaccination because of fear, fuelled by stories on social media. Explore and address these fears. Some key messages are: vaccines protect against serious diseases; they are rigorously tested and monitored for safety; they can cause short-lived side effects including feeling unwell or a sore arm but, overall, vaccinating is safer than not vaccinating. Vaccines do not cause autism or allergies; they do not overload or weaken the immune system; and they do not contain mercury or any other ingredients in harmful amounts. Advise individuals given a live vaccine to avoid close contact with immunosuppressed people for 1–2 weeks after vaccination. For people concerned that immunoglobulin is prepared from human blood, reassure them that it is tested rigorously for infections.
Monitoring and stopping	In people with a history of anaphylaxis, consider observing for 30 minutes post-vaccination. Report suspected adverse reactions to the Medicines and Healthcare Products Regulatory Agency (MHRA) via the Yellow Card scheme.
Cost	Although individual doses are relatively inexpensive (e.g. injectable influenza vaccine £6–12), widespread vaccination (e.g. influenza ~12 million doses/year) is costly for the health service. This is offset by reduced healthcare use and sick days.

Clinical tip—It is important to ascertain tetanus vaccination status following injuries. In intermediate-risk scenarios (e.g. puncture injury while gardening; vaccinated >10 years ago), an immediate reinforcing dose of tetanus *vaccine* should be offered. In high-risk scenarios (e.g. wound heavily contaminated with soil, or an unvaccinated person), tetanus *immunoglobulin* should also be offered. Normal immunoglobulin is an acceptable alternative if tetanus immunoglobulin is unavailable.

Valproate (valproic acid)

CLINICAL PHARMACOLOGY

Common indications	❶ Seizure prophylaxis in **epilepsy.** Valproate has a broad spectrum of antiepileptic activity, so is effective in most seizure types. In people who cannot become pregnant, it is a first-line option for generalised tonic–clonic seizures. It is also an option for focal seizures, but toxicity (particularly in women and girls) limits its use. ❷ Selected cases of **established convulsive status epilepticus** that have not responded to adequate treatment with a **benzodiazepine.** ❸ **Bipolar disorder,** for the acute treatment of manic episodes and prophylaxis against recurrence. ❹ As an option to prevent frequent **migraine** attacks.
Mechanisms of action	Valproate has multiple actions. It **increases** activity of **glutamic acid decarboxylase (GAD),** which increases production of γ-**aminobutyric acid (GABA),** the principal inhibitory neurotransmitter in the brain. It also appears to be a weak inhibitor of voltage-dependent sodium channels. Together these effects, and others, reduce neuronal excitability, suppressing both initial seizure discharges and their propagation.
Important adverse effects	The most common dose-related adverse events are **GI upset, neurological and psychiatric** effects (including tremor, ataxia, and behavioural disturbances), **thrombocytopenia** and transient increase in **liver enzymes.** Hypersensitivity reactions include **hair loss,** with subsequent regrowth being curlier than original hair. Rare, **life-threatening, idiosyncratic** adverse effects include severe liver injury, pancreatitis, bone marrow failure, and antiepileptic hypersensitivity syndrome (see **Carbamazepine**).
Warnings	Unless there is no alternative, valproate should be avoided in ✖ **girls and women who could become pregnant** particularly around the time of ✖ **conception** and in the ✖ **first trimester of pregnancy.** It is the antiepileptic drug associated with the greatest risk of **fetal abnormalities,** including neural tube defects, craniofacial, cardiac and limb abnormalities, and developmental delay. If use is unavoidable, highly effective contraception is essential. It should be avoided in ▲ **hepatic impairment** and dose reduction is required in ▲ **severe renal impairment.**
Important interactions	Valproate inhibits hepatic enzymes, increasing plasma concentration and risk of toxicity with ▲ **lamotrigine** (by inhibition of glucuronidation) and ▲ **drugs metabolised by cytochrome P450 (CYP) enzymes,** such as **warfarin.** Valproate is itself metabolised by CYP enzymes, so its concentration is reduced (and risk of seizures increased) by ▲ **CYP inducers** (e.g. **carbamazepine,** phenytoin) and, through an uncertain mechanism, ▲ **carbapenems** (see CLINICAL TIP). Adverse effects are increased by ▲ **CYP inhibitors** (e.g. **macrolides,** protease inhibitors). The efficacy of antiepileptic drugs is reduced by ▲ **drugs that lower the seizure threshold** (e.g. **antipsychotics, tramadol**).

PRACTICAL PRESCRIBING

Prescription	Valproate is formulated as a sodium salt, licensed for epilepsy, and as valproic acid, licensed for bipolar disorder. A typical starting prescription for adults with **epilepsy** is sodium valproate 300 mg orally 12-hrly, or for **bipolar disease**, valproic acid 250 mg orally 8-hrly. The dose is increased to a usual total daily dose of 1–2 g.
Administration	Valproate is available in a bewildering array of normal or enteric-coated tablets, capsules, granules, and oral solutions. Some formulations can be crushed (tablets) or mixed with food (granules), whereas modified-release and enteric-coated formulations must be swallowed whole. Give appropriate instructions for the formulation chosen. Valproate can be given IV if oral administration is not possible.
Communication	For epilepsy, explain that the aim of treatment is to reduce frequency of seizures. Warn that they may have indigestion or tummy upset when starting valproate, but that these will settle in a few days and can be reduced by taking tablets with food. As the most serious potential adverse effects are unpredictable, they should seek urgent medical advice for unexpected symptoms such as lethargy, loss of appetite, vomiting or abdominal pain or bruising, a high temperature or mouth ulcers. For women and girls of childbearing potential, if treatment with valproate is unavoidable, UK regulations require that they are enrolled on a pregnancy prevention programme. Advise that driving is prohibited unless they have been seizure-free for 12 months, and for 6 months after changing or stopping treatment.
Monitoring and stopping	Monitor **efficacy** by comparing seizure frequency before and after starting treatment or dose adjustment. Monitor **safety** by symptom enquiry. Measurement of liver function before and during the first 6 months of treatment is advisable. Plasma valproate concentrations (usually 40–100 mg/L) do not correlate well with therapeutic effect. They should therefore only be measured to check for adherence or toxicity. Withdrawal of antiseizure therapy is a specialist area that requires careful consideration of individual risks and benefits. Generally, it is considered after the person has been seizure-free for at least 2 years. The dosage should be tapered over 2–3 months. In bipolar disease, the dosage should be tapered over at least 4 weeks.
Cost	Generic valproate/valproic acid tablets are inexpensive, but cost increases with complexity of the formulation.

Clinical tip—An important interaction exists between valproate and **carbapenems** (e.g. meropenem, ertapenem). Valproate concentrations fall rapidly and profoundly if a carbapenem is introduced, with a corresponding high risk of seizures. It is not feasible to manage this interaction by dosage adjustment, so it is best to avoid the combination. If a carbapenem is essential, alternative antiseizure treatment should be considered.

Vitamins

CLINICAL PHARMACOLOGY

Common indications	❶ Thiamine (vitamin B_1) is used in the treatment and prevention of **Wernicke's encephalopathy** and **Korsakoff's psychosis,** which are manifestations of severe thiamine deficiency. ❷ Folic acid (the synthetic form of folate or vitamin B_9) is used in **megaloblastic anaemia** due to folate deficiency, and in the first trimester of pregnancy to **reduce the risk of neural tube defects.** ❸ Hydroxocobalamin and cyanocobalamin (synthetic forms of cobalamin or vitamin B_{12}) are used in the treatment of **megaloblastic anaemia** and **subacute combined degeneration of the cord** as a result of vitamin B_{12} deficiency. ❹ Phytomenadione (the plant form of vitamin K) is recommended for all newborn babies to prevent **vitamin K deficiency bleeding** and is used for **reversal of warfarin anticoagulation** (prothrombin complex concentrate should also be given in cases of major bleeding).
Mechanisms of action	Vitamins are organic substances required in small amounts for normal metabolic processes. Vitamin deficiencies and their associated clinical manifestations may be treated with a pharmaceutical form of the relevant vitamin (see INDICATIONS). In pregnancy and the preconception period, folic acid reduces the risk of congenital neural tube defects. As it is required for normal cell division, it may work by facilitating cell proliferation involved in neural tube closure, but this is not completely understood. Phytomenadione reverses warfarin by providing a fresh supply of vitamin K for the synthesis of vitamin K-dependent clotting factors by the liver.
Important adverse effects	When given IV, phytomenadione and high-dose thiamine may rarely cause **anaphylaxis.** Most other vitamin preparations are relatively non-toxic.
Warnings	If there is ▲ **co-existing vitamin B_{12} and folate deficiency,** both vitamins should be replaced simultaneously. This is because replacing folate alone may be associated with (and perhaps hasten) progression of the neurological manifestations of vitamin B_{12} deficiency. The major concern is the risk of provoking subacute combined degeneration of the cord. Phytomenadione is less effective in reversing warfarin in **severe liver disease,** as clotting factors are synthesised in the liver.
Important interactions	As noted earlier, vitamin K and warfarin have an antagonistic interaction which, in the context of over-warfarinisation, is desirable. However, if warfarin is restarted after vitamin K has been given, dosing requirements may initially be erratic.

PRACTICAL PRESCRIBING

Prescription	In the hospital setting, people at high risk of **thiamine deficiency** are treated initially with a compound preparation of B and C vitamins, given by injection. Pabrinex® is the usual choice. It is prescribed in 'pairs' of ampules: for *prophylaxis* in high-risk groups the dose is 1 pair 12-hrly IV for 3 days; *treatment* doses are higher. Oral thiamine (e.g. 200 mg daily) is used in the longer term. To prevent **neural tube defects**, folic acid 400 micrograms daily should be started before conception ideally, or otherwise at the diagnosis of pregnancy, and continued until week 12. This can be purchased without prescription. Where there is high risk of neural tube defect (e.g. in epilepsy), a higher dose of 5 mg daily is used. This is also the dose used in **folate deficiency anaemia**. In **vitamin B$_{12}$ deficiency**, hydroxocobalamin is given by IM injection. Oral cyanocobalamin is an alternative, but it may be less effective if there is defective vitamin B$_{12}$ absorption. To prevent **vitamin K deficiency bleeding** in neonates, phytomenadione 1 mg IM is given once only (lower doses in preterm neonates). To treat **over-warfarinisation,** it is best to give a low dose of phytomenadione (e.g. 1 mg orally or IV). In cases of major bleeding, 10 mg IV is given. Consult local specialist guidance and the BNF.
Administration	Each carton of Pabrinex® contains 2 ampules labelled No 1 and No 2. The contents of both ampules are added to a small bag (50–100 mL) of 0.9% sodium chloride or 5% glucose, mixed, and infused over 30 minutes. Phytomenadione, when given IV, should be injected very slowly.
Communication	It is always worth raising the issue of folic acid supplementation in consultations with woman who could become pregnant, due to the benefits of starting this in the preconception period.
Monitoring and stopping	Treatment of thiamine deficiency is monitored clinically. Treatment of folate and vitamin B$_{12}$ deficiency is monitored clinically and with full blood counts. The effect of phytomenadione on the international normalised ratio (INR) is evident 12–24 hours after administration. No monitoring is required after prophylactic use in neonates. Decisions about stopping therapy depend on whether the indication for treatment is acute (e.g. phytomenadione in neonates), chronic but reversible (e.g. dietary insufficiency) or chronic and lifelong (e.g. pernicious anaemia).
Cost	Most vitamin preparations are inexpensive.

Clinical tip—In over-warfarinisation with no bleeding, a low dose of vitamin K (e.g. 0.5–1 mg) is recommended. However, the oral formulation of vitamin K (menadiol phosphate) is available only as 10-mg tablets. An unlicensed but acceptable alternative is to prescribe the IV formulation of phytomenadione solution for oral administration. It can be diluted (e.g. with sterile water) to allow the required dose to be measured out.

Warfarin

CLINICAL PHARMACOLOGY

Common indications	❶ To treat and prevent recurrence of **venous thromboembolism** (VTE, the collective term for **deep vein thrombosis** and **pulmonary embolism**). However, **direct oral anticoagulants** (DOACs) are usually preferred. ❷ To prevent arterial embolism from **atrial fibrillation** (AF). **DOACs** are usually preferred in non-valvular AF, but warfarin is the first-line option for AF associated with mechanical heart valves, bioprosthetic valves (within 3–6 months of insertion) and rheumatic mitral stenosis. ❸ To prevent arterial embolism from **mechanical heart valves,** whether or not this is associated with atrial fibrillation.
Mechanisms of action	Production of clotting factors II, VII, IX, and X (termed the 'vitamin K-dependent clotting factors') requires vitamin K in its reduced form to act as a cofactor. Oxidised vitamin K generated from this reaction is then recycled into its reduced form by the enzyme **vitamin K epoxide reductase,** which is **inhibited by warfarin.** This reduces production of vitamin K-dependent clotting factors (and proteins C and S) which, over several days, produces an anticoagulant effect.
Important adverse effects	**Bleeding** is the main adverse effect. In therapeutic use or minor over-warfarinisation, there is increased risk of bleeding from minor trauma (e.g. intracerebral haemorrhage after minor head injury) and existing abnormalities such as peptic ulcers. Severe over-warfarinisation can trigger apparently spontaneous bleeding, such as epistaxis or retroperitoneal haemorrhage. The effect of warfarin can be reversed with **phytomenadione** (vitamin K_1) or dried prothrombin complex.
Warnings	The benefits of preventing clots must be carefully balanced against the risks of bleeding. Warfarin is obviously contraindicated if there is ✖ **active bleeding** or an immediate risk of this, including after trauma and peri-operatively. ▲ **Liver disease** impairs both warfarin metabolism and clotting factor synthesis. Warfarin should be avoided in the first trimester of ✖ **pregnancy** due to teratogenicity (cardiac and cranial abnormalities) and near term due to the risk of peripartum haemorrhage. **Heparins** are preferred in this context.
Important interactions	The concentration of warfarin required to prevent clotting is close to the concentration that causes bleeding (low therapeutic index). Small changes in warfarin metabolism by cytochrome P450 (CYP) enzymes can cause clinically significant changes in anticoagulation. ▲ **CYP inducers** (e.g. phenytoin, **carbamazepine**, rifampicin) increase warfarin metabolism and risk of clots. ▲ **CYP inhibitors** (e.g. **fluconazole**, **macrolides**) decrease warfarin metabolism and increase bleeding risk. Other antibiotics can increase the effect of warfarin by killing the gut flora that synthesise vitamin K, but this is rarely a problem clinically.

PRACTICAL PRESCRIBING

Prescription	A loading dose of 10 mg orally daily is often given on days 1–3, or 5 mg daily in older people and those with low body weight or higher bleeding risk (e.g. due to interacting medicines). Subsequent doses are guided by the international normalised ratio (INR) (see MONITORING AND STOPPING). After starting warfarin, it takes several days for anticoagulation to be achieved. If immediate anticoagulation is needed, **heparin** may be started concurrently, then stopped once the target INR is reached.
Administration	Traditionally, warfarin is taken each day at around 18:00 for consistent effects on the INR taken the following morning. This may also help people to remember when to take it (around tea time).
Communication	Explain that anti-clotting treatment is a balance between benefits (preventing harm from clots) and risks (bleeding). Emphasise that food, alcohol, and other drugs can affect warfarin treatment. Provide an anticoagulant book ('Yellow Book'). This is used to record warfarin doses, blood test results, treatment indication, and duration, and should be brought to consultations with healthcare practitioners.
Monitoring and stopping	The INR is a ratio expressing the intensity of anticoagulation. It is calculated from the prothrombin time of the individual divided by that of a normal control sample. The target INR range depends on the indication (e.g. 2.0–3.0 in AF and VTE; higher for mechanical heart valves). When commencing warfarin, the INR is measured daily in hospital inpatients and every few days in outpatients. Once a stable dose of warfarin has been established, INR measurement is less frequent. Warfarin treatment duration is 3–6 months for a single episode of VTE that was unprovoked, or if the associated condition/risk factor has receded. Long-term anticoagulation is required for AF, recurrent VTE, or VTE associated with an enduring precipitant (e.g. prothrombotic tendency), but the risk–benefit balance should be reviewed periodically.
Cost	Warfarin drug costs are about £1/month per patient, but associated monitoring costs add to this. The drug costs of **DOACs** are higher, but these are offset by lower monitoring costs. Decisions should be based primarily on the clinical needs of the individual.

Clinical tip—Dosing warfarin can be a challenge. Follow local guidelines if available and applicable, and if in doubt seek advice from the anticoagulation service. Changes in INR lag behind changes in the warfarin dose. Look back over the last 48–72 hours to see what doses have led to the current INR. Avoid large dose changes wherever possible.

Z-drugs

CLINICAL PHARMACOLOGY

Common indications	Short-term treatment of **insomnia** which is debilitating or distressing, although non-pharmacological treatment (or treatment of the underlying cause, if applicable) is invariably preferable.
Mechanisms of action	The 'Z-drugs' have a similar mechanism of action to **benzodiazepines**, although they are chemically distinct. Their target is the **γ-aminobutyric acid type A (GABA$_A$) receptor**. The GABA$_A$ receptor is a chloride (Cl⁻) channel that opens in response to binding by GABA, the main inhibitory neurotransmitter in the brain. Opening the channel allows chloride to flow into the cell, making the cell more resistant to depolarisation. Like benzodiazepines, Z-drugs facilitate and enhance binding of GABA to the GABA$_A$ receptor (**allosteric modulation**). This has a widespread depressant effect on synaptic transmission. The clinical manifestations of this include reduced anxiety, sleepiness, and sedation. Note that Z-drugs are not useful anticonvulsants, as they cannot be given by injection. Z-drugs have a shorter duration of action than most benzodiazepines.
Important adverse effects	All Z-drugs can cause **daytime sleepiness,** which may affect ability to drive or perform complex tasks the day after taking the medication. **Rebound insomnia** may occur when the drugs are stopped. Other **neurological effects** include headache, confusion, nightmares, and (rarely) amnesia. As Z-drugs differ chemically from one another, their adverse effects are also different. Zopiclone can cause **taste disturbance,** whereas zolpidem more commonly causes **GI upset.** Prolonged use of Z-drugs beyond 4 weeks can lead to **dependence,** with **withdrawal symptoms** on stopping, including headaches, muscle pains, and anxiety. In **overdose,** Z-drugs cause **drowsiness, coma, and respiratory depression.**
Warnings	Z-drugs should be used with caution in ▲ **older people,** who are often more sensitive to drugs with neurological effects. They should not be prescribed for people with ✖ **obstructive sleep apnoea,** ✖ **respiratory muscle weakness** or ✖ **respiratory depression,** in whom they may worsen respiratory failure during sleep.
Important interactions	Z-drugs enhance the sedative effects of alcohol, **antihistamines** and **benzodiazepines**. They enhance the hypotensive effect of antihypertensive medications. As Z-drugs are metabolised by cytochrome P450 (CYP) enzymes, ▲ **CYP inhibitors** (e.g. **macrolides**) can enhance sedation, whereas **CYP inducers** (e.g. phenytoin, rifampicin) can impair sedation.

PRACTICAL PRESCRIBING

Prescription	Z-drugs should be prescribed at the lowest effective dose for the shortest possible period (generally no longer than 2 weeks). Typical doses are zopiclone 7.5 mg or zolpidem 10 mg orally, to be taken at bedtime. Starting doses should be halved for older people.
Administration	Z-drugs are available for oral administration only, as tablets or capsules.
Communication	When treating insomnia, explain that 'sleeping tablets' should only be used as a short-term measure to help them get over a bad patch. Discuss reasons why they are not sleeping and offer advice on 'sleep hygiene'. Advise them to take tablets only when really needed, as the body can get used to them if taken regularly. Warn that they should not use them for longer than 2–4 weeks, as otherwise they may become dependent on them and may feel unwell when they stop taking them. Warn them not to drive or operate complex or heavy machinery after taking the drug and explain that sometimes sleepiness may persist the following day.
Monitoring and stopping	In insomnia and anxiety, enquiry about symptoms and side effects is the best form of monitoring. Treatment should be for no longer than 4 weeks, with dosage reduction starting at 2 weeks. If taken for longer than this, gradual tapering is important to avoid a withdrawal reaction.
Cost	Both zopiclone and zolpidem are available in non-proprietary preparations and are relatively inexpensive.

Clinical tip—Routine prescription of hypnotics, such as Z-drugs, is not recommended for the treatment of insomnia because of the potential for tolerance and dependence and because it does not address the underlying cause of insomnia. However, hypnotics can be useful as short-term treatment in *specific* circumstances: e.g. for an anxious person in need of a single good night's sleep prior to surgery, or for recently bereaved people for whom insomnia is a significant, acute problem.

Emergency drugs

Adenosine

CLINICAL PHARMACOLOGY

Common indications	As a first-line diagnostic and therapeutic agent in **supraventricular tachycardia (SVT)** without life-threatening features. If life-threatening features (e.g. shock) are present, electrical cardioversion is preferred.
Mechanisms of action	Adenosine is an **agonist** of **adenosine receptors** on cell surfaces. In the heart, activation of these G protein-coupled receptors induces several effects, including reducing the frequency of spontaneous depolarisations *(automaticity)* and increasing resistance to depolarisation *(refractoriness)*. In turn, this transiently slows the sinus rate and conduction velocity and increases the refractory period in the atrioventricular (AV) node. SVT is usually evident on the electrocardiogram (ECG) as a regular, narrow-complex tachycardia, and often it is caused by a self-perpetuating electrical (re-entry) circuit that includes the AV node. Increasing refractoriness in the AV node temporarily breaks the re-entry circuit, which allows normal depolarisations from the sinoatrial (SA) node to resume control of heart rhythm *(cardioversion).* Where the circuit does not involve the AV node (e.g. in atrial flutter), adenosine will not induce cardioversion. However, by blocking conduction to the ventricles, it allows closer inspection of the atrial rhythm on the ECG. This may reveal the diagnosis. The duration of effect of adenosine is very short because it is rapidly taken up by cells (e.g. red cells). Its half-life in plasma is less than 10 seconds.
Important adverse effects	By interfering with the functions of the SA and AV nodes, adenosine can induce **bradycardia** and even **asystole**. Inevitably, this is accompanied by a deeply unpleasant sensation. It is said to feel like a **sinking feeling** in the chest, often accompanied by **breathlessness** and a **sense of 'impending doom'**. Fortunately, due to the drug's short-lived effect, this feeling is only brief.
Warnings	Adenosine is contraindicated in ✖ **hypotension,** ✖ **coronary ischaemia** or ✖ **decompensated heart failure,** where its transient haemodynamic effects may be intolerable. Adenosine may induce bronchospasm in susceptible individuals, so should be avoided in ✖ **asthma** and ▲ **COPD.** People with a ▲ **heart transplant** are very sensitive to the effects of adenosine, because in the absence of vagal innervation, the sinus and AV nodes show an exaggerated response to neurotransmitter stimulation. Lower doses should be used, and under specialist direction only.
Important interactions	▲ Dipyridamole, an antiplatelet agent, blocks cellular uptake of adenosine. This prolongs and potentiates its effect, so the dose of adenosine should be halved. Theophylline and aminophylline (systemic bronchodilators) are competitive antagonists of adenosine receptors and reduce its effect. People who have taken these drugs respond poorly and may require higher doses.

PRACTICAL PRESCRIBING

Prescription	Adenosine is always given IV. The initial dose is usually 6 mg IV once only. If this is ineffective, 12 mg may be given, followed if necessary by 18 mg. Lower doses (e.g. 3 mg initially) are preferred if given via a central line or to a person taking dipyridamole or with a transplanted heart.
Administration	Adenosine should be administered only by doctors experienced in its use, or under their direct supervision, in a suitably equipped high-dependency environment. It is important that adenosine reaches the heart quickly to minimise cellular uptake *en route*. This requires a large-bore cannula (e.g. 18 G [green] or bigger), sited as proximally as possible (e.g. in the antecubital fossa). Administer the dose as a rapid injection and then immediately follow it with a flush, e.g. 20 mL of 0.9% sodium chloride. The effect will usually be evident on the cardiac monitor within 10–15 seconds, and then dissipate over about 30–60 seconds.
Communication	Explain that you are offering treatment with a medicine that will hopefully 'reset' their heart into a normal rhythm. Explain that it will briefly make them feel terrible, but this sensation will only last for about 30 seconds. Talk to the patient during its administration, acknowledging the unpleasant sensation and reassuring them it will go away quickly. Observing profound bradycardia or transient asystole on the cardiac monitor may induce some anxiety on your part too. Try not to convey this externally!
Monitoring and stopping	Administration of adenosine requires very close monitoring. This *must* include a continuous cardiac rhythm strip (preferably multiple leads), recorded for subsequent inspection. If cardioversion is not achieved after following the escalating dose ladder (see PRESCRIPTION), it should generally be stopped and other options considered.
Cost	Adenosine is inexpensive.

Clinical tip—Advance preparation is invaluable in the administration of adenosine. Plan what doses you will give and draw these up away from the bedside. Use small syringes (e.g. 2 mL) for adenosine, as this will make it easier to administer rapidly. Draw up one 20 mL 0.9% sodium chloride flush for each planned dose, plus one spare. *Label all the syringes carefully.* To administer the drug, first attach a three-way tap to the cannula. Use your spare flush to check its patency. Next, replace this with a new, full flush, and attach the first dose of adenosine to the other port. Start the continuous ECG recording, then (after warning the patient) administer the adenosine and the flush in rapid succession. Stop the ECG recording once a stable cardiac rhythm resumes, print it out and annotate it to indicate when and how much adenosine was administered.

Adrenaline (epinephrine)

CLINICAL PHARMACOLOGY

Common indications	**❶** In **cardiac arrest** (given IV) as part of the Advanced Life Support (ALS) treatment algorithm for shockable and non-shockable rhythms. **❷** In **anaphylaxis** (given IM) for immediate management. **❸** In **croup** (by nebuliser) if response to initial treatment with a **corticosteroid** is insufficient (see CLINICAL TIP). **❹** Adrenaline may be injected directly into tissues to induce **local vasoconstriction,** e.g. during endoscopy to control mucosal bleeding, or premixed with **local anaesthetics** to prolong their effect.
Mechanisms of action	Adrenaline is a potent **agonist** of the α_1-, α_2-, β_1- and β_2-**adrenoceptors,** and correspondingly has a multitude of sympathetic ('fight or flight') effects. These include vasoconstriction of vessels supplying skin, mucosa, and abdominal viscera (mainly α_1 mediated); increases in heart rate, force of contraction, and myocardial excitability (β_1); and vasodilation of vessels supplying the heart and muscles (β_2). These explain its use in cardiac arrest, where the redistribution of blood flow in favour of the heart is desirable, at least theoretically. However, clinical trials have shown mixed results, and there is some evidence of harm if adrenaline is administered too early in those with shockable rhythms (see PRESCRIPTION). In anaphylaxis, where widespread release of inflammatory mediators from mast cells produces generalised vasodilatation, profound hypotension and often bronchoconstriction, the vasoconstrictor effects of adrenaline may be life-saving. In addition, via β_2-receptors, it causes bronchodilatation and suppresses inflammatory mediator release from mast cells.
Important adverse effects	Adrenaline is a dangerous drug, but its risks are balanced against the severity of the condition being treated. In cardiac arrest, restoration of output is often followed by adrenaline-induced **hypertension.** It may cause **anxiety, tremor, headache,** and **palpitations.** It may also precipitate **angina, myocardial infarction,** and **arrhythmias,** particularly in people with existing heart disease.
Warnings	There are no contraindications to the use of adrenaline for life-threatening conditions. When given to induce local vasoconstriction, it should be used with caution in ▲ **heart disease.** Combination adrenaline–anaesthetic preparations should not be used in ✖ **areas supplied by an end-artery** (i.e. with poor collateral supply), such as fingers and toes, where vasoconstriction can cause tissue necrosis.
Important interactions	Co-administration with ▲ β-**blockers** may induce widespread vasoconstriction, because the α_1-mediated vasoconstricting effects cannot be opposed by β_2-mediated vasodilatation.

PRACTICAL PRESCRIBING

Prescription	In life-threatening situations, adrenaline is administered first then prescribed later. The name 'adrenaline' is still used for prescribing in the UK, although the international non-proprietary name (epinephrine) is also printed on product packaging. In adult cardiac arrest with a shockable rhythm (ventricular fibrillation (VF) or pulseless ventricular tachycardia (VT)), adrenaline 1 mg IV is given after the third shock, and repeated every 3–5 minutes thereafter (i.e. every other cycle of cardiopulmonary resuscitation (CPR)). If the rhythm is not shockable (asystole or pulseless electrical activity), adrenaline 1 mg IV is given as soon as IV access is available, and then repeated every 3–5 minutes. In anaphylaxis, the adult dose is 500 micrograms administered IM to the anterolateral thigh. This may be repeated after 5 minutes if necessary. Most practitioners should *not* administer IV adrenaline in anaphylaxis, unless cardiac arrest supervenes. However, it may be used by specialists in high-dependency environments (e.g. critical or peri-operative care).
Administration	In cardiac arrest, adrenaline is administered from a pre-filled syringe containing a 1:10,000 (1 mg in 10 mL) solution. For adults, administer the whole 10 mL, followed by a flush (e.g. 10 mL of 0.9% sodium chloride). In anaphylaxis, give 0.5 mL of a 1:1000 (1 mg in 1 mL) adrenaline solution by IM injection. Inject this into the anterolateral aspect of the thigh halfway between the knee and the hip, from where it should be rapidly absorbed. If there is thick subcutaneous tissue (e.g. in obesity), you may need to inject deeply in order to be confident of IM administration.
Communication	In anaphylaxis, simultaneously with providing treatment, explain that they are experiencing a severe allergic reaction and that you are giving them an injection of adrenaline to treat this.
Monitoring and stopping	In the context of cardiac arrest and anaphylaxis, intensive clinical and haemodynamic monitoring should be instituted as soon as practical. Adrenaline injections are for immediate life-saving treatment only.
Cost	Cost is not a consideration at the bedside.

Clinical tip—In children with croup (laryngotracheitis), nebulised adrenaline is an unlicensed but widely recommended treatment for those whose condition has not responded adequately to a **systemic corticosteroid**. The dose is 400 micrograms/kg (to a maximum of 5 mg), prepared from the 1:1000 (1 mg/mL) solution. Doses less than 3 mg should be diluted to 3 mL using 0.9% sodium chloride to ensure effective nebulisation. It is important to note that this is a symptomatic treatment only, which does not alter the course of the underlying disease. Its effect lasts 1–2 hours.

Fibrinolytic drugs

CLINICAL PHARMACOLOGY

Common indications	❶ In **acute ischaemic stroke,** alteplase increases the chance of living independently if it is given within 4.5 hours of the onset of the stroke, alone or in combination with mechanical thrombectomy (see CLINICAL TIP). ❷ In **ST-elevation acute coronary syndrome,** fibrinolytic drugs can reduce mortality when they are given within 12 hours of the onset of symptoms in combination with antiplatelet agents and anticoagulants. However, primary percutaneous coronary intervention (where available) has largely superseded fibrinolytics in this context. ❸ For **massive pulmonary embolism (PE)** with haemodynamic instability, fibrinolytic drugs reduce clot size and pulmonary artery pressures, but there is no clear evidence that they improve mortality.
Mechanisms of action	Fibrinolytic drugs, also known as thrombolytic drugs, **catalyse the conversion of plasminogen to plasmin,** which acts to dissolve fibrinous clots and re-canalise occluded vessels. This allows reperfusion of affected tissue, preventing or limiting tissue infarction and cell death and improving outcomes.
Important adverse effects	Common adverse effects include **nausea** and **vomiting, bruising** around the injection site, and **hypotension**. Adverse effects that require treatment to be stopped include **serious bleeding, allergic reaction, cardiogenic shock,** and **cardiac arrest.** Serious bleeding may require treatment with coagulation factors and antifibrinolytic drugs, e.g. **tranexamic acid,** but this is usually avoidable as fibrinolytic agents have a very short half-life. Reperfusion of infarcted brain or heart tissue can lead to **cerebral oedema** and **arrhythmias,** respectively.
Warnings	There are many contraindications to thrombolysis, which are mostly factors that predispose to ✖ **bleeding,** including recent haemorrhage, recent trauma or surgery, bleeding disorders, severe hypertension, and peptic ulcers. In acute stroke, ✖ **intracranial haemorrhage** must be excluded with a computed tomography (CT) scan before treatment. ✖ **Previous streptokinase treatment** is a contraindication to repeat dosing (although other fibrinolytics can be used), as development of antistreptokinase antibodies can block its effect.
Important interactions	The risk of haemorrhage is increased in people taking **anticoagulants** and **antiplatelet** agents. **Angiotensin-converting enzyme (ACE) inhibitors** appear to increase the risk of anaphylactoid reactions.

PRACTICAL PRESCRIBING

Prescription	Fibrinolytic drugs should be prescribed only by clinicians with expertise in their use. The dose varies depending on the indication, timing from the onset of symptoms, and body weight. They are available as injectable preparations only. A bolus dose is usually given first, followed by an IV infusion.
Administration	Fibrinolytic drugs should be administered in a high-dependency area such as the emergency department, hyperacute stroke unit or coronary care unit, by staff with expertise in their use. Alteplase comes as a powder, which is reconstituted with sterile water (also provided in the package), and then either given directly as an IV bolus injection or diluted further in 0.9% sodium chloride and given as an IV infusion.
Communication	The decision to 'thrombolyse' (prescribe fibrinolytic therapy) should be made by an expert clinician, and the risks and benefits carefully explained. For example, in acute stroke, explain that part of the brain is being starved of blood and oxygen due to a blocked artery, which will cause long-term damage. Giving a 'clot-busting drug' can reduce damage to the brain by dissolving the blood clot and restoring blood flow. However, it works only if given soon after the onset of the stroke. With or without treatment, people may show some improvement, but symptoms may also get worse. On average, among every three people with a stroke, one will die. Although the chance of death is increased initially after receiving a clot-busting drug (due to bleeding), after the first week the chances of living independently are increased. For licensed indications, written consent is not essential but verbal consent should be obtained. If neurological impairment prevents consent, treatment can still be given if judged to be in the individual's best interests.
Monitoring and stopping	Management should be in a high-dependency area, with vital signs checked every 15 minutes for the first 2 hours. This should include observation for signs of bleeding, anaphylaxis and, particularly in the case of acute stroke, neurological deterioration. If there are any signs of adverse effects treatment should be stopped immediately.
Cost	Fibrinolytic agents are currently available as branded products only. A typical dose of alteplase costs around £300–£600 and streptokinase costs around £80.

Clinical tip—In acute ischaemic stroke, the benefits of thrombolysis diminish rapidly with time. Compared with untreated patients, the chance of being alive and independent at 6 months is increased by 10% if thrombolysis is given within 3 hours of symptom onset, but only 2% at 3–6 hours. Endovascular clot removal (mechanical thrombectomy) is increasingly superseding thrombolysis for large, proximal, anterior circulation strokes—in which it may be superior, and the window for intervention is wider (up to 24 hours in some cases).

Naloxone

CLINICAL PHARMACOLOGY

Common indications	Acute treatment of **opioid toxicity** associated with respiratory and/or neurological depression. A pre-filled syringe formulation, suitable for administration in the community, may be indicated for individuals at high risk of recurrent opioid toxicity due to drug misuse. It is intended for administration (after appropriate training) by someone close to that person as a life-saving intervention.
Mechanisms of action	Naloxone binds to opioid receptors, particularly the pharmacologically important **opioid μ-receptors,** where it acts as a **competitive antagonist.** It has little or no effect in the absence of an exogenous opioid (e.g. morphine). However, if an opioid is present, naloxone displaces it from receptors and reverses its effects. In opioid toxicity, this is used to restore an adequate level of consciousness and respiratory rate.
Important adverse effects	Naloxone has few intrinsic adverse effects. However, the effect of opioid reversal in an opioid-dependent individual may be a significant **opioid withdrawal reaction**. This presents with pain (if the opioid was being taken for its analgesic effect), restlessness, nausea and vomiting, dilated pupils, and cold, dry skin with piloerection ('cold turkey').
Warnings	There are no specific contraindications to the use of naloxone. However, caution should be exercised in people with ▲ **opioid dependence** (whether from therapeutic or recreational use) because of the risk of precipitating opioid withdrawal. Lower doses should be used in ▲ **palliative care** to reduce the risk of complete reversal of analgesia.
Important interactions	Naloxone has no clinically important drug interactions other than its interaction with opioids, which is central to its pharmacological and therapeutic effects.

PRACTICAL PRESCRIBING

Prescription	Acute opioid toxicity can usually be adequately reversed with naloxone 400–1200 micrograms IV, titrated to effect (see ADMINISTRATION). Lower doses, and smaller increments, should be used in palliative care settings. If IV access is impractical, it can be given IM, SC or intranasally. In an emergency it is reasonable to treat first and prescribe later. The pre-filled syringe formulation (Prenoxad®), for individuals at high risk of opioid overdose, should be prescribed only after careful assessment and training. The practicalities of this will depend on local pathways; this should be overseen by a specialist drugs misuse service.
Administration	In hospital, naloxone is usually administered by the prescriber or under their direct supervision. Incremental doses (e.g. 200–400 micrograms IV) are given every 2–3 minutes until satisfactory reversal is achieved (rousable with adequate respiration). For opioid toxicity in the context of chronic use (especially in palliative care), smaller incremental doses (e.g. 40–100 micrograms) should be used. The form of naloxone intended for use by members of the public is given by IM injection in doses of 400 micrograms (0.4 mL of the 1 mg/mL solution) every 2–3 minutes until professional help arrives.
Communication	Once consciousness returns, you can, as appropriate for the situation, explain that they required life-saving treatment for the overdose. Depending on the clinical context, you may need to discuss how this situation arose and how to avoid it in future. For individuals at high risk of recurrent overdose due to opioid misuse, it may be appropriate to discuss supplying naloxone for them to keep on their person, for emergency life-saving use by someone close to them.
Monitoring and stopping	Close monitoring is essential, as the dose is titrated to effect. Once adequate reversal is achieved, monitoring should continue for at least an hour. This is because the duration of action of naloxone (about 20–60 minutes, depending on route of administration) is shorter than that of most opioids. Consequently, opioid toxicity can recur when the effect of naloxone has dissipated, necessitating repeated doses or, occasionally, an infusion. If an infusion is used, the appropriate duration of therapy will depend on the half-life of the opioid and the absorption characteristics of the formulation (e.g. longer if a modified-release formulation). Expert advice (e.g. from critical care) is essential.
Cost	Naloxone is available in non-proprietary form and is inexpensive.

Clinical tip—When giving very small doses of naloxone (e.g. 40 micrograms), it is impractical to use the 400 microgram/mL solution that is usually available on the wards. Therefore take 1 mL (400 micrograms) of this solution in a 10-mL syringe and add 9 mL of 0.9% sodium chloride. Label the syringe immediately. The resulting 40-microgram/mL solution can then be administered in more practical 1-mL increments.

Oxygen

CLINICAL PHARMACOLOGY

Common indications	❶ To increase tissue oxygen delivery in **acute hypoxaemia.** It is also used for *long-term oxygen therapy* (LTOT) in **chronic hypoxaemia,** but this is outside the scope of this monograph. ❷ To accelerate reabsorption of pleural gas in **pneumothorax.** ❸ To reduce carboxyhaemoglobin half-life in **carbon monoxide (CO) poisoning.**
Mechanisms of action	An abnormally low partial pressure of oxygen (PO_2) in arterial blood (PaO_2), termed *hypoxaemia,* may be a consequence of a wide range of disease processes. It reduces delivery of oxygen to tissues *(hypoxia)*, increasing their reliance on anaerobic metabolism for energy generation. Supplemental oxygen therapy increases PO_2 in alveolar gas (P_AO_2), driving more rapid diffusion of oxygen into blood. The resulting rise in PaO_2 increases delivery of oxygen to the tissues (but note CLINICAL TIP), which in effect 'buys time' while the underlying disease is corrected. In *pneumothorax,* supplemental oxygen has an additional benefit of reducing the fraction of nitrogen in alveolar gas. This accelerates the diffusion of nitrogen out of the body. Since pleural air is composed mostly of nitrogen, this increases its rate of reabsorption. In *CO poisoning,* oxygen competes with CO to bind with haemoglobin and thereby shortens the half-life of carboxyhaemoglobin, returning haemoglobin to a form that can transport oxygen to tissues.
Important adverse effects	The most common adverse effects of oxygen are related to the delivery device (e.g. the **discomfort of a face mask**; nasal cannulae may be more comfortable) or its lack of water vapour (**dry throat**; humidification may improve this). Except in pneumothorax and CO poisoning, there is little to be gained from an *abnormally high* PaO_2 and, indeed, there is some evidence that **hyperoxaemia may be harmful**. Routine oxygen administration to *non-hypoxaemic* patients with stroke and myocardial infarction does not improve, and may worsen, outcomes. This may be because hyperoxaemia induces vasoconstriction in systemic arteries.
Warnings	People with **chronic type 2 respiratory failure** (e.g. those with severe COPD) exhibit several adaptive changes in response to persistent hypoxaemia and hypercapnia. If exposed to high inspired oxygen concentrations, this finely balanced adaptive state may be disturbed, resulting in a rise in $PaCO_2$. This may lead to respiratory acidosis, depressed consciousness, and worsened tissue hypoxia. This necessitates a different approach to oxygen therapy (see PRESCRIPTION and ADMINISTRATION). Oxygen accelerates combustion and therefore presents a fire risk if exposed to a **heat source or naked flame,** including from smoking.
Important interactions	There are no clinically important interactions.

PRACTICAL PRESCRIBING

Prescription	Oxygen therapy should always be guided by a written prescription, except in emergencies when it may be administered first and prescribed later. The key feature of the oxygen prescription is the specification of a **target oxygen saturation (SpO$_2$) range,** as measured by pulse oximetry. The target SpO$_2$ should be 94%–98% in most people and 88%–92% in those with chronic type 2 respiratory failure. For the initial delivery device, in general, prescribe a reservoir ('non-rebreathing') mask for emergency treatment of critical illness or profound hypoxia, a Venturi mask (28%) for those in chronic type 2 respiratory failure, and nasal cannulae for everyone else.
Administration	*Reservoir masks* have a bag (reservoir) that is continuously filled by the incoming oxygen supply. Inspired gas is drawn from the bag and so contains a high oxygen concentration (at least 60%–80%). The oxygen flow rate should be 15 L/min. *Venturi devices* blend oxygen with air in a fixed ratio. These devices may be colour-coded nozzles attached to masks (delivering a fixed FiO$_2$) or wall-mounted devices (adjustable FiO$_2$, usually with humidification). *Nasal cannulae* deliver a variable oxygen concentration (roughly 24%–50% at flow rates of 2–6 L/min). *Simple face masks* are also variable-performance devices; they have few advantages over nasal cannulae and are less comfortable. *Humidified high-flow nasal oxygen* is an advanced therapy in which a warmed, humidified air/oxygen mixture (with specified FiO$_2$) is delivered at a high flow rate (typically >40 L/min). This can provide high FiO$_2$ (up to 100%), together with a low level of positive end-expiratory pressure. It may be a better option than a reservoir mask in non-hypercapnic (type 1) respiratory failure.
Communication	Explain that oxygen should generally be administered continuously, although face masks may briefly be removed to allow eating and drinking. Ask them to report any discomfort, as it may be possible to improve this with a different device or the addition of humidification.
Monitoring and stopping	Frequent SpO$_2$ monitoring is essential when supplemental oxygen is required in acute illness. The device and/or flow rate should be adjusted as necessary to keep the SpO$_2$ within the target range. Additionally, arterial blood gas measurement is informative in critical illness; people who may also have hypercapnoea (i.e. type 2 respiratory failure); and those with hypoxaemia that is unexpected or progressive. Unless hyperoxia is required (pneumothorax, CO poisoning), oxygen is stopped if the target SpO$_2$ range is achieved breathing air.
Cost	Cost of oxygen therapy is not a consideration at the bedside.

Clinical tip—Remember that SpO$_2$ is only one determinant of the amount of oxygen reaching the tissues. The others are cardiac output and haemoglobin concentration. Neglecting these, if they are significantly abnormal, may render oxygen therapy worthless.

Fluids

Colloids (plasma substitutes)

CLINICAL PHARMACOLOGY

Common indications	❶ To expand circulating volume in states of **impaired tissue perfusion** (including **shock**). However, compound sodium lactate and sodium chloride 0.9% are preferred. ❷ In **cirrhotic liver disease,** albumin is used to mitigate haemodynamic effects from large-volume **paracentesis** (ascitic fluid drainage).
Mechanisms of action	Colloid fluid preparations contain comparatively large, **osmotically active molecules,** such as albumin or modified gelatin. These do not readily cross semipermeable membranes, such as vascular endothelium, so in principle, their osmotic effect should 'hold' the infused volume in the intravascular compartment. Their effect in **expanding circulating volume** is therefore potentially greater than that of a crystalloid (a solution of small, water-soluble molecules, e.g. sodium chloride). Under experimental conditions, 70%–80% of a gelatin-based colloid remains in the plasma. However, in pathological states in which volume expansion is required (e.g. sepsis), the capillaries are 'leaky', and the colloid is lost into the interstitium more rapidly than predicted. On balance, evidence suggests that colloids are no better than crystalloids, and trials using starch-based colloids have demonstrated harm. Sodium-based crystalloids (e.g. compound sodium lactate, sodium chloride 0.9%) are therefore usually preferred. In people with ascites due to cirrhotic liver disease, large-volume paracentesis (generally defined as >5 L) can abruptly lower intraabdominal pressure. This reduces systemic vascular resistance, increases the capacitance of abdominal veins, and encourages fluid shifts from the intravascular to extracellular compartment. The resulting haemodynamic effects can be mitigated by plasma volume expansion, for which albumin is recommended.
Important adverse effects	Infusion of colloid solutions promotes **oedema**. Excessive plasma volume expansion may increase left ventricular filling beyond the point of maximal contractility on the Starling curve, **worsening cardiac output** and potentially precipitating **pulmonary oedema**. Gelatins may cause **hypersensitivity reactions,** including anaphylaxis—another reason to prefer crystalloids, which are non-allergenic.
Warnings	Caution is required in ▲ **heart failure,** due to the risk of worsening cardiac output (see ADVERSE EFFECTS). If fluid resuscitation is required, it is best to reduce the *volume* of fluid challenges, but still to infuse them *rapidly* so that the effect of transient volume expansion is appreciated. In ▲ **renal impairment,** monitor fluid balance closely to avoid volume overload.
Important interactions	There are no clinically important interactions.

PRACTICAL PRESCRIBING

Prescription	Synthetic colloids are usually prescribed by brand name. Specify the volume to be infused and the rate at which it is to be given. The rate may be stated either in mL/hr or as the intended duration for infusion of the total volume. For example, in the unusual situation that at colloid is used for **shock,** Gelofusine® 250 mL to be given IV over 5 minutes might be prescribed. For **large-volume paracentesis,** consult with local specialists regarding the need for albumin. A common regimen is to give 100 mL of albumin 20% solution IV for every 2 L of ascitic fluid drained.
Administration	Infusions may be administered simply through a giving set, in which case the flow is controlled with a roller valve. A pressure bag can be applied to infuse the fluid more quickly if required. An infusion pump can be used to control the rate and volume precisely, although the maximum infusion rate is usually too slow for an effective fluid challenge. An alternative is to use a 50-mL syringe and a three-way tap to give the desired volume by successive injection of aliquots.
Communication	Explain that you advise treatment with fluid through a drip to (for example) improve blood pressure. Ask them to report any irritation, swelling, or wetness around the cannula site, as this may indicate that the cannula is not functioning correctly.
Monitoring and stopping	By definition, the need for fluid resuscitation identifies patients who are sick and require close monitoring. Assess haemodynamic status (e.g. pulse, blood pressure, capillary refill time, urine output, lactate) before and after infusion as a guide to further therapy. Fluid resuscitation should be stopped once acceptable haemodynamic endpoints are achieved, or if adverse effects outweigh benefits. Similarly, close monitoring is required in the context of large-volume paracentesis to detect adverse haemodynamic consequences, whether due to ascitic fluid drainage or albumin administration.
Cost	Colloid solutions are considerably more expensive than crystalloids.

Clinical tip—In managing a severely ill patient requiring large-volume fluid therapy, it is a good idea to use warmed fluids if possible, to avoid causing hypothermia. A fluid-warming device can usually be found in the operating department, emergency department or intensive care unit.

Compound sodium lactate (Hartmann's solution)

CLINICAL PHARMACOLOGY

Common indications	❶ To provide sodium and water for **people unable to meet their water and electrolyte requirements** orally (or by enteral tube). ❷ To expand circulating volume in states of **impaired tissue perfusion** (including **shock**). This may be done as a 'fluid challenge', where a bolus of fluid (e.g. 500 mL) is infused rapidly. Sodium chloride 0.9% and colloids are alternatives.
Mechanisms of action	Compound sodium lactate (more commonly known by its eponymous name, Hartmann's solution) is a balanced crystalloid solution. Its electrolyte composition approximates serum: 1 L contains Na^+ 131 mmol, Cl^- 111 mmol, K^+ 5 mmol, Ca^{2+} 2 mmol, and lactate 29 mmol. The infused lactate is readily metabolised, generating bicarbonate. This makes it a suitable choice for providing sodium and water in patients unable to take enough orally. As compound sodium lactate contains sodium in a concentration similar to extracellular fluid, the infused volume is largely retained in the extracellular water compartment. As intravascular water accounts for about 20% of extracellular water, about 20% of the infused volume will remain in vessels to expand circulating volume (a transiently greater increase may occur before distribution is complete). This makes it a viable choice for use in fluid resuscitation. Its main advantage over sodium chloride 0.9% is its lower chloride content, making it less likely to cause hyperchloraemic acidosis.
Important adverse effects	Compound sodium lactate contains sodium, diffusion of which into the interstitium promotes **oedema.** Excessive plasma volume expansion may increase left ventricular filling beyond the point of maximal contractility on the Starling curve, **worsening cardiac output** and potentially precipitating **pulmonary oedema**.
Warnings	Exercise caution during rapid infusion of IV fluid in patients with ▲ **heart failure,** due to the risk of pulmonary oedema (see Colloids). In **renal** impairment, monitor fluid balance closely to avoid overload. Compound sodium lactate contains potassium 5 mmol/L; this does not cause hyperkalaemia, but the serum potassium concentration should be monitored as part of overall disease management. Conventional advice is to avoid compound sodium lactate in ▲ **severe liver disease** because of reduced capacity to metabolise lactate. However, as lactate (the conjugate base) does not itself cause acidosis, the clinical implications of this are debatable.
Important interactions	Compound sodium lactate should not be mixed or infused with **ceftriaxone**, as its calcium content may cause precipitation.

PRACTICAL PRESCRIBING

Prescription	Compound sodium lactate is prescribed as an infusion. Specify the volume to be infused and the rate at which it is to be given. The rate may be described either in mL/hr or as the intended duration for infusion of the total volume. The typical adult maintenance requirement for sodium is 1 mmol/kg/day, which may be approximated with 500–1000 mL/day of compound sodium lactate. The remaining water requirement (to provide a total of 25–30 mL/kg/day) may be provided with glucose 5%. To expand circulating volume, compound sodium lactate is given as a 'fluid challenge' (e.g. 500 mL over 5 minutes in adults).
Administration	Infusions may be administered simply through a giving set, in which case the flow is controlled with a roller valve and the rate estimated from the number of drips per minute. A pressure bag can be applied to infuse fluid more quickly if required. Preferably, however, an infusion pump should be used to control the rate precisely. The maximum rate of infusion using a pump is usually too slow for an effective fluid challenge. An alternative is to use a 50-mL syringe and a three-way tap to give the desired volume by successive injection of aliquots.
Communication	Explain that you are offering treatment with a drip because (for example) they are unable to take enough fluid by mouth. As appropriate, encourage oral fluid intake, explaining that this is much better than giving fluid artificially. Ask them to report any irritation, swelling, or wetness around the cannula site, as this may indicate that the cannula is not functioning correctly.
Monitoring and stopping	Fluid balance must be monitored and recorded (see Glucose for further discussion). Stop IV fluids once requirements can be met orally. When administering fluid to expand circulating volume, assess haemodynamic status (e.g. pulse, blood pressure, capillary refill time, urine output, lactate) before and after infusion as a guide to further therapy.
Cost	Compound sodium lactate is inexpensive. However, the associated costs (including infusion equipment, consumables, staff time, and treatment of complications) are considerable.

Clinical tip—As it has a slightly lower sodium content and a substantially lower chloride content, compound sodium lactate is often preferable to sodium chloride 0.9%. There is much to be said for using it as your 'standard' sodium-based crystalloid solution. The main caveat is that it cannot be used for potassium replacement (whereas sodium chloride and glucose are routinely available in combination with potassium chloride in concentrations of 20 and 40 mmol/L).

Glucose (dextrose)

CLINICAL PHARMACOLOGY

Common indications	❶ To provide water for **people unable to meet their water requirements** orally (or by enteral tube). ❷ **Severe hypoglycaemia.** Glucagon is an alternative (see CLINICAL TIP). ❸ As a **substrate fluid** in people receiving IV **insulin** infusions. ❹ With **insulin** to treat **hyperkalaemia. Calcium gluconate** may also be given to stabilise the myocardium, and an ion-exchange agent (e.g. sodium zirconium cyclosilicate) to bind potassium in the gut. ❺ **Reconstitution and dilution of drugs** administered by injection or infusion. Sodium chloride 0.9% and sterile water are alternatives.
Mechanisms of action	Glucose ($C_6H_{12}O_6$) is a monosaccharide that is the principal source of energy for cellular metabolism. Of its several isomeric configurations, D-glucose (dextrose) is most relevant in mammalian biology. Glucose 5% is given by IV infusion as a means of providing water and may be used in the reconstitution and dilution of drugs. Its glucose content ensures it is *initially* isotonic with serum, so that it does not induce osmotic lysis of cells in the immediate vicinity of infusion. Glucose is rapidly taken up by cells and metabolised, leaving 'free' *(hypotonic)* water that distributes across all body water compartments. Higher-concentration glucose solutions are used to treat **hypoglycaemia;** the mechanism for this is self-explanatory. In **hyperkalaemia,** soluble **insulin** is given to stimulate Na^+/K^+-ATPase and shift potassium into cells. In this context, glucose is given to prevent hypoglycaemia.
Important adverse effects	**Glucose 50% is highly irritant to veins** and may cause local pain, phlebitis and thrombosis. Its use is now discouraged, unless it can be given via a central line. Glucose 20% is also irritant, but less so. **Hyperglycaemia** will occur if glucose administration exceeds its utilisation (more likely in people with diabetes mellitus).
Warnings	Giving IV glucose in ▲ **thiamine deficiency** can cause **Wernicke's encephalopathy**. If glucose is required for hypoglycaemia, thiamine (as Pabrinex®; see **Vitamins**) must also be given. In ▲ **renal failure,** close monitoring of fluid balance is essential to avoid overload. Administering hypotonic fluid in ▲ **hyponatraemia** (or in people more susceptible to its effects, e.g. ▲ **children** and those with ▲ **acute brain injuries**) may precipitate hyponatraemic encephalopathy.
Important interactions	Glucose and **insulin** have antagonistic effects, but are often administered concurrently (e.g. as a *substrate* for IV insulin, see INDICATIONS). The rate of glucose infusion should be kept constant unless treatment for hypoglycaemia is required.

PRACTICAL PRESCRIBING

Prescription	Glucose (*not* dextrose) is the approved name for prescribing. Specify the volume to be infused and the rate at which it is to be given. Rate may be specified either in mL/hr or as the duration for infusion of the total volume. The typical adult **maintenance requirement** for water is 25–30 mL/kg/day, some of which may be provided with a sodium-containing fluid (e.g. compound sodium lactate or sodium chloride 0.9%, to provide the daily sodium requirement) and the rest made up with glucose 5%. Write a separate prescription for each bag of fluid to be administered (see ADMINISTRATION). Potassium may be prescribed as a constituent of the glucose solution (e.g. 20 mmol per 1 L bag, 0.15%; see Potassium chloride). For treatment of **severe hypoglycaemia**, a typical prescription is for glucose 10% 200 mL IV over 15 minutes. In **hyperkalaemia,** glucose (e.g. glucose 50% 50 mL, or glucose 20% 125 mL) is infused with soluble **insulin** (Actrapid®) 10 units over 30 minutes.
Administration	IV fluids are provided in bags of various volumes, the largest of which is 1 L. Infusions may be administered simply through a giving set, in which case the flow is controlled with a roller valve, and the rate estimated from the number of drips per minute. It is preferable, though, to use an infusion pump to control the rate and volume precisely.
Communication	If providing IV fluids to supplement or replace oral intake, explain (if appropriate) that they should still try to take fluid by mouth, as this is much better than artificial hydration though a drip. Hypoglycaemia may result in uncooperativeness, but the person should be strongly encouraged to accept treatment before unconsciousness supervenes.
Monitoring and stopping	Fluid balance should be monitored carefully in all patients receiving IV fluid therapy. This consists of measuring fluid input (including oral intake and infusions) and output (urine output and additional losses, e.g. from surgical drains) and calculating the net fluid balance (input minus output) for each 24-hour period. Stop IV fluids once oral intake is sufficient. In the treatment of hypoglycaemia and hyperkalaemia, the serum glucose and potassium concentrations should be monitored.
Cost	Glucose solutions are inexpensive, but associated costs (e.g. equipment, consumables, staff time) are considerable.

Clinical tip—An alternative option for severe hypoglycaemia is **glucagon.** The dose is 1 mg and this can be conveniently given by IM injection if IV access is not available. Glucagon is a natural hormone that stimulates hepatic glycogenolysis and gluconeogenesis. However, it is poorly effective if hepatic glycogen stores are depleted, e.g. in malnutrition. If response is inadequate at 10 minutes, glucose should be given.

Potassium chloride

CLINICAL PHARMACOLOGY

Common indications	❶ Prevention of potassium depletion in **people unable to meet their electrolyte requirements** orally (see also **Potassium, oral**). ❷ Treatment of established **potassium depletion** and **hypokalaemia**. IV administration is necessary when this is severe (<2.5 mmol/L), symptomatic or associated with electrocardiogram (ECG) changes.
Mechanisms of action	The normal requirement to prevent potassium depletion is about 1 mmol/kg/day in adults with normal renal function. In people unable to tolerate dietary intake, who are instead receiving their sodium and water requirement by IV infusion, potassium may be provided intravenously. Established potassium depletion and hypokalaemia may be caused, for example, by diarrhoea, vomiting, drugs (e.g. **loop** and **thiazide diuretics**), and secondary hyperaldosteronism. In severe cases, hypokalaemia may result in arrhythmias (which may be life-threatening) and muscle weakness. IV potassium repletion in these scenarios may be life-saving. For best effect, IV potassium is given with sodium chloride rather than glucose. This is because infusion of negatively charged Cl⁻ ions promotes retention of K⁺ in the serum, whereas glucose may promote insulin release with resultant stimulation of Na^+/K^+-ATPase, shifting potassium into cells. Hypokalaemia is often associated with hypomagnesaemia. When it is, it may be difficult to correct unless magnesium is also replaced. Always check the magnesium level and prescribe magnesium replacement if necessary (seek advice on how to do this).
Important adverse effects	The major risk of IV potassium infusion is overcorrection leading to **hyperkalaemia** and a resultant risk of **arrhythmias.** Close monitoring is essential to avoid this. Potassium-containing solutions are **irritant to veins** if infused rapidly or in too high concentration. For this reason, the infusion rate in a peripheral vein should generally not exceed 10 mmol/hr.
Warnings	It is generally unnecessary and potentially dangerous to prescribe potassium in ▲ **renal impairment** or ▲ **oliguria,** as potassium losses are minimal and susceptibility to hyperkalaemia is high.
Important interactions	IV potassium has an additive effect with other **potassium-elevating drugs**, including **oral potassium, aldosterone antagonists**, potassium-sparing diuretics, **angiotensin-converting enzyme (ACE) inhibitors**, and **angiotensin-receptor blockers**.

potassium chloride 0.15% (20 mmol/L), 0.3% (40 mmol/L)

PRACTICAL PRESCRIBING

Prescription	Potassium chloride is not available as a 'stand-alone' solution on general wards. Instead, it is prescribed as an ingredient in sodium chloride and glucose solutions, in concentrations of 20 or 40 mmol/L.
Administration	Potassium should be infused at a rate no higher than 10 mmol/hr, due to the risks of venous irritation and cardiac toxicity. For routine use in prevention of potassium depletion, the other considerations for the administration of potassium are the same as those for fluid replacement in general. In the treatment of established potassium depletion and hypokalaemia, when the patient may be at heightened risk of arrhythmias, IV potassium should ideally be given into a large vein and under close monitoring. In intensive care units, higher concentrations may be given via a central venous catheter.
Communication	In maintenance fluid and electrolyte replacement, explain (as appropriate) that they should still try to take fluid by mouth, as this is much better than receiving it artificially though a drip. In established potassium depletion and hypokalaemia, advise that potassium replacement through a drip is required because a low potassium level in the blood can upset their heart rhythm, which is potentially very dangerous. Explain the need for close monitoring during this, including with blood tests. This is to ensure the low potassium level is corrected, but not overcorrected, because that too can be risky.
Monitoring and stopping	In maintenance fluid and electrolyte replacement, the serum potassium concentration should be monitored. The intensity of this depends on the clinical context. Close monitoring is necessary when treating established potassium depletion and hypokalaemia. IV potassium replacement should be stopped once the serum potassium concentration is normalised and oral intake is sufficient, or if hyperkalaemia or renal impairment develop.
Cost	Cost is not a factor in prescribing decisions for hypokalaemia.

Clinical tip—Although potassium chloride is added at the manufacturing stage, some prescribing systems require it to be specified as an 'additive'. Others require you to specify it as a concentration, either in mmol/L or as a percentage. Unfortunately, therefore, you need to be familiar with all three. For example, if you need to prescribe 10 mmol potassium in 500 mL of 0.9% sodium chloride, you might specify this as the *total amount* of potassium chloride in the bag (10 mmol), the *concentration per litre* (20 mmol/L) or the *concentration as a percentage* (0.15%). Which you use will depend on the requirements of the prescribing interface.

Red cells

CLINICAL PHARMACOLOGY

Common indications	To increase the oxygen-carrying capacity of blood in **anaemia** and **acute haemorrhage.** Depending on the indication, alternatives to transfusion include **iron** (for anaemia), erythropoietin (in renal disease), and cell salvage (during surgery). Decisions are informed by holistic assessment of the person's condition (symptomatic anaemia, acute bleeding), physiological reserves, markers of tissue oxygen delivery (e.g. lactate), and haemoglobin concentration (most evidence favours a 'restrictive' transfusion trigger of 70–80 g/L).
Mechanisms of action	The oxygen content of arterial blood (CaO_2) is determined primarily by its oxygen saturation and haemoglobin concentration. In severe anaemia causing adverse clinical effects (e.g. altered consciousness, myocardial ischaemia) and/or with markers of inadequate tissue oxygen delivery (e.g. lactic acidosis), there is rationale in transfusing red cells to improve CaO_2. Transfusion is also rational in acute major haemorrhage where, prior to haemodilution, haemoglobin concentration may initially be normal. It must be appreciated, though, that red cell transfusion has risks (see ADVERSE EFFECTS), and transfused red cells behave differently to native red cells. These factors may explain the *blood transfusion–anaemia paradox*: anaemia is associated with adverse outcomes, but transfusion to correct anaemia does not necessarily improve outcomes.
Important adverse effects	Immunological adverse effects include **haemolytic reactions** (e.g. life-threatening acute haemolysis due to ABO incompatibility) and non-haemolytic reactions (e.g. **febrile reactions, anaphylactic reactions,** and **transfusion-related acute lung injury (TRALI)**). Red cell transfusion can cause volume overload and pulmonary oedema (**transfusion-associated circulatory overload (TACO)**). It can also cause a variety of metabolic effects, including **hypocalcaemia** and **hypoglycaemia** (both due to citrate in the preservative solution), **hyperkalaemia** (due to cell lysis), and **iron overload** (after multiple transfusions for chronic anaemia). Although donated blood is carefully screened, **infection** (bacteria, viruses, prions) may very rarely be transmitted.
Warnings	▲ **Cardiac or renal disease** increases risk of TACO. ▲ **Immune suppression** increases risk of adverse effects from transfused mononuclear leucocytes, which may transmit latent cytomegalovirus (CMV). This may be mitigated by requesting irradiated, CMV-negative preparations (seek expert advice).
Important interactions	Calcium-containing infusions must not mix with red cell transfusions, as calcium chelates the citrate anticoagulant, which may cause clotting.

PRACTICAL PRESCRIBING

Prescription	Red cell units have an average volume of 280 mL (UK specifications 220–340 mL) and haemoglobin content of 53 g. They contain minimal plasma, platelets, granulocytes and clotting factors. Red cell units are typically prescribed for IV infusion over 1–2 hours, extended to 3 hours in patients at risk of TACO (when a **loop diuretic** may also be given—seek advice). Transfusion must be completed within 4 hours of removal from temperature-controlled storage. It is recommended that, unless there is active bleeding, one unit be prescribed at a time, with reassessment before giving further units (see MONITORING). In acute massive haemorrhage, multiple units may be administered rapidly, usually with other blood products (e.g. platelets, fresh frozen plasma), IV fluids and **tranexamic acid**.
Administration	The administration process begins with the collection of a pre-trans-fusion sample for cross-matching (or 'group and save' if transfusion is not required immediately). The person taking the sample must ask the patient (if able) to state their full name and date of birth, and cross-check this against the request form and identification (ID) wristband. They should label the sample at the bedside. It is best practice for the red cell pack to be collected by the person who is going to administer it, who should take it directly to the bedside. Before commencing transfusion they should perform final checks, including of name, date of birth, ID wristband and the unit's label and compatibility tag. A blood administration set is used for infusion.
Communication	Careful explanation is essential for informed decision-making. Explain the reason for transfusion; its benefits, risks, and practicalities; and any alternative options. Explain that they will no longer be eligible to donate blood. Provide written information if available, and document the discussion in the clinical notes.
Monitoring and stopping	Observations depend on the clinical context. At minimum, basic physiological observations should be checked before commencing the infusion, 15 minutes after starting it, and on completion. Symptoms and haemoglobin concentration should then be reassessed to determine whether further units are needed.
Cost	Blood products are costly and, more importantly, a scarce resource.

Clinical tip—The management of suspected adverse reactions to transfusions varies according to their nature and severity. However, the initial action is always the same: **stop the transfusion immediately.** Cross-check the patient's identity, compatibility tag, and label. If there is a mismatch, **alert the laboratory immediately,** because there may be another person in the hospital about to receive the unit intended for your patient.

Sodium chloride

CLINICAL PHARMACOLOGY

Common indications	❶ To provide sodium and water for **people unable to meet their water and electrolyte requirements** orally (or by enteral tube). ❷ To expand circulating volume in states of **impaired tissue perfusion** (including **shock**). Compound sodium lactate and colloids are alternatives. ❸ **Reconstitution and dilution of drugs** administered by injection or infusion. Glucose solutions and sterile water are alternatives.
Mechanisms of action	Extracellular fluid (ECF) is made up of intravascular water (about 20%) and interstitial water (about 80%). Sodium is partitioned into ECF by Na^+/K^+-ATPase on cell membranes, which pumps sodium out of cells in exchange for potassium. As sodium is the main cation in ECF, it is the principal determinant of its osmolality. Osmolality is tightly regulated within a narrow range, so an increase in body sodium content (e.g. due to administration of a sodium-containing fluid) leads to an increase in ECF volume. The amount by which a fluid expands ECF depends on its sodium concentration. Sodium chloride 0.9% contains sodium 154 mmol/L, similar to ECF. Accordingly, ECF expands by approximately the same amount as the volume of sodium chloride 0.9% administered. This distributes between the intravascular and interstitial compartments, so about 20% of the volume administered remains in vessels to expand circulating volume. Sodium chloride solutions are also used to provide sodium and water if oral intake is insufficient.
Important adverse effects	Diffusion of sodium and water into the interstitium promotes **oedema.** The concentration of chloride in sodium chloride 0.9% (154 mmol/L) is significantly higher than that of ECF (about 100 mmol/L). This may cause **hyperchloraemia** which, in turn, promotes **acidaemia.** Probably the best explanation for this (among the several proposed) is that as Cl^- concentration rises, so HCO_3^- concentration must fall (and/or H^+ and K^+ rise) to maintain electroneutrality. Excessive plasma volume expansion may increase left ventricular filling beyond the point of maximal contractility on the Starling curve, **worsening cardiac output** and potentially precipitating **pulmonary oedema**.
Warnings	Caution is required with rapid IV infusions in ▲ **heart failure,** due to the risk of pulmonary oedema (see Colloids for further discussion). In **renal impairment,** monitor fluid balance closely to avoid overload.
Important interactions	When reconstituting drugs, it is important to check its compatibility with the diluent. For example, **amiodarone** is incompatible with sodium chloride. Refer to local policies and product information.

PRACTICAL PRESCRIBING

Prescription	Prescribe 'sodium chloride 0.9%' rather than 'normal saline', since the latter is not the approved name, and gives a misleading impression of its constituents (its electrolyte content is not 'normal'). Specify the volume to be infused and the rate at which it is to be given. Rate may be specified either in mL/hr or as the duration for infusion of the total volume. The typical adult maintenance requirement for sodium is 1 mmol/kg/day, which may be approximated with 500–1000 mL/day of 0.9% sodium chloride. The remaining water requirement (making up to a total of 25–30 mL/kg/day, see CLINICAL TIP) may be provided with glucose 5%. To expand circulating volume, 0.9% sodium chloride is given as a 'fluid challenge' (e.g. 500 mL over 5 minutes in adults).
Administration	Infusions may be administered through a giving set, in which case the flow is controlled with a roller valve, and the rate estimated from the number of drips per minute. Preferably, though, an infusion pump should be used to control the rate and volume precisely. The maximum rate of infusion using a pump is usually too slow for an effective fluid challenge. An alternative is to use a 50-mL syringe and a three-way tap to give the desired volume by successive injection of aliquots.
Communication	Explain that you are offering treatment with a drip because (for example) they are unable to take enough fluid by mouth. If appropriate, encourage oral intake, explaining that this is much better than giving fluid artificially. Ask them to report any irritation, swelling or wetness around the cannula, as this may indicate that the cannula is not functioning correctly.
Monitoring and stopping	Fluid balance must be monitored and recorded (see Glucose). Stop IV fluids once oral intake is sufficient. When administering fluid to expand circulating volume, assess haemodynamic status (e.g. pulse, blood pressure, capillary refill time, urine output, lactate) before and after infusion as a guide to further therapy.
Cost	Sodium chloride itself is inexpensive. However, associated costs (e.g. equipment, consumables, staff time) are considerable.

Clinical tip—When estimating maintenance fluid requirement, a simple rule of thumb is to infuse fluid at an hourly rate (in mL/hr) equal to body weight. This will provide 24 mL/kg/day of water, which is close to the 25–30 mL/kg/day recommended in guidelines. For example, for a 75-kg adult, you might prescribe sodium chloride 0.9% (1 × 500 mL bag) and glucose 5% (2 × 1 L bags), each infused at 75 mL/hr.

Self assessment and knowledge integration

Single best answer questions

Cardiovascular medicine

Common Indications

1. A 68-year-old man is discharged from hospital following treatment for a non-ST-elevation myocardial infarction. He has made a good recovery and has no symptoms. His current medications are aspirin, clopidogrel, bisoprolol, and atorvastatin.

What additional drug is most likely to reduce the risk of further cardiovascular events?

A. Amiloride
B. Digoxin
C. Glyceryl trinitrate
D. Ramipril
E. Warfarin

Cardiovascular medicine

Common Indications

2. A 72-year-old woman with a previous diagnosis of heart failure (New York Heart Association class III) complains of ankle swelling and is slightly more breathless than usual. Her current medications are bisoprolol, bumetanide, and ramipril. Recent blood tests show mild hypokalaemia with a serum potassium concentration around 3.1 mmol/L (normal 3.5–4.7).

What drug should be added to her treatment?

A. Amiloride
B. Furosemide
C. Indapamide
D. Isosorbide mononitrate
E. Spironolactone

Cardiovascular medicine

Common Indications

3. A 76-year-old man is found to have atrial fibrillation. He is asymptomatic. He has a past medical history of hypertension, hypercholesterolaemia and heart failure (New York Heart Association class II). He takes furosemide, ramipril, and simvastatin and has no allergies. Physical examination is normal except for a heart rate of approximately 120 beats/min with an irregular rhythm.

What is the most appropriate drug for ventricular rate control?

A. Amiodarone
B. Bisoprolol
C. Digoxin
D. Doxazosin
E. Verapamil

Cardiovascular medicine

Mechanisms of action

4. An 82-year-old woman with ischaemic heart disease and cardiac failure is treated with bisoprolol, furosemide, ramipril, simvastatin, and spironolactone.

Which of her medications acts by inhibiting a membrane transport protein?

A. Bisoprolol
B. Furosemide
C. Ramipril
D. Simvastatin
E. Spironolactone

Cardiovascular medicine

Mechanisms of action

5. A 54-year-old man is found to have supraventricular tachycardia. Metoprolol is given in an effort to restore sinus rhythm.

What receptor is the main target of metoprolol?

A. α_1-adrenoceptor
B. α_2-adrenoceptor
C. β_1-adrenoceptor
D. β_2-adrenoceptor
E. β_3-adrenoceptor

Cardiovascular medicine

Important adverse effects

6. A 63-year-old woman presents to the practice nurse complaining of swollen ankles. Her past medical history includes hypertension, type 2 diabetes, and COPD. Her medication includes amlodipine, chlortalidone, metformin, gliclazide, and tiotropium. Examination is unremarkable save for slight pitting oedema of her ankles. The practice nurse suspects an adverse drug reaction.

What drug is most likely to be contributing to her peripheral oedema?

A. Amlodipine
B. Chlortalidone
C. Gliclazide
D. Metformin
E. Tiotropium

Cardiovascular medicine

Important adverse effects

7. A 42-year-old woman is admitted to hospital after collapsing on the train. The ambulance service recorded broad-complex tachycardia on an electrocardiogram (ECG), which spontaneously terminated. The pharmacist is concerned that her hospital admission may be due to an adverse effect of her medication, which includes amitriptyline.

To whom should this event be reported?

A. British National Formulary (BNF)
B. Care Quality Commission (CQC)
C. Manufacturer of the drug
D. Medicines and Healthcare Products Regulatory Agency (MHRA)
E. National Institute for Health and Care Excellence (NICE)

Cardiovascular medicine

Warnings

8. A 59-year-old woman is attending the pre-operative assessment clinic before having a hysterectomy. Her past medical history includes hypercholesterolaemia, hypertension, and a transient ischaemic attack (TIA). Her regular medications are amlodipine, atorvastatin, clopidogrel, indapamide, and ramipril.

What medicine should she be advised to stop taking 1 week before the procedure?

A. Amlodipine
B. Atorvastatin
C. Clopidogrel
D. Indapamide
E. Ramipril

Cardiovascular medicine

Important interactions

9. An 81-year-old man presents with syncope. He has a past medical history of hypertension, angina, and chronic obstructive pulmonary disease (COPD). His usual oral medications are amlodipine, diltiazem, indapamide, ramipril, and simvastatin. Two days ago, he saw a doctor who did not have access to his full medical records, but advised him that he should be taking a β-blocker. Bisoprolol was prescribed.

On examination, his heart rate is 45 beats/min. His blood pressure is 96/60 mmHg. The ECG shows third-degree heart block.

What medication is most likely to interact with bisoprolol to cause heart block?

A. Amlodipine
B. Diltiazem
C. Indapamide
D. Ramipril
E. Simvastatin

Cardiovascular medicine

Administration

10. A 48-year-old man has started taking isosorbide mononitrate immediate-release tablets 20 mg twice daily for prevention of angina symptoms.

What are the most appropriate times of day for him to take the tablets?

A. 8 am and 12 pm
B. 8 am and 3 pm
C. 8 am and 8 pm
D. 12 pm and 12 am
E. 12 pm and 8 pm

Cardiovascular medicine

Administration

11. A young man collapses at a wedding reception. He was seen fumbling with a cartridge-like device before he collapsed, but had not been able to use it. On examination, he is unresponsive. His breathing is noisy; this improves slightly with a head-tilt-chin-lift manoeuvre. His face appears flushed and his lips are swollen. A carotid pulse is palpable but it is thready.

An ambulance has been called but has not arrived. The cartridge-like device is handed to you. It is labelled 'EpiPen Auto-Injector'.

How should this be administered?

A. Intramuscularly into the anterolateral thigh
B. Intramuscularly into the triceps muscle
C. Intravenously into any available peripheral vein
D. Subcutaneously into the anterior abdominal wall
E. Subcutaneously into the tissue overlying the triceps muscle

Cardiovascular medicine

Communication

12. A 50-year-old White man attends a blood pressure check with his practice nurse. He was noted to have high blood pressure at a routine health check last month. As his blood pressure remains high, a decision is made to start antihypertensive treatment with ramipril.

What common side effect should the nurse discuss with him?

A. Blurred vision
B. Diarrhoea
C. Dry cough
D. Headache
E. Urinary retention

Cardiovascular medicine

Monitoring and stopping

13. A 58-year-old woman who started taking simvastatin 3 months ago is asked to attend a follow-up visit with her GP.

What blood test should be performed to monitor for side effects of statins?

A. Creatine kinase
B. Liver profile
C. Fasting lipid profile
D. Full blood count
E. Thyroid function tests

Cardiovascular medicine

Monitoring and stopping

14. A 68-year-old man has started taking eplerenone for heart failure following a myocardial infarction.

What test should be performed in the first 1–2 weeks of therapy to identify possible adverse effects?

A. Echocardiogram
B. Electrocardiogram
C. Serum brain natriuretic peptide
D. Serum potassium
E. Serum troponin

Critical care, peri-operative medicine, and pain

Mechanisms of action

15. A 66-year-old woman with severe chronic pain takes amitriptyline, ibuprofen, morphine, omeprazole, and senna.

Which of her medications acts by inhibiting synthetic enzyme function?

A. Amitriptyline
B. Ibuprofen
C. Morphine
D. Omeprazole
E. Senna

Critical care, peri-operative medicine, and pain

Important interactions

16. A 24-year-old woman is vomiting following an evacuation of retained products of conception, performed under general anaesthesia. She was given cyclizine 50 mg IV 30 minutes ago but this has not improved her symptoms.

Her past medical history is notable for a severe illness involving fever and muscles spasms, which was thought to have been precipitated by a prochlorperazine injection.

What is the most appropriate treatment for her nausea and vomiting?

A. Chlorpromazine
B. Cyclizine
C. Haloperidol
D. Metoclopramide
E. Ondansetron

Endocrinology and metabolic medicine

Mechanisms of action

17. A 45-year-old man with type 2 diabetes is taking metformin.

What is the main mechanism by which metformin lowers blood glucose concentration?

A. Increased pancreatic insulin secretion
B. Increased peripheral insulin sensitivity
C. Increased urinary glucose excretion
D. Reduced hepatic glucose output
E. Reduced intestinal glucose absorption

Endocrinology and metabolic medicine

Important adverse effects

18. A 78-year-old man is admitted to the emergency department with loss of consciousness and is found to have a blood glucose concentration of 1.2 mmol/L. His usual medications are bendroflumethiazide, bisoprolol, gliclazide, metformin, and prednisolone.

What drug is most likely to have caused his hypoglycaemic attack?

A. Bendroflumethiazide
B. Bisoprolol
C. Gliclazide
D. Metformin
E. Prednisolone

Endocrinology and metabolic medicine

Important adverse effects

19. A 59-year-old man with type 2 diabetes is found to have suboptimal glycaemic control. He takes metformin 1 g orally twice daily. He is content to start a second medication, but says he cannot accept an increased risk of hypoglycaemia.

What drug is most likely to increase the risk of hypoglycaemic attacks?

A. Empagliflozin
B. Gliclazide
C. Metformin
D. Pioglitazone
E. Sitagliptin

Endocrinology and metabolic medicine

Important adverse effects

20. A 70-year-old woman presents with abdominal pain and shock. A surgical cause is suspected, and she is placed 'nil by mouth' while arrangements for an emergency laparotomy are made. She has a past medical history of polymyalgia rheumatica. She has taken prednisolone 5 mg daily for several years, but none in the last 3 days because of nausea.

What is the most appropriate option for immediate steroid replacement?

A. Budesonide
B. Fludrocortisone
C. Fluticasone
D. Hydrocortisone
E. Prednisolone

21. A 28-year-old woman starts taking tamoxifen for locally advanced oestrogen-receptor positive breast cancer.

What is the most appropriate advice to give her regarding potential side effects?

A. It can stimulate milk production from her breasts

B. It causes infertility

C. It is safe to take during pregnancy

D. There is an increased risk of cancer of the lining of the womb

E. There is an increased risk of ovarian cancer

22. A 34-year-old woman is taking tamoxifen following a mastectomy for locally advanced oestrogen-receptor positive breast cancer. Her past medical history includes anxiety, hay fever, and schizophrenia. Her current medications are codeine, fluoxetine, loratadine, propranolol, and risperidone.

What drug is most likely to reduce the efficacy of tamoxifen?

A. Codeine

B. Fluoxetine

C. Loratadine

D. Propranolol

E. Risperidone

23. A 50-year-old man presents for a review of results of recent blood tests. He has a past medical history of type 2 diabetes and hypertension. He takes metformin 1 g orally twice daily and ramipril 10 mg orally daily.

Investigations: Creatinine 148 µmol/L (60–110), estimated glomerular filtration (eGFR) 44 mL/min/1.73 m^2 (>60)

What is the principle concern with metformin if taken in the context of renal impairment?

A. GI upset

B. Hypersensitivity reaction

C. Lactic acidosis

D. Megaloblastic anaemia

E. Taste disturbance

24. A 55-year-old man attends the general practice for a planned review. Three months ago, he was found to have type 2 diabetes, and has since made concerted efforts to follow lifestyle advice. You advise him to have a blood test to measure the haemoglobin A_{1c} (HbA$_{1c}$) level.

What HbA$_{1c}$ threshold best describes the level at which pharmacological therapy should be offered?

A. 28 mmol/mol (4.7%)
B. 48 mmol/mol (6.5%)
C. 53 mmol/mol (7.0%)
D. 58 mmol/mol (7.5%)
E. 64 mmol/mol (8.0%)

GI and liver

Common indications

25. A 48-year-old woman who has peptic ulcers caused by *Helicobacter pylori* infection presents to her GP to commence treatment. She is allergic to benzylpenicillin, which caused an anaphylactic reaction.

What is the most appropriate 1-week oral treatment regimen?

A. Lansoprazole, amoxicillin, and clarithromycin
B. Lansoprazole, amoxicillin, and metronidazole
C. Omeprazole and clarithromycin
D. Omeprazole and metronidazole
E. Omeprazole, clarithromycin, and metronidazole

GI and liver

Common indications

26. An 86-year-old woman has been taking codeine phosphate following a sprained wrist. Co-incidentally, she has noticed that this has improved the diarrhoea she usually suffers from as a result of diverticular disease.

Although her wrist has now healed, she is keen to continue taking the codeine, as not having to open her bowels so regularly has considerably improved her quality of life. However, the codeine does make her feel a little 'light headed', which she finds unpleasant.

What alternative opioid would be better to treat her diarrhoea?

A. Loperamide
B. Morphine (immediate release)
C. Morphine (modified release)
D. Oxycodone (modified release)
E. Pethidine

GI and liver

Important adverse effects

27. A 55-year-old woman with psoriatic arthritis was admitted to hospital 12 days ago with severe cellulitis. On admission, her liver function was normal but she has now developed cholestatic jaundice.

Her medications are flucloxacillin, methotrexate, morphine, paracetamol, and simvastatin.

Which drug is most likely to have caused cholestatic jaundice?

A. Flucloxacillin
B. Methotrexate
C. Morphine
D. Paracetamol
E. Simvastatin

GI and liver

Important interactions

28. A 44-year-old man complains of heartburn. His past medical history includes asthma, epilepsy, and hypothyroidism. His current medications are beclomethasone, carbamazepine, levothyroxine, montelukast, and salbutamol. His GP recommends a trial of Gaviscon in the first instance.

What medicine should he be advised to separate from Gaviscon by at least 2 hours?

A. Beclomethasone
B. Carbamazepine
C. Levothyroxine
D. Montelukast
E. Salbutamol

Haematology & immunology

Important interactions

29. A 77-year-old woman has persistent epistaxis (nose-bleeding). She was admitted to hospital 5 days ago with an exacerbation of COPD, for which she is being treated with clarithromycin, ipratropium, prednisolone, and salbutamol, together with controlled oxygen therapy. Her past medical history includes atrial fibrillation, for which she takes dabigatran.

What drug is most likely to increase the anticoagulant effect of dabigatran?

A. Clarithromycin
B. Ipratropium
C. Oxygen
D. Prednisolone
E. Salbutamol

Haematology & immunology

Important adverse effects

30. An 86-year-old man is admitted to the emergency department with shock after a major gastrointestinal bleed. His wife advises that he is taking dabigatran for atrial fibrillation.

What drug reverses the anticoagulant effect of dabigatran?

A. Andexanet α
B. Dried prothrombin complex
C. Idarucizumab
D. Phytomenadione (vitamin K_1)
E. Protamine

Haematology & immunology

Warnings

31. A 75-year-old man is found to have acute haemolytic anaemia. He has a past medical history of glucose-6-phosphate dehydrogenase (G6PD) deficiency. It emerges that he has inadvertently been taking medicines from his wife's blister pack instead of his own. Her medications include allopurinol, levothyroxine, metformin, quinine, and sitagliptin.

What drug is most likely to have precipitated haemolysis?

A. Allopurinol
B. Levothyroxine
C. Metformin
D. Quinine
E. Sitagliptin

Haematology & immunology

Monitoring and stopping

32. A 31-year-old woman develops a DVT when she is 16 weeks' pregnant and requires anticoagulation with a low-molecular-weight heparin for the rest of her pregnancy.

What test would be most useful to determine if her anticoagulation is adequate?

A. Activated partial thromboplastin time ratio
B. Antifactor Xa assay
C. INR
D. Plasma fibrinogen concentration
E. Platelet count

Infection

Common indications

33. A 22-year-old woman complains of dysuria. Her GP diagnoses an uncomplicated UTI. Her only medication is the combined oral contraceptive pill and she has not missed any doses of this. She has no allergies.

What is the most appropriate treatment?

A. Cefotaxime
B. Ciprofloxacin
C. Clarithromycin
D. Gentamicin
E. Trimethoprim

Infectious diseases

Common indications

34. A 72-year-old woman is admitted to hospital with severe cellulitis of her right leg. She has no allergies.

What is the most appropriate treatment?

A. Amoxicillin and clarithromycin
B. Benzylpenicillin and flucloxacillin
C. Cefotaxime and aciclovir
D. Co-amoxiclav and metronidazole
E. Co-amoxiclav and gentamicin

Infectious diseases

Common indications

35. An 83-year-old woman is admitted to the acute medical unit with mild community-acquired pneumonia (CURB-65 score 1). Her mobility is poor, but she has no active co-morbidities, does not usually take any medications, and has no allergies.

What is the most appropriate antibiotic treatment?

A. Cefotaxime
B. Ciprofloxacin
C. Doxycycline
D. Ertapenem
E. Flucloxacillin

36. A 77-year-old man with multiple sclerosis is admitted as an emergency with urinary sepsis. He has a long-term suprapubic catheter for the treatment of urinary retention. Urine cultures have grown *Pseudomonas aeruginosa*.

What antibiotic is most likely to be active against this organism?

A. Amoxicillin with clavulanic acid
B. Cefalexin
C. Nitrofurantoin
D. Piperacillin with tazobactam
E. Trimethoprim with sulfamethoxazole

37. A 75-year-old man is being treated for a UTI. He has no other medical problems, takes no regular medicines, and has no allergies. The results of his urine culture and sensitivity analyses suggest any β-lactam antibiotic would be suitable.

What antibiotic should be offered?

A. Amoxicillin
B. Ciprofloxacin
C. Clarithromycin
D. Doxycycline
E. Metronidazole

38. A 44-year-old man needs antibiotic treatment for an infection caused by a penicillinase-producing strain of *Staphylococcus aureus*.

What antibiotic is this organism most likely to be resistant to?

A. Benzylpenicillin
B. Co-amoxiclav
C. Flucloxacillin
D. Piperacillin with tazobactam
E. Vancomycin

39. A hospital antimicrobial guideline recommends use of the narrow-spectrum penicillin benzylpenicillin, rather than the broad-spectrum penicillin amoxicillin, as first-line antibiotic therapy for community-acquired pneumonia. It further recommends that this should be prescribed with doxycycline.

In general, what is the main advantage of narrow-spectrum over broad-spectrum antibiotics?

A. Easier to administer
B. Less likely to give rise to antibiotic resistance
C. Less likely to trigger an allergic reaction
D. More likely to be effective against β-lactamase-producing organisms
E. More likely to be effective where the pathogen is unknown

Infectious diseases

Important adverse effects

40. A 56-year-old man notices tinnitus and dizziness after discharge from hospital where he was treated for severe pneumonia. During this admission (which included a spell in the intensive care unit), his antibiotic treatment included courses of doxycycline, co-amoxiclav, clarithromycin, piperacillin with tazobactam, and gentamicin.

Which antibiotic is most likely to have caused this adverse effect?

A. Clarithromycin
B. Co-amoxiclav
C. Doxycycline
D. Gentamicin
E. Piperacillin with tazobactam

Infectious diseases

Important adverse effects

41. A 68-year-old woman is found to have cellulitis. She has a past medical history of hypertension, leg cramps and urge incontinence. Her medication comprises bendroflumethiazide, oxybutynin, and quinine sulfate. She is allergic to penicillin, which causes a rash. The doctor begins to prescribe clarithromycin, but is alerted to a possible interaction by the electronic prescribing system.

What is the main risk of prescribing clarithromycin in this case?

A. Hyperkalaemia
B. QT-interval prolongation
C. Renal impairment
D. Myopathy
E. Seizures

Infectious diseases

Important interactions

42. A 72-year-old woman is advised to take doxycycline 100 mg orally daily and prednisolone 30 mg orally daily for an exacerbation of COPD. Her usual medications are aspirin 75 mg daily, ferrous sulfate 200 mg twice daily, furosemide 40 mg daily, lansoprazole 30 mg daily and ramipril 5 mg daily, all taken orally.

What medicine should she be advised to separate from doxycycline by at least 2 hours?

A. Aspirin
B. Ferrous sulfate
C. Furosemide
D. Lansoprazole
E. Ramipril

Infectious diseases

Important interactions

43. A 58-year-old man attends his GP with a 2-day history of cough productive of green sputum, fever, and shortness of breath on exertion. His medical history includes atrial fibrillation, hypertension, and hypercholesterolaemia. His regular medications are bisoprolol, indapamide, ramipril, simvastatin, and warfarin. He is allergic to penicillin and doxycycline. His GP diagnoses a lower respiratory tract infection (LRTI) and prescribes clarithromycin.

What drug should be held while he is taking clarithromycin to avoid a significant drug interaction?

A. Bisoprolol
B. Indapamide
C. Ramipril
D. Simvastatin
E. Warfarin

Infectious diseases

Warnings

44. A 54-year-old man has a history of a severe anaphylactic reaction to penicillin. He now requires antibiotics for treatment of sepsis of uncertain cause.

What antibiotic is most likely to be safe in the context of a severe penicillin allergy?

A. Cefotaxime
B. Ciprofloxacin
C. Co-amoxiclav
D. Ertapenem
E. Piperacillin with tazobactam

Infectious diseases

Warnings

45. A 4-year-old boy is found to have pneumonia.

What antibiotic is contraindicated at this age?

A. Amoxicillin
B. Cefotaxime
C. Co-amoxiclav
D. Clarithromycin
E. Doxycycline

Infectious diseases

Warnings

46. A 33-year-old man with severe renal impairment requires antibiotic treatment for sepsis.

What antibiotic can generally be used without dosage reduction in severe renal impairment?

A. Benzylpenicillin
B. Co-amoxiclav
C. Gentamicin
D. Metronidazole
E. Vancomycin

Infectious diseases

Communication

47. A 29-year-old man who has been advised to take antibiotics asks his doctor if he can drink alcohol while on treatment.

What antibiotic should not be taken with alcohol?

A. Amoxicillin
B. Clarithromycin
C. Doxycycline
D. Metronidazole
E. Trimethoprim

Infectious diseases

Communication

48. A 19-year-old man has had seven episodes of genital herpes in the past year. He asks if he can start aciclovir tablets to reduce the frequency of attacks.

What is the most appropriate advice to give him regarding suppressive treatment with aciclovir?

A. He should take the treatment as soon as he notices the onset of symptoms
B. He should wash his hands before and after handling the tablets
C. He will need to continue the treatment indefinitely
D. It will clear his body of the virus within 6 months
E. It will not completely stop spread of infection to sexual partners

Infectious diseases

Monitoring and stopping

49. A 53-year-old man with severe *Haemophilus influenzae* epiglottitis, who has a history of severe allergy to all β-lactam antibiotics, is started on IV chloramphenicol.

Which test should be performed regularly to monitor treatment safety?

A. Audiometry
B. C-reactive protein
C. Full blood count
D. Liver function
E. Renal function

Infectious diseases

Monitoring and stopping

50. A 47-year-old woman is being treated with once-daily gentamicin for pyelonephritis. She received her first dose 21 hours ago. Her next dose is due in 3 hours and the nurse has called you to ask if any tests need to be performed before it is given.

What test is most useful in the first 48 hours of therapy to guide gentamicin dosing?

A. Audiometry
B. C-reactive protein (CRP) concentration
C. Estimated glomerular filtration rate (eGFR)
D. Serum creatinine concentration
E. Serum gentamicin concentration

51. A 54-year-old woman who presented with fever and left flank pain is found to have pyelonephritis. Co-amoxiclav 1.2 g IV 8-hrly is started. After 48 hours of antibiotics, her pain has improved and her temperature is 37.2°C.

Her blood tests show CRP 88 mg/L (admission 206, normal <4), white cell count (WCC) 10 × 10⁹/L (admission 15, normal 4–11) and normal renal function. *Escherichia coli* was cultured from urine, sensitive to nitrofurantoin, co-amoxiclav and piperacillin–tazobactam, but resistant to trimethoprim. Renal ultrasound showed no obstruction or collection.

What is the most appropriate next step in management?

A. Continue IV co-amoxiclav
B. Stop antibiotics
C. Switch to oral co-amoxiclav
D. Switch to oral nitrofurantoin
E. Switch to IV piperacillin with tazobactam

52. A 25-year-old woman presents to her GP to request a combined oral contraceptive pill. She has a past medical history of epilepsy, which is well controlled on lamotrigine 200 mg daily and levetiracetam 1 g 12-hrly. After appropriate assessment and counselling, a preparation containing ethinylestradiol 30 micrograms and levonorgestrel 150 micrograms per tablet (Microgynon 30) is prescribed.

What modification, if any, is most likely to be needed to her antiepileptic treatment?

A. Decrease levetiracetam dosage
B. Decrease lamotrigine dosage
C. Increase levetiracetam dosage
D. Increase lamotrigine dosage
E. No changes required to antiepileptic therapy

53. A 45-year-old woman is seen in her GP surgery with a 6-month history of moderate depression. Attempts to treat this with cognitive behavioural therapy have proved unsuccessful. There are no psychotic features and she is assessed to be at low risk of self-harm. She has no other medical problems.

What is the most appropriate treatment?

A. Amitriptyline
B. Citalopram
C. Mirtazapine
D. Olanzapine
E. Psychological interventions only

Neurology and psychiatry

Common indications

54. A 31-year-old woman with a past psychiatric history of bipolar disorder presents with a 2-month history of tiredness, reduced appetite, and general dissatisfaction with life. The psychiatrist makes a diagnosis of moderate bipolar depression and recommends pharmacological treatment. She is not currently taking any mood-stabilising medication and is concerned about the risk of precipitating a manic episode.

What is the most appropriate treatment?

A. Gabapentin
B. Lamotrigine
C. Lithium
D. Sertraline
E. Valproate

Neurology and psychiatry

Common indications

55. A 55-year-old man attends his GP complaining that he has been unable to sleep for weeks. He has recently lost his job and is worried about his finances. He would like to take something to help him sleep as he has a job interview in a few days.

What drug may be offered as a short-term measure to treat his insomnia?

A. Diazepam
B. Midazolam
C. Propofol
D. St John's wort
E. Zopiclone

Neurology and psychiatry

Common indications

56. A 55-year-old man presents to his GP complaining of pain in his right foot. He describes a prickling, burning sensation that has been present for some weeks, particularly at night, and is interfering with sleep. He has a past medical history of type 2 diabetes, for which he takes metformin. He also takes paracetamol regularly but this is insufficient.

What is the most appropriate treatment at this stage?

A. Amitriptyline
B. Carbamazepine
C. Ibuprofen
D. Morphine
E. Tramadol

Neurology and psychiatry

Mechanisms of action

57. A 75-year-old man with generalised tonic–clonic seizures secondary to cerebrovascular disease is advised to take levetiracetam.

What is the most likely molecular site of action of levetiracetam?

A. Calcium channels
B. γ-aminobutyric acid (GABA) receptors
C. Potassium channels
D. Sodium channels
E. Synaptic vesicles

58. A 20-year-old woman with epilepsy, who suffers from generalised tonic–clonic seizures of undetermined aetiology, is advised to take lamotrigine.

What symptom should prompt her to seek urgent medical attention?

A. Difficulty concentrating
B. Headache
C. Nausea
D. Rash
E. Tiredness

59. A 72-year-old woman has become aggressive on a general medical ward after being admitted with a significant urinary tract infection and delirium. Her medical problems include hypertension and type 2 diabetes. On admission, it was noted that her corrected QT interval was slightly prolonged. As she has been hitting the nursing staff with her walking stick repeatedly and is endangering herself and other patients, a decision is made to administer a drug to calm her.

What drug should be avoided because of her prolonged QT interval?

A. Diazepam
B. Haloperidol
C. Lorazepam
D. Propofol
E. Zopiclone

60. A 34-year-old man presents to the emergency department following a tonic–clonic seizure. In the course of this, he knocked over a kettle of boiling water and sustained a significant burn injury to his right arm, which will need to be cleaned once adequate analgesia is established. He has a past medical history of focal epilepsy, for which he takes carbamazepine.

What analgesic is most strongly contraindicated in this setting?

A. Codeine
B. Morphine
C. Naproxen
D. Paracetamol
E. Tramadol

Neurology and psychiatry

Warnings

61. A 58-year-old woman complains of fizzing shapes in her vision, followed by a headache and nausea. Her past medical history includes asthma, ischaemic heart disease, osteoporosis, psoriasis, and type 2 diabetes. Her doctor diagnoses migraine with aura and considers prescribing sumatriptan.

What is the main contraindication to prescribing sumatriptan in this case?

A. Asthma
B. Ischaemic heart disease
C. Osteoporosis
D. Psoriasis
E. Type 2 diabetes

Neurology and psychiatry

Important interactions

62. A 56-year-old man, who is an inpatient, has a 2-minute generalised tonic–clonic seizure. He was admitted 1 week ago with chest pain caused by a pulmonary embolus. Dalteparin, warfarin, paracetamol, and ibuprofen had been started. Three days ago, he was found to have hospital-acquired pneumonia, and meropenem was added. He has a past medical history of epilepsy. He takes sodium valproate (Epilim Chrono) 500 mg 12-hrly. He is allergic to penicillin (it brings him out in hives).

What medication is most likely to have interacted with valproate to increase the risk of seizures?

A. Dalteparin
B. Ibuprofen
C. Meropenem
D. Paracetamol
E. Warfarin

Neurology and psychiatry

Monitoring and stopping

63. A 46-year-old woman with bipolar disorder is advised to take olanzapine and fluoxetine.

What monitoring option should be assessed at baseline and intermittently during therapy?

A. Albumin, bilirubin, and INR
B. Haemoglobin and white cell count
C. Serum sodium and potassium
D. Thyroid stimulating hormone (TSH), triiodothyronine (T_3) and thyroxine (T_4)
E. Weight, lipid profile, and haemoglobin A_{1c} (HbA$_{1c}$)

64. A 32-year-old woman presents to her GP with a 6-month history of heavy menstruation. Her periods last 8 days and she has to use both tampons and sanitary towels, which she changes up to every 2 hours. She is awaiting a review by a gynaecologist for treatment of fibroids but would like treatment in the meantime. She does not take any regular medicines. Previously, she has been unable to tolerate insertion of a levonorgestrel intrauterine device. Her GP recommends a trial of tranexamic acid.

What is the most appropriate advice to give her regarding tranexamic acid?

A. Deep vein thrombosis is a common side effect
B. It reduces the effectiveness of the combined oral contraceptive pill
C. It works by helping your body to break down blood clots
D. She should take it every day, even when not on her period
E. Tablets can take up to 24 hours to reach full effect

65. An 84-year-old woman has started taking anastrozole, after being found to have advanced breast cancer.

What best describes the mechanism of action of anastrozole?

A. 5α-reductase inhibition
B. Aromatase inhibition
C. Inhibition of ergosterol synthesis
D. Luteinising hormone (LH)/follicle-stimulating hormone (FSH) suppression
E. Selective oestrogen receptor modulation

66. A 73-year-old woman is advised to take oxybutynin to improve her symptoms of urinary urgency and urge incontinence.

What best describes the mechanism by which oxybutynin should improve her symptoms?

A. Agonism at the β_2-adrenoceptor
B. Antagonism at the α_1-adrenoceptor
C. Antagonism at the muscarinic M_3 receptor
D. Antagonism at the nicotinic acetylcholine receptor
E. Inhibition of 5α-reductase

Renal medicine
and urology

Important
interactions

67. A 60-year-old man is advised to take sildenafil as required for erectile dysfunction. His medical problems include hypertension and COPD. His medication includes doxazosin, indapamide, ramipril, salbutamol taken orally, and tiotropium by inhalation.

What drug should he avoid taking at the same time of day as sildenafil?

A. Doxazosin
B. Indapamide
C. Ramipril
D. Salbutamol
E. Tiotropium

Renal medicine
and urology

Important
adverse effects

68. A 48-year-old man is found to be hyperkalaemic. One month ago he was admitted to hospital with a non-ST-elevation myocardial infarction, for which he underwent percutaneous intervention. His medications, which were all started during the recent hospital admission, comprise aspirin, clopidogrel, atorvastatin, bisoprolol, and ramipril.

What drug is most likely to cause hyperkalaemia?

A. Aspirin
B. Atorvastatin
C. Bisoprolol
D. Clopidogrel
E. Ramipril

Renal medicine
and urology

Important
adverse effects

69. A 92-year-old woman, who lives in a residential home for people with dementia, is found confused and wandering. Her caregivers think that this was precipitated by a medicine for 'overactive bladder', which was started last week. Unfortunately, they cannot find the drug in her room as she has been hiding things, and the GP surgery is closed.

What drug is most likely to have caused her confusion?

A. Finasteride
B. Furosemide
C. Solifenacin
D. Tamsulosin
E. Trimethoprim

Renal medicine and urology

Important adverse effects

70. A 61-year-old man with benign prostatic enlargement is advised to take tamsulosin to improve urinary flow.

What side effect is most likely to occur when starting this drug?

A. Bronchospasm
B. Postural hypotension
C. Erectile dysfunction
D. Gynaecomastia
E. Prostate cancer

Renal medicine and urology

Important interactions

71. A 67-year-old man presents to the GP to discuss his medication. For several years he has been taking sildenafil for erectile dysfunction. He has previously found this to be an effective and tolerable treatment, but says it has recently been causing headaches.

He has a past medical history of COPD. In addition, he was recently found to have atrial fibrillation. His treatment has been adjusted frequently over the past few weeks. His regular treatment now comprises digoxin, diltiazem, simvastatin, tiotropium, and warfarin. Examination is normal other than for an irregular pulse at a rate of 80–90 beats/min.

What drug is most likely to interact with sildenafil to provoke side effects?

A. Digoxin
B. Diltiazem
C. Simvastatin
D. Tiotropium
E. Warfarin

Respiratory medicine

Warnings

72. A 63-year-old man with gout, hypertension, and hypercholesterolaemia complains of swelling and pain in his left big toe. His GP makes a diagnosis of acute gout. His regular medications are allopurinol, amlodipine, indapamide, ramipril, and simvastatin.

What drug could be stopped or substituted to reduce the risk of future attacks of gout?

A. Allopurinol
B. Amlodipine
C. Indapamide
D. Ramipril
E. Simvastatin

Respiratory medicine

Mechanisms of action

73. A 72-year-old man with hypertension, COPD, and irritable bowel syndrome sees his GP for a medication review. His medicines are amlodipine, doxazosin, fluticasone, hyoscine butylbromide, ipratropium, and salmeterol.

What receptors are most likely to have been activated by this treatment?

A. α_1-adrenoceptors
B. α_2-adrenoceptors
C. β_1-adrenoceptors
D. β_2-adrenoceptors
E. Muscarinic receptors

Respiratory medicine

Important adverse effects

74. A 62-year-old man with COPD complains that one of his medications is causing a dry mouth. He is taking aminophylline, fluticasone, salbutamol, salmeterol orally, and tiotropium by inhalation.

What is the most likely cause of his dry mouth?

A. Aminophylline
B. Fluticasone
C. Salbutamol
D. Salmeterol
E. Tiotropium

Respiratory medicine

Warnings

75. An 82-year-old man with COPD is breathless and has recurrent exacerbations. His past medical history includes an episode of urinary retention secondary to benign prostatic enlargement.

What treatment should be used with caution in people with a history of urinary retention?

A. Salbutamol
B. Salmeterol
C. Seretide
D. Symbicort
E. Tiotropium

Rheumatology

Warnings

76. A 62-year-old woman is found to have gout. Her past medical history includes asthma and hypertension. Her current medications are bendroflumethiazide orally, and salbutamol and Symbicort (budesonide with formoterol) inhaled. She is intolerant of aspirin as it exacerbates her asthma.

What treatment for gout is most strongly contraindicated in this case?

A. Codeine
B. Colchicine
C. Naproxen
D. Paracetamol
E. Prednisolone

Toxicology

Common indications

77. A 31-year-old man presents 7 hours after a paracetamol overdose. His only symptoms are nausea and epigastric discomfort. He has no relevant past medical history and takes no regular medication. The serum paracetamol concentration is above the treatment line on the paracetamol poisoning treatment graph.

What is the most appropriate treatment?

A. Acetylcysteine
B. Activated charcoal
C. Cyclizine
D. Omeprazole
E. Naloxone

Toxicology

Common indications

78. A 68-year-old man is brought to the emergency department because he has become increasingly drowsy over the past 24 hours. He has had diarrhoea for the preceding week. His medical problems include chronic back pain, epilepsy, and depression. Regular medications include diazepam, morphine, fluoxetine, paracetamol, and sodium valproate. On examination, he has a Glasgow Coma Scale (GCS) score of 9 (scale range 3–15) and a respiratory rate of 8 breaths/min. His pupils are pinpoint. He appears dehydrated and blood tests reveal an acute kidney injury. Drug toxicity is suspected.

What is the most appropriate initial treatment?

A. Acetylcysteine
B. Activated charcoal
C. Flumazenil
D. Naloxone
E. Sodium bicarbonate

Toxicology

Mechanisms of action

79. A 63-year-old woman, who is an inpatient, complains of headache, nausea, and sore mouth. She was admitted 2 weeks ago with a fracture of her left femoral neck. She has a past medical history of rheumatoid arthritis.

Blood tests reveal new renal and liver impairment and pancytopenia. Reviewing her inpatient prescriptions, you notice that methotrexate has been prescribed daily instead of weekly.

What is the most appropriate immediate treatment for her methotrexate toxicity?

A. Activated charcoal
B. Folic acid
C. Folinic acid
D. Granulocyte colony-stimulating factor (G-CSF)
E. Haemodialysis

Toxicology

Important adverse effects

80. A 24-year-old woman is receiving an IV infusion of acetylcysteine for paracetamol poisoning. Thirty minutes into the infusion, she develops a rash. On examination, her heart rate is 95 beats/min and her blood pressure is 117/78 mmHg. She has a widespread urticarial rash.

What is the most appropriate immediate management?

A. Continue acetylcysteine and give chlorphenamine
B. Continue acetylcysteine and give ranitidine
C. Temporarily stop acetylcysteine and give adrenaline
D. Temporarily stop acetylcysteine and give chlorphenamine
E. Temporarily stop acetylcysteine and give ranitidine

Prescribing questions

Cardiovascular medicine

Prescription

81. A 52-year-old man sees his GP with episodic chest pain that occurs on exertion. His GP makes a diagnosis of stable angina and advises him to start bisoprolol 5 mg orally daily to reduce the risk of attacks, pending further investigation.

Write a prescription for an additional medicine, to be taken as 'rescue' treatment if an angina attack occurs.

Drug	
Dose	
Route	
Frequency	

Endocrinology and metabolic medicine

Prescription

82. A 56-year-old woman attends a planned follow-up review for type 2 diabetes, which was diagnosed 3 months ago. She has a body mass index (BMI) of 27 kg/m^2 and no known allergies. Despite lifestyle changes, her haemoglobin A_{1c} remains above target. She has normal renal function. Her GP advises her to start pharmacological therapy.

Write a prescription for initial treatment of type 2 diabetes.

Drug	
Dose	
Route	
Frequency	

GI and liver

Prescription

83. A 62-year-old man with a background of alcoholic cirrhosis is admitted to the acute medical unit with confusion. A diagnosis of hepatic encephalopathy is made. His wife reports that he had been complaining of constipation in the days leading up to admission.

Write a prescription for one drug to treat hepatic encephalopathy.

Drug	
Dose	
Route	
Frequency	

Haematology & immunology

Prescription

84. An 85-year-old woman is admitted to the acute medical unit with a urinary tract infection (UTI). Her past medical history includes a left-leg deep vein thrombosis (DVT) 5 years ago, for which she was treated with warfarin for 3 months. She has no risk factors for bleeding and her renal function is normal.

Write a prescription for one drug to reduce the risk of venous thromboembolism.

Drug	
Dose	
Route	
Frequency	

Infectious diseases

Prescription

85. A 60-year-old woman is admitted with fever, confusion, and seizures. A decision is made to treat her empirically for herpes simplex encephalitis. Her body weight is 75 kg.

Write a prescription for one drug to treat suspected herpes simplex encephalitis.

Drug	
Dose	
Route	
Frequency	
Duration	
Indication	

Critical care, peri-operative medicine, and pain

Prescription

86. A 35-year-old woman is found to be hypotensive. She was admitted 6 hours ago with acute pancreatitis. Analgesia and IV fluids were administered and she was transferred to the ward. Over the past hour, her heart rate has been 100–110 beats/min and her blood pressure around 85/50 mmHg. She has not passed any urine since admission. Her serum potassium concentration is 5.1 mmol/L (normal 3.5–4.7).

Write a prescription for initial fluid resuscitation.

Fluid (including any additives)	Volume	Rate/duration

Critical care, peri-operative medicine, and pain

Prescription

87. A 75-year-old man who has long-term hypoxic brain injury is admitted to hospital because his gastrostomy feeding tube has become blocked. It is due to be replaced sometime the next day. You are asked to prescribe 'maintenance' IV fluid.

He weighs 85 kg. He is not dehydrated. His serum potassium concentration and renal function are normal. In the past 24 hours, he has already received two 1 L bags of glucose 5% with potassium chloride 0.3% (40 mmol/L), each given over 8 hours.

Write a prescription to meet his remaining maintenance requirements for the current 24-hour period.

Fluid (including any additives)	Volume	Rate/duration

Critical care, peri-operative medicine, and pain

Prescription

88. A 72-year-old woman is found to be hypokalaemic. She had an elective right knee arthroplasty 3 days ago. Over the last 24 hours she has developed vomiting and abdominal pain. Viral gastroenteritis is suspected, as other patients on the ward have been affected by the same symptoms.

On examination, her pulse is 88 beats/min and her blood pressure is 156/90 mmHg. Her mucous membranes are dry. Her serum potassium concentration is 2.3 mmol/L (3.5–4.7). The rest of her serum biochemistry is normal. The ECG shows small T waves.

Write a prescription to provide initial treatment for the most urgent problem.

Fluid (including any additives)	Volume	Rate/duration

Neurology and psychiatry

Prescription

89. A 40-year-old man is brought to the emergency department because of a fit. He is accompanied by a friend who says the fit started about 25 minutes ago. On examination, there are findings consistent with an ongoing clonic seizure. The capillary blood glucose concentration is 5.9 mmol/L. No antiepileptic treatment has been administered so far.

Write a prescription for immediate treatment of this seizure.

Drug	
Dose	
Route	
Frequency	

Respiratory medicine

Prescription

90. A 12-year-old boy sees his GP following an emergency department visit for an acute asthma attack. Following a short course of a systemic corticosteroid, he has made a good recovery. His current treatment is salbutamol 100–200 micrograms inhaled as required up to four times daily, which he uses about three times a week.

Write a prescription for one drug to reduce the risk of future asthma attacks.

Drug	
Dose	
Route	
Frequency	

Calculation questions

Cardiovascular medicine

Prescription

91. A 73-year-old woman requires an infusion of glyceryl trinitrate to treat acute coronary syndrome.

The recommended dosage is 10–200 micrograms/min, to be adjusted according to response. However, the rate of infusion is to be set in units of mL/hr. Glyceryl trinitrate is available in vials containing a 50 mg/50 mL solution for infusion, which is to be administered without further dilution.

What is the maximum rate (in mL/hr) at which glyceryl trinitrate can be infused?

Infusion rate (mL/hr)	

Critical care, peri-operative medicine, and pain

Prescription

92. A 24-year-old man requires local anaesthesia for insertion of a chest drain. You are asked to calculate the maximum volume of lidocaine 1% solution that can be injected subcutaneously. His body weight is 75 kg.

The local protocol specifies a maximum dose of 3 mg/kg of body weight, or 200 mg, whichever is lower.

Calculate the maximum volume (in mL) of lidocaine 1% solution that can be injected.

Volume (mL)	

Critical care, peri-operative medicine, and pain

Prescription

93. A 76-year-old woman is recovering from emergency abdominal surgery for diverticular perforation. She has type 2 diabetes, usually treated with insulin. While she is unable to eat, this has been substituted with an IV insulin infusion. In accordance with the local protocol, sodium chloride 0.45% with glucose 5% and potassium chloride 0.15% is being infused concurrently, at a constant rate of 85 mL/hr. This has been running for 14 hours.

How much glucose (in g) has been administered in the past 14 hours?

Mass (g)	

Critical care, peri-operative medicine, and pain

Administration

94. An 8-year-old girl requires fluid resuscitation for sepsis. She is to be given an initial bolus of 20 mL/kg of sodium chloride 0.9%, to be infused over 10 minutes. She weighs 24 kg.

At what rate (in mL/hr) will this fluid bolus need to be infused?

Rate (mL/hr)	

Haematology & immunology

Prescription

95. A 29-year-old woman is found to have iron-deficiency anaemia. Following discussion, it is agreed that she will try a liquid formulation in the first instance. She requires 200 mg of elemental iron per day, to be taken in two divided doses.

Ferrous fumarate is available as a 140 mg/5 mL oral solution, which is dosed in 5-mL spoonfuls. Ferrous fumarate 200 mg contains 65 mg of elemental iron.

How many 5-mL spoonfuls should be taken for each dose?

Spoonfuls	

Infectious diseases

Prescription

96. A 54-year-old woman requires treatment with gentamicin for sepsis. You are asked to calculate an initial dose of 5 mg/kg IV, based on adjusted body weight. For practical purposes, you are asked to round the calculated dose to the nearest 40 mg.

For the purpose of gentamicin dosing, adjusted body weight is calculated as:

Adjusted body weight

= [ideal body weight] + 0.4 × ([actual body weight] − [ideal body weight])

Her actual body weight is 94 kg and her ideal body weight is 68 kg.

Calculate the initial dose of gentamicin in mg.

Dose (mg)	

Infectious diseases

Prescription

97. A 4-year-old girl requires amoxicillin for acute otitis media with spontaneous tympanic membrane perforation. She is to take 250 mg three times a day for 5 days.

Amoxicillin is available in 100-mL bottles containing a 125 mg/5 mL oral suspension.

How many 100-mL bottles (rounded up to a whole number) will be required for this course of treatment?

Whole bottles	

Infectious diseases

Administration

98. A 3-year-old boy requires nebulised adrenaline (epinephrine) for severe croup. His body weight is 12 kg.

The local protocol specifies that the dose is 400 micrograms/kg (to a maximum of 5 mg), prepared from the 1:1000 solution.

Calculate the volume (in mL) of adrenaline 1:1000 solution required.

Volume (mL)	

Infectious diseases

Administration

99. A 33-year-old man, who has late-stage HIV infection, requires oral co-trimoxazole for treatment of *Pneumocystis jirovecii* pneumonia. His body weight is 63 kg.

The dosage required is 120 mg/kg per day, to be given in two divided doses. Co-trimoxazole is available in 480-mg tablets, which can be halved.

How many 480-mg tablets should be given at each dose (rounded to the nearest whole or half tablet)?

Number of tablets	

Neurology and psychiatry

Administration

100. A 65-year-old woman is found to have hyperchloraemic metabolic acidosis. She was admitted 2 days ago with a left anterior circulation stroke and has required IV maintenance fluid due to dysphagia. Due to her acute brain injury, hypotonic fluids (e.g. glucose 5%) are relatively contraindicated.

Over the past 48 hours, she has received 5000 mL of sodium chloride 0.9% with potassium chloride 0.15%. This solution contains sodium chloride 154 mmol/L and potassium chloride 20 mmol/L.

How much chloride (in mmol) has been administered in the last 48 hours?

Amount (mmol)	

Answers and explanations

Single best answer questions

1. D. Ramipril. Clinical trials have shown that **angiotensin-converting enzyme (ACE) inhibitors** (e.g. ramipril), antiplatelet agents (e.g. **aspirin**, **clopidogrel**), β-blockers, and **statins** significantly reduce the risk of major adverse cardiovascular events following a myocardial infarction.

The other drugs have no role in secondary prevention following myocardial infarction. Amiloride is a potassium-sparing diuretic, used to reduce potassium losses caused by other diuretics (**loop** or **thiazide diuretics**). **Digoxin** is a cardiac glycoside. It is an option for rate control in atrial fibrillation (AF), particularly in people with heart failure. Glyceryl trinitrate is a **nitrate** which is used to relieve angina by reducing myocardial work and oxygen demand; however, it does not prevent myocardial infarction. **Warfarin** is an anticoagulant. It is used to reduce the risk of intracardiac thrombus formation and therefore of systemic embolism in AF.

2. E. Spironolactone. This woman needs treatment to control her symptoms of heart failure (ankle swelling and shortness of breath), and to normalise her serum potassium concentration, since hypokalaemia is associated with a risk of dangerous arrhythmias. Spironolactone is an **aldosterone antagonist** which competitively blocks the aldosterone receptor, causing increased sodium and water excretion and potassium retention in the distal renal tubules. Although aldosterone antagonists are relatively weak diuretics, they can improve symptoms and reduce mortality in moderate heart failure. They also increase the serum potassium concentration. Eplerenone is an alternative aldosterone antagonist; it is more expensive but is a useful option if spironolactone is not tolerated due to endocrine side effects.

Furosemide (a **loop diuretic**, like bumetanide which she is already taking) and indapamide (a **thiazide-like diuretic**) could improve symptoms by increasing sodium and water excretion. However, both drugs may further reduce the serum potassium concentration by increasing renal potassium excretion. **Nitrates** are used in the treatment of acute, but not chronic, heart failure and will not address the hypokalaemia. Amiloride (a potassium-sparing diuretic) can increase the serum potassium concentration but is a weak diuretic that will have little impact on symptoms and offers no prognostic benefits in heart failure.

3. B. Bisoprolol. There are two basic approaches to managing chronic atrial fibrillation (AF). One is 'rhythm control', which seeks to restore normal sinus rhythm either by electrical cardioversion, antiarrhythmic drugs or both. The other is 'rate control', in which the abnormal heart rhythm is accepted as permanent, and efforts are focused simply on preventing ventricular rate from running too fast. In most cases, rate control is just as effective as rhythm control and considerably simpler.

The ideal agent for ventricular rate control in AF is either a **β-blocker** (e.g. bisoprolol) or a non-dihydropyridine **calcium channel blocker** (e.g. verapamil or diltiazem). In practice, a β-blocker is used in most cases. This would be a particularly appropriate choice for this man because of his history of heart failure: β-blockers are indicated in heart failure to improve prognosis, whereas verapamil and diltiazem should be avoided.

Digoxin can be used for rate control in AF but, on its own, it is less effective than a β-blocker or calcium channel blocker and potentially more toxic. Likewise, although **amiodarone** is an effective agent for both rate and rhythm control in AF, it is much too toxic for first-line use. Doxazosin is an **α-blocker** used in hypertension and benign prostatic enlargement; it has no role in AF.

4. B. Furosemide. Furosemide is a **loop diuretic** which inhibits the $Na^+/K^+/2Cl^-$ co-transporter in the ascending limb of the loop of Henle, preventing transport of sodium, potassium, and chloride ions from the renal tubular lumen into the epithelial cell.

Bisoprolol and spironolactone are receptor antagonists that block $β_1$-adrenoceptors and aldosterone receptors, respectively (see **β-blockers** and **Aldosterone antagonists**). Ramipril and simvastatin are enzyme inhibitors. Ramipril is an **ACE inhibitor**, preventing conversion of angiotensin I to angiotensin II. Simvastatin, a **statin**, inhibits 3-hydroxy-3-methyl-glutaryl coenzyme A (HMG CoA) reductase, preventing the synthesis of cholesterol.

5. C. $β_1$-adrenoceptor. Metoprolol is a **β-blocker** that is relatively selective for the $β_1$-adrenoceptor. Blockade of this receptor reduces the force of myocardial contraction and decreases the speed of electrical conduction in the heart. By prolonging the refractory period of the atrioventricular (AV) node and slowing conduction in the atria, it can terminate some supraventricular tachycardias and reduce the ventricular rate in atrial fibrillation.

$β_2$-adrenoceptors are found in smooth muscle, such as in the bronchial tree; $β_3$-adrenoceptors are found in adipose tissue. Blockade of these receptors is not clinically useful in the management of supraventricular tachycardias. Metoprolol does not have any effect on α-adrenoceptors.

6. A. Amlodipine. Ankle swelling is a common adverse effect of treatment with dihydropyridine **calcium channel blockers**. It is understood to be due to preferential dilatation of the pre-capillary arterioles, relative to post-capillary venules, causing increased pressure in the capillary bed and therefore greater filtration of fluid from vessels to the interstitium. Chlortalidone is a **thiazide-like diuretic**. It does not cause oedema and, in other situations, might be expected to improve it. However, calcium channel blocker-induced oedema does not respond well to diuresis, because it is not due to increased extracellular fluid (ECF) volume. Drugs with a venodilation effect, notably **ACE inhibitors** and **angiotensin receptor antagonists**, may help. The oral diabetes agents gliclazide (a **sulphonylurea**) and **metformin**, and the **inhaled antimuscarinic** drug tiotropium, do not cause oedema.

7. D. Medicines and Healthcare Products Regulatory Agency (MHRA). In the UK, suspected adverse effects of medicines should be reported to the medicines regulator (the MHRA) by health professionals or the public using the Yellow Card scheme. All serious suspected adverse drug reactions should be reported. In this context, 'serious' is defined as a reaction that caused death or was life threatening, caused or prolonged hospital admission, resulted in significant disability or incapacity or was considered in any other way 'medically significant'. In addition, all reactions (regardless of seriousness) to drugs undergoing intensive surveillance (identified by a ▼ black triangle) should be reported, as should all reactions occurring in children.

The Care Quality Commission (CQC) is the UK regulator of health and social care organisations. The National Institute for Health and Care Excellence (NICE) is a non-departmental public body that provides guidance and advice on health and social care matters (notably the use of medicines and other medical technologies) in the UK. The British National Formulary (BNF) is a prescribing reference manual published jointly by the BMJ Group and the Pharmaceutical Press.

8. C. Clopidogrel. Clopidogrel is an antiplatelet agent. It is used in cerebrovascular disease to reduce the risk of future events. As it irreversibly inhibits platelet aggregation, its effect takes 7–10 days to wear off (reflecting the lifespan of circulating platelets). If surgery is planned for a person who takes antiplatelet or anticoagulant medications, an assessment should be made about their risk of bleeding from surgery and their risk of thrombosis. In this case, it is probably advisable to withhold the antiplatelet drug for the week before surgery, assuming her other vascular risk factors are well controlled. Antiplatelet drugs should not be stopped within 6–12 months of insertion of a coronary artery stent without first discussing this with a cardiologist.

9. B. Diltiazem. ** Diltiazem, like verapamil, is a non-dihydropyridine **calcium channel blocker. Non-dihydropyridine calcium channel blockers are relatively cardioselective: they reduce the rate and force of cardiac contraction and interfere with conduction at the atrioventricular (AV) node. These effects are similar to those of β-**blockers**. Non-dihydropyridine calcium channel blockers and β-blockers should not be combined except under the close supervision of a specialist, as their effects on the heart are additive. Together, they can cause heart block, cardiogenic shock, and even asystole. This man has third-degree heart block: that is, transmission between the atria and ventricles is completely blocked and the chambers are now beating independently. This serious interaction highlights the dangers of prescribing drugs without a full and accurate medication history.

10. D. 8 am and 3 pm. ** Isosorbide mononitrate is a **nitrate that is used to control angina. Nitrates are associated with tachyphylaxis, a phenomenon in which they become less effective with continued use. To minimise this, it is helpful to have a 'nitrate-free period' overnight, when need for its effect should be low. In this example, dosing at 8 am and 3 pm ensures he receives peak activity of the drug during active daytime hours, with a nitrate-free period overnight. An alternative strategy could be to use a modified-release preparation, taken once daily in the morning.

11. A. Intramuscularly into the anterolateral thigh. Adrenaline (epinephrine) is the most important treatment for anaphylaxis. People who have experienced an anaphylactic reaction should be provided with an adrenaline auto-injector for self-administration in the event of a recurrent attack. The EpiPen (adult form) is designed to deliver 300 micrograms of adrenaline as an intramuscular (IM) injection. It should be administered into the anterolateral thigh. You do this by removing the blue safety cap then jabbing the orange end of the device firmly against the outer thigh, holding it there for about 10 seconds. It can be given through clothing if necessary. Of note, not all the contents of the glass cartridge will be injected; the device contains 2 mg of adrenaline (as a 1 mg/mL solution) and delivers only 0.3 mg (0.3 mL) of this.

Injection into smaller muscles is less desirable, as absorption is not as reliable, but they can be used if necessary. The SC route should not be used, as absorption is too slow. Adrenaline must not be administered IV, except by clinicians experienced in its use by this route, or unless cardiac arrest supervenes.

12. C. Dry cough. Dry cough is a common side effect associated with **ACE inhibitor** therapy. It is due to increased levels of bradykinin, which is usually inactivated by ACE. Where it is problematic, an **angiotensin receptor blocker** may be offered as an alternative. These drugs do not inhibit ACE, so have no effect on bradykinin degradation.

13. B. Liver profile. Around 1 in 200 people taking a **statin** will develop elevated liver enzymes. Early detection of this allows treatment to be adjusted, minimising the risk of long-term harm. A liver profile should be measured before starting statin treatment and again at 3 months. The statin should be stopped if liver transaminase levels increase to greater than three times the upper limit of normal.

There is no need to check creatine kinase levels routinely, but they may be measured in people who develop new muscle aches and pains. Thyroid function should be checked *before* a statin is started, as untreated hypothyroidism is a reversible cause of hyperlipidaemia and can increase the risk of adverse effects from statins. A lipid profile may be a useful marker of *efficacy*, rather than safety.

14. D. Serum potassium. Eplerenone is an **aldosterone antagonist**. It acts by inhibiting the effects of aldosterone. This leads to increased sodium and water excretion and potassium retention, which can cause hyperkalaemia. Serum potassium concentrations should be checked before and within 1–2 weeks of starting aldosterone antagonists, and whenever a dose adjustment is made.

15. B. Ibuprofen. Ibuprofen is a **non-steroidal antiinflammatory drug** (NSAID) that inhibits the enzyme cyclooxygenase, preventing conversion of arachidonic acid to prostaglandins.

Amitriptyline and omeprazole inhibit membrane transport proteins. Amitriptyline is a **tricyclic antidepressant** that inhibits transporters responsible for removing serotonin and noradrenaline from the synaptic cleft. Omeprazole is a **proton pump inhibitor** that inhibits H^+/K^+-ATPase in gastric parietal cells, preventing the secretion of gastric acid. Morphine is a strong **opioid** that activates opioid μ (mu) receptors in the central nervous system. Senna is an orally administered **laxative** that acts as an irritant in the gut, stimulating increased water and electrolyte secretion from the colonic mucosa.

16. E. Ondansetron. Predicting which antiemetic will work in which situation is not easy. In practice, drug selection is often based on pragmatic considerations such as familiarity and availability, and then adjusted according to clinical response. With this person having already had cyclizine (see **Antiemetics, histamine H₁-receptor antagonists**), it would now be best to offer her a drug from a different class. This choice is influenced by her past reaction to prochlorperazine (see **Antiemetics, dopamine D₂-receptor antagonists**), which sounds like neuroleptic malignant syndrome (NMS). NMS is a serious condition that may be precipitated by drugs that have an antidopaminergic effect, including phenothiazine antiemetics (e.g. prochlorperazine, chlorpromazine), dopamine antagonist antiemetics (e.g. metoclopramide), and **antipsychotics** (including haloperidol, which is sometimes also used as an antiemetic). The risk of recurrence of NMS with re-exposure is unclear, but it would be prudent to avoid these drug classes where suitable alternatives exist. A suitable alternative might be ondansetron (see **Antiemetics, serotonin 5-HT3-receptor antagonists**) which is not associated with NMS.

17. D. Reduced hepatic glucose output. The main mechanism by which **metformin** lowers blood glucose is through a reduction in hepatic glucose output (from gluconeogenesis). It may also improve peripheral insulin sensitivity (and therefore glucose uptake) but this is probably less important to its glucose-lowering effect. Other minor contributors to its glucose-lowering effect include weight loss and reduced dietary intake.

18. C. Gliclazide. Sulphonylureas (e.g. gliclazide) lower blood glucose by stimulating pancreatic insulin secretion. Hypoglycaemia is a potentially serious adverse effect, which is more likely with high treatment doses or if multiple glucose-lowering medications are prescribed.

Metformin lowers blood glucose by reducing hepatic glucose output and doesn't usually cause hypoglycaemia. Bendroflumethiazide (a **thiazide diuretic**) and prednisolone (a **systemic corticosteroid**) both raise blood glucose and can reduce the efficacy of glucose-lowering agents. **β-blockers** may mask symptoms of hypoglycaemia such as sweating, shaking, tachycardia, and anxiety, which are mediated by sympathoadrenal activation.

19. B. Gliclazide. Gliclazide, a **sulphonylurea**, acts by stimulating pancreatic insulin secretion. Its adverse effects are predictable from the actions of insulin, including hypoglycaemia and weight gain. All the other drugs are oral antihyperglycaemic agents with a low risk of hypoglycaemia. Empagliflozin is a **sodium–glucose co-transporter 2 (SGLT-2) inhibitor**, which inhibits reabsorption of glucose from the proximal renal tubule. This lowers blood glucose, but as insulin secretion is not stimulated, and normal homeostatic responses to hypoglycaemia are intact, the risk of hypoglycaemia is low. **Metformin** acts mainly by reducing hepatic glucose output and, to a lesser extent, improving peripheral insulin sensitivity. Pioglitazone is a thiazolidinedione. It activates the γ subclass of nuclear peroxisome proliferator-activated receptors (PPARγ), promoting expression of genes which enhance insulin sensitivity. It does not increase insulin secretion and so does not increase the risk of hypoglycaemia, but it does promote weight gain. Thiazolidinediones increase the risk and severity of heart failure. This concern, among other factors, has been associated with reduced prescribing of this drug class. Sitagliptin, a **DPP-4 inhibitor**, targets the enzyme that inactivates incretins. Incretins promote insulin secretion, but only when the blood glucose concentration is normal or elevated, so hypoglycaemia is not induced.

20. D. Hydrocortisone. Medically administered **systemic corticosteroids**, like endogenous corticosteroids, suppress hypothalamic secretion of corticotropin-releasing hormone (CRH) and pituitary secretion of adrenocorticotropic hormone (ACTH). When taken chronically, prolonged suppression of ACTH release leads to adrenocortical atrophy. If the exogenous steroid is then stopped abruptly, or if the stress of an intercurrent illness necessitates increased corticosteroid secretion, the atrophied adrenal glands may be unable to meet this need. The resulting state of acute adrenal insufficiency (an 'Addisonian crisis') may cause hypotension and various non-specific symptoms (e.g. confusion, weakness, nausea, abdominal pain).

It is possible that acute adrenal insufficiency explains this presentation. Parenteral corticosteroid replacement must be given urgently. If she does have a 'surgical abdomen', she still requires intensified corticosteroid therapy to cover the associated physiological stress. A typical choice for immediate steroid replacement is **hydrocortisone 100 mg IV**. Fludrocortisone is a mineralocorticoid that will not address the acute need for glucocorticoid replacement. Budesonide and fluticasone (see **Corticosteroids, inhaled**) and prednisolone are glucocorticoids, but they cannot be administered IV. Fluid resuscitation (e.g. with **sodium chloride 0.9%**) should also be given urgently.

21. D. There is an increased risk of cancer of the lining of the womb. Tamoxifen is a **sex hormone antagonist**, which can lead to endometrial changes including a small risk of endometrial cancer, but not ovarian cancer. Those starting tamoxifen should be advised to report vaginal bleeding to their doctor. Other side effects include *suppression* of lactation and increased risk of venous thromboembolism. Tamoxifen does not cause infertility and is in fact a treatment option in anovulatory infertility. It is not safe in pregnancy, as it increases the risk of abnormal fetal development.

22. B. Fluoxetine. Tamoxifen is a **sex hormone antagonist**. It is a prodrug that requires activation by a cytochrome P450 (CYP) enzyme, CYP2D6. CYP2D6 is also involved in the metabolism of other drugs, including codeine (also a prodrug, which is metabolised by CYP2D6 to more active metabolites), loratadine, propranolol, and risperidone. Fluoxetine, a **selective serotonin reuptake inhibitor (SSRI)**, is a potent inhibitor of CYP2D6. For the prodrugs tamoxifen and codeine, inhibition of CYP2D6 results in lower plasma levels of active metabolites. This can result in reduced efficacy. For drugs that are inactivated by CYP2D6, such as propranolol (a β-blocker), risperidone (a **second-generation antipsychotic**), and loratadine (an **antihistamine**), the interaction may increase the risk of adverse effects.

23. C. Lactic acidosis. Rarely, **metformin** is associated with a state of severe metabolic acidosis and high serum lactate concentration, termed **lactic acidosis**.

This is a serious condition that may be life threatening. The extent to which this is *caused by*, as opposed to *associated with*, metformin is controversial. Clinical trial and population data suggest that metformin does not increase the risk in people taking standard doses. However, in supratherapeutic concentrations (due to overdose or renal impairment, since metformin is eliminated by the kidneys), metformin may be a contributory factor.

The other effects listed may be caused by metformin, but are not the main concern in renal impairment. Megaloblastic anaemia with metformin therapy is understood to be caused by impaired vitamin B_{12} absorption, due to altered transport of the vitamin B_{12}-intrinsic factor complex across cell membranes in the intestine.

24. B. 48 mmol/mol (6.5%). Haemoglobin A_{1c} (HbA$_{1c}$) is used in three main ways:
1. To diagnose diabetes mellitus.
2. To set a target level of glycaemic control with an existing therapeutic regimen (e.g. to guide dosage titration).
3. To trigger intensification of treatment, by offering another agent.

Diagnostic and therapeutic decisions are commonly made at three key HbA$_{1c}$ levels (48, 53, and 58 mmol/mol), which are therefore worth committing to memory. Remember these in units of mmol/mol because percentage values are no longer quoted routinely (because of a drive for international harmonisation).

HbA$_{1c}$ ≥48 mmol/mol can support a diagnosis of diabetes mellitus. People treated by lifestyle measures should target HbA$_{1c}$ levels <48 mmol/mol, and drug treatment should be started if this is not achieved. Those taking a single agent should also target HbA$_{1c}$ <48 mmol/mol, but in people on two or more agents the target is <53 mmol/mol (recognising that treatment with two agents carries more risks and burdens, which may offset the benefits of glycaemic control). The trigger for intensification of pharmacological treatment (i.e. adding another agent) is HbA$_{1c}$ ≥58 mmol/mol.

25. E. Omeprazole, clarithromycin, and metronidazole. *Helicobacter pylori* is a Gram-negative bacterium which causes peptic ulcer disease. Effective treatment requires combination therapy with two antibiotics and a **proton pump inhibitor** (PPI) for 1 week. Treatment with a single antibiotic may be ineffective and may cause the bacteria to develop resistance.

The various regimens considered acceptable for *H. pylori* eradication, including recommended drug doses, are helpfully set out in a treatment summary in the BNF. Options for proton pump inhibition include lansoprazole, omeprazole, and pantoprazole. The antibiotics are selected from amoxicillin (a **broad-spectrum penicillin**), clarithromycin (a **macrolide**), and **metronidazole**. As this person has previously had an anaphylactic reaction to benzylpenicillin, amoxicillin is contraindicated and clarithromycin with metronidazole should be used. Note that the doses recommended for antibiotics when used in *H. pylori* eradication may differ from those used in other indications.

26. A. Loperamide. Loperamide is an antimotility drug used in selected cases of diarrhoea. Pharmacologically, it is an **opioid** similar to pethidine, but unlike other opioids it does not cross the blood–brain barrier. This means it is devoid of central nervous system (CNS) effects, including analgesia, but retains the peripheral effects such as reducing gut motility. The antimotility effects are mediated by opioid μ-receptor agonism in the myenteric plexus of the GI tract.

While the other opioids in this list will have similar antimotility effects, they are likely also to cause CNS effects which, in this context, are undesirable.

27. A. Flucloxacillin. Cholestatic jaundice is a rare, but potentially serious, adverse effect of flucloxacillin (see **Penicillins, narrow-spectrum**). It can occur even when treatment has been completed and is a contraindication to future use of this drug.

Although **paracetamol**, **methotrexate,** and simvastatin (a **statin**) can all cause liver toxicity, they do not generally cause cholestatic jaundice. Paracetamol in overdose causes hepatocellular necrosis, which can be fatal if untreated. Methotrexate can cause hepatitis as part of a hypersensitivity reaction or if taken in overdose. Chronic use of methotrexate can cause hepatic cirrhosis. Statins can cause a rise in liver enzymes (transaminases) and, less frequently, drug-induced hepatitis. Morphine (an **opioid**) does not cause hepatotoxicity, but it is metabolised in the liver so dose reduction is required in people with liver failure.

28. C. Levothyroxine. Gaviscon is a compound **alginate and antacid** preparation that contains calcium carbonate. The divalent cation (Ca^{2+}) in calcium carbonate can bind many drugs in the gut and reduce their absorption. Examples include **tetracyclines**, **digoxin**, **iron**, **bisphosphonates,** and **thyroid hormones** such as levothyroxine. To minimise this interaction, a 2-hour gap is advised between taking Gaviscon and other medicines.

29. A. Clarithromycin. Dabigatran is a **direct oral anticoagulant**. It is susceptible to interactions with drugs that inhibit its metabolism (cytochrome P450 (CYP) inhibitors) and/or its transport across cell membrane (P-glycoprotein inhibitors). Clarithromycin is a **macrolide** antibiotic which is a strong CYP inhibitor and moderate P-glycoprotein inhibitor, and therefore can increase the effect of dabigatran. The other drugs listed do not interact with dabigatran.

30. C. Idarucizumab. Dabigatran is a **direct oral anticoagulant** (DOAC) that directly inhibits thrombin, preventing conversion of fibrinogen to fibrin. Idarucizumab is a humanised monoclonal antibody fragment that binds to dabigatran and its metabolites, reversing its effects.

Andexanet α is a recombinant, modified form of human factor Xa that reverses drugs that inhibit factor Xa, whether directly (e.g. rivaroxaban) or indirectly (e.g. **Heparins and fondaparinux**). Anticoagulation with **warfarin** can be reversed by phytomenadione (see **Vitamins**), which replenishes vitamin K_1 for the synthesis of new clotting factors. In major bleeding, dried prothrombin complex can be used to replace factors IX, VII, and X directly. Protamine is a highly cationic peptide that forms a stable complex with heparin molecules, reversing their anticoagulant effect. It is most effective against unfractionated heparin but also binds low molecular weight heparins. It is ineffective against fondaparinux.

31. D. Quinine. While glucose-6-phosphate dehydrogenase (G6PD) deficiency is rare in northern Europe, it is common in southern Europe, parts of Africa, Asia and Oceania. Because of its X-linked inheritance pattern, it is more common in men. G6PD is an oxidative enzyme, which if inhibited (in the context of a deficiency state) leads to haemolysis of red blood cells. Food triggers of acute haemolysis classically include fava beans. Drug causes in the top 100 list include **aspirin, nitrofurantoin, quinolones, sulfonylureas**, and **quinine**. There is significant variation between individuals in their response to different drugs, and many other drugs have not been tested for their effects on G6PD.

32. B. Antifactor Xa assay. Low molecular weight **heparins** (LMWHs), e.g. dalteparin, promote binding of antithrombin to factor Xa, inhibiting the final part of the clotting cascade to prevent production of a fibrin clot. LMWH-related anticoagulation can be quantified with an antifactor Xa assay. This is not required routinely, but it may be useful when the LMWH effect is less predictable, such as in pregnancy, renal impairment, and significantly abnormal body weight. Platelet count and serum potassium should be measured in those receiving LMWH for >4 days to monitor for side effects (heparin-induced thrombocytopenia, hyperkalaemia), but this is not an indicator of anticoagulation.

In people receiving IV unfractionated **heparin** (UFH), careful monitoring of the activated partial thromboplastin time (APTT) is required. This is expressed as the activated partial thromboplastin ratio (APTR), calculated as the individual's APTT divided by that of a normal control. The rate of infusion is adjusted to achieve a target APTR of 1.5–2.5, representing sufficient but not excessive anticoagulation. **Warfarin** is monitored using the international normalised ratio (INR), the ratio of the person's prothrombin time to that from a normal control. The target INR in most indications is 2.0–3.0. Fibrinogen is an acute phase protein and a marker of disseminated intravascular coagulation (a disordered clotting state usually associated with severe acute illness). It is not a useful measure of therapeutic anticoagulation.

33. E. Trimethoprim. First-line options for an uncomplicated urinary tract infection (UTI) include **trimethoprim, nitrofurantoin,** and amoxicillin (a **broad-spectrum penicillin**). Remember that when prescribing trimethoprim, you must always consider whether there is a possibility of pregnancy. Trimethoprim is potentially teratogenic in the first trimester. Nitrofurantoin should be avoided in the latter stages of pregnancy.

Cefotaxime, a third-generation **cephalosporin**, and gentamicin, an **aminoglycoside**, have to be given intravenously, so are not suitable for treatment of uncomplicated UTI outside hospital. However, cefaclor, an orally active second-generation cephalosporin, can be used as second- or third-line oral treatment for UTI (i.e. where first-line antibiotics do not work), and is an option for UTIs occurring in pregnancy. Ciprofloxacin is a **quinolone** that can be used as a second- or third-line oral treatment for UTI or for complicated UTIs, but should not be used as a first-line treatment, as bacteria can easily become resistant to it. Unless their use is essential, quinolones should be avoided in pregnancy and in children as they may cause arthropathy. **Macrolides**, such as clarithromycin, have little activity against the Gram-negative organisms that commonly cause UTI, such as *Escherichia coli*. They are not known to be harmful in pregnancy.

34. B. Benzylpenicillin and flucloxacillin. In the clinical setting, antibiotics are chosen based on a 'best guess' as to the likely causative organism and antibiotic sensitivities (referred to as 'empirical' treatment). When infection is severe, being wrong with this guess and prescribing inadequate antibiotic treatment can be life threatening, so combination antibiotics are often prescribed to cover all likely eventualities.

Skin and soft tissue infections are most commonly caused by *Staphylococcus aureus* and group A streptococci (e.g. *Streptococcus pyogenes*). These bacteria are usually sensitive to flucloxacillin and benzylpenicillin (see **Penicillins, narrow-spectrum**), respectively. As such, this combination is appropriate for severe cellulitis.

35. C. Doxycycline. A wide spectrum of organisms can cause community-acquired pneumonia, including *Streptococcus pneumoniae* (Gram positive), *Haemophilus influenzae* (Gram negative), and 'atypical' organisms such as *Mycoplasma pneumoniae* and *Legionella pneumophila*. The 'best guess' antibiotic for pneumonia therefore should ideally have a broad spectrum of activity to cover all these possibilities. Doxycycline (a **tetracycline**) is suitable because it covers Gram-positive, Gram-negative, and atypical organisms.

Flucloxacillin is incorrect because it is a **narrow-spectrum penicillin**, principally focused against *S. aureus*. The **quinolone** antibiotics, including ciprofloxacin, are generally reserved for second- or third-line therapy to preserve their usefulness, as bacteria easily acquire resistance to them. Ciprofloxacin is mostly effective against Gram-negative organisms, including *Pseudomonas aeruginosa*. Moxifloxacin and levofloxacin have greater activity against Gram-positive organisms so are preferred if a quinolone is required for pneumonia. Cefotaxime and ertapenem (a **cephalosporin and carbapenem**, respectively) are broad-spectrum antibiotics given by injection. They are reserved for severe infections and where organisms are expected to be resistant to other options, for example in critical illness.

36. D. Piperacillin with tazobactam. UTIs are most commonly caused by *Escherichia coli* and other Gram-negative organisms (*Klebsiella* and *Proteus* species) and Gram-positive *Staphylococcus saprophyticus*. First-line antibiotic choice is usually **nitrofurantoin** or **trimethoprim**, and second-line options include **amoxicillin** and **cefalexin**.

People with long-term catheters have reduced bladder defence against infection. This facilitates growth of organisms that don't usually infect healthy bladders. *Pseudomonas aeruginosa* is a Gram-negative organism well suited to colonising catheters. It forms biofilms that enable the bacteria to evade the host's defence and survive in environments where they wouldn't otherwise be successful.

Piperacillin with the β-lactamase inhibitor tazobactam is an **antipseudomonal penicillin**. It is reserved for severe or complicated infection in which *P. aeruginosa* is suspected. Other options are **cephalosporins and carbapenems** and some **quinolones**. An **aminoglycoside** may be added in selected cases, particularly in critical illness.

37. A. Amoxicillin. Penicillins, **cephalosporins**, **and carbapenems** are all β-lactam antibiotics, so-called because they share a common 'β-lactam ring' in their chemical structure. Of the drugs listed as options here, only amoxicillin is a β-lactam. Ciprofloxacin is a **quinolone**, clarithromycin is a **macrolide**, doxycycline is a **tetracycline**, and **metronidazole** is a nitroimidazole (it is the only commonly used example from this class).

38. A. Benzylpenicillin. Penicillinases are a type of β-lactamase enzyme produced by most staphylococci. They inactivate penicillins (e.g. benzylpenicillin) by breaking their β-lactam ring.

Flucloxacillin (see **Penicillins, narrow-spectrum**) is more likely to be active against penicillinase-producing staphylococci because it has an acyl side chain that protects its β-lactam ring. It is the antibiotic of choice for straightforward staphylococcal infections. **Vancomycin** does not contain a β-lactam ring, so is naturally resistant to penicillinases. It is reserved for more severe Gram-positive infections or those resistant to penicillins (e.g. meticillin-resistant *S. aureus* (MRSA)). The compound preparations co-amoxiclav (see **Penicillins, broad-spectrum**) and piperacillin–tazobactam (**Penicillins, antipseudomonal**) contain β-lactamase inhibitors. This improves their activity against penicillinase-producing staphylococci and, more importantly, β-lactamase-producing Gram-negative organisms.

39. B. Less likely to give rise to antibiotic resistance. Narrow-spectrum antibiotics are active against a narrow group of bacteria, e.g. benzylpenicillin against certain Gram-positive organisms and Gram-negative cocci. They are prescribed for infections where the organism has been identified and its sensitivity demonstrated on bacterial culture. They can also be used as part of an empirical (best guess) regimen where the organism is very likely to be susceptible to the antibiotic: e.g. community-acquired pneumonia is commonly caused by *Streptococcus pneumoniae*, which is commonly sensitive to benzylpenicillin (see **Penicillins, narrow-spectrum**).

Broad-spectrum antibiotics are active against a wide range of bacterial types: e.g. amoxicillin (see **Penicillins, broad-spectrum**) against a wide range of Gram-positive and Gram-negative organisms, including Gram-negative bacilli. They are prescribed empirically where the causative organism is unknown and diverse bacteria may be implicated. They are particularly useful in severe infections requiring urgent effective treatment.

As narrow-spectrum antibiotics kill fewer normal microorganisms in the body than broad-spectrum antibiotics, they are less likely to generate new antibiotic resistance and less likely to cause superinfection, e.g. *Clostridium difficile* colitis. The spectrum of action doesn't affect the ease of administration or likelihood of allergy (e.g. if someone is penicillin allergic they will react to both benzylpenicillin and amoxicillin, as their allergy is to the basic penicillin structure).

40. D. Gentamicin. Aminoglycosides (e.g. gentamicin) accumulate in cochlear and vestibular hair cells where they trigger apoptosis and cell death. This can cause deafness, tinnitus, and vertigo. **Macrolides** (e.g. clarithromycin) can also cause tinnitus and hearing loss, but this is rare and is usually associated with long-term therapy. Other drugs that cause ototoxicity include **vancomycin** and **loop diuretics**.

41. B. QT-interval prolongation. The QT interval is the time between the beginning of the QRS complex and the end of the T-wave. It mostly reflects the time taken for the ventricles to repolarise. The QT interval is said to be prolonged if, after correction for heart rate (by dividing the QT interval by the square root of the RR interval), it exceeds 0.44 seconds in men or 0.46 seconds in women. This is associated with an increased risk of a life-threatening arrhythmia called torsades de pointes, a form of ventricular tachycardia.

There are several causes of a prolonged QT interval. Drug causes include antiarrhythmics (e.g. **amiodarone**), antipsychotics (e.g. haloperidol, see **Antipsychotics, first generation**), **macrolide antibiotics** (e.g. clarithromycin), and **quinine**. Combining drugs with QT-prolonging effects can be dangerous (clarithromycin with quinine sulfate in this case) and should be avoided. A resource for checking which drugs prolong the QT interval can be found at https://crediblemeds.org/ (Note: free registration required; last checked 16/06/2022).

This person is not taking any drugs that increase the potassium concentration and is not at risk of seizures. Had she been taking a **statin**, there would have been a risk that clarithromycin could precipitate myopathy.

42. B. Ferrous sulfate. Tetracyclines bind to divalent cations. They should therefore be separated by at least 2 hours from doses of **calcium**, **antacids** or **iron** (e.g. ferrous sulfate). The interaction reduces absorption of both drugs, although the risk of subtherapeutic antibiotic concentrations is generally the greatest concern.

43. D. Simvastatin. The metabolism of statins is reduced by cytochrome P450 inhibitors, such as **amiodarone**, diltiazem (see **Calcium channel blockers**), itraconazole (see **Antifungal drugs**), **macrolides**, and protease inhibitors (see **Antiviral drugs, other**). This leads to accumulation of the statin in the body, which may increase the risk of adverse effects. To mitigate this, simvastatin can be safely held for 1 week. There is also a potential interaction with warfarin, although the risk of stroke from atrial fibrillation precludes stopping it. The international normalised ratio (INR) should be checked more often during treatment.

44. B. Ciprofloxacin. Immunoglobulin E (IgE)-mediated anaphylactic reactions to penicillins are rare, affecting around 0.05% of people exposed to these drug classes. However, they are potentially life threatening, including some or all of hypotension, bronchial, and laryngeal oedema and oropharyngeal angioedema. As the reaction is to the basic penicillin structure, people who are allergic to one penicillin will be allergic to all. This man should therefore not receive co-amoxiclav (containing amoxicillin, see **Penicillins, broad-spectrum**) or piperacillin–tazobactam (often referred to by a trade name, Tazocin, see **Penicillins, antipseudomonal**). As **cephalosporins and carbapenems** share structural similarities to penicillins, cross-reactivity can occur. The risk of this is difficult to estimate, and probably lower than the 10% figure often quoted. However, cefotaxime and ertapenem should also be avoided in those with a history of anaphylactic reaction to penicillins. They may be used with caution in people with a history of less severe penicillin allergy (e.g. rash), or after a negative penicillin skin test.

Ciprofloxacin is a **quinolone** antibiotic. There is no cross-sensitivity between quinolones and penicillins; therefore ciprofloxacin is the least likely to precipitate further anaphylaxis.

45. E. Doxycycline. Tetracyclines (e.g. doxycycline) bind to calcium in developing teeth and bone. This can cause discolouration and/or hypoplasia of tooth enamel and, theoretically, could affect the developing skeleton. They should not be prescribed for women who are pregnant or breastfeeding or to children who have not yet formed their secondary dentition (under 12 years of age). The other antibiotics listed in this question can be used in children if clinically indicated.

46. D. Metronidazole. Metronidazole is metabolised and eliminated by the liver. Dosage reduction is therefore required in severe hepatic impairment rather than renal impairment.

Many other antibiotics are eliminated by the kidney. In renal impairment, antibiotics may therefore accumulate, increasing the risk of adverse effects. However, there is always a balance to be struck between the risk of drug toxicity and the risk of undertreating the infection. As such, renal impairment does not necessarily contraindicate the drug's use, but it does mandate a more cautious approach to drug selection and dosing regimens.

In severe renal impairment, dose reductions are required with penicillins such as benzylpenicillin (see **Penicillins, narrow-spectrum**) and co-amoxiclav (see **Penicillins, broad-spectrum**) because of the risk of neurological toxicity, including fits; **aminoglycosides** such as gentamicin, which may cause ototoxicity and nephrotoxicity; and **vancomycin**, which may also cause ototoxicity and nephrotoxicity, as well as blood disorders such as neutropenia and thrombocytopenia.

47. D. Metronidazole. People taking **metronidazole** who drink alcohol may experience an unpleasant reaction, including flushing, headache, nausea, and vomiting. This reaction is thought to be due to inhibition of the enzyme acetaldehyde dehydrogenase, preventing clearance of the intermediate alcohol metabolite—acetaldehyde—from the body. Alcohol should be avoided during and for 48 hours after metronidazole treatment.

Chronic excessive alcohol consumption can reduce absorption of doxycycline (a **tetracycline**), but this is less likely and less severe than the interaction with metronidazole. The other antibiotics listed here do not interact with alcohol. Nevertheless, this might be a good opportunity to discuss 'safe' alcohol consumption.

48. E. It will not completely stop spread of infection to sexual partners. Suppressive treatment with aciclovir, an **antiviral** drug, aims to prevent recurrences of genital herpes. It should be considered in patients suffering from six or more episodes a year. It should be taken daily, rather than just when symptomatic. The treatment is usually continued for 1–2 years, after which it is stopped and the patient is monitored for recurrence. Aciclovir acts by inhibiting viral replication, but it does not clear the virus from the body completely. Consequently, there is always a risk of spreading infection to sexual partners, including 'asymptomatic shedding'. People using *topical* aciclovir should be advised about the importance of handwashing before and after administering the cream.

49. C. Full blood count. Patients taking systemic **chloramphenicol** commonly develop dose-dependent bone marrow suppression, which is fully reversible if the drug is withdrawn. Idiosyncratic aplastic anaemia is a rare adverse effect of systemic chloramphenicol, which can be fatal. During systemic therapy, blood counts should be monitored closely and a change in treatment considered if there is any change indicative of marrow suppression.

Prolonged chloramphenicol therapy can cause optic neuritis but does not affect hearing (unlike **aminoglycoside** treatment, which may be ototoxic). C-reactive protein (CRP) is a marker of severity of infection and can be used to monitor treatment efficacy, but not safety. Neither hepatotoxicity nor nephrotoxicity are recognised side effects of chloramphenicol treatment, so liver and renal function do not need to be monitored to ascertain safety. However, chloramphenicol is metabolised by the liver, so dose reduction and serum concentration measurement may be required in hepatic impairment.

50. E. Serum gentamicin concentration. Gentamicin, an **aminoglycoside**, is a potentially dangerous drug. Its dosing should be guided by measurement of the serum gentamicin concentration. There are several approaches to monitoring once-daily gentamicin therapy and you should consult local policies. Two methods are in common use. One is to measure the 'trough' concentration: that is, the lowest concentration expected during the dosage interval. This is taken 18–24 hours after the last dose, and should be <1 mg/L to minimise the risk of toxicity. The other is to measure a mid-interval concentration (6–14 hours after the last dose) and refer to a chart ('nomogram') to determine when the next dose should be given.

The other tests are less likely to be informative in the first 48 hours of therapy. Audiometry may be used in prolonged aminoglycoside therapy to monitor its effects on hearing, since aminoglycosides are ototoxic. C-reactive protein (CRP) is an inflammatory marker which can be used to monitor for resolution of infection. Impaired renal function is common in severe infections and influences gentamicin dosing regimens. It is assessed using the estimated glomerular filtration rate (eGFR) and the serum creatinine concentration, from which eGFR is derived. The eGFR may be more informative than serum creatinine concentration, but it can be misleading when the renal function is unstable.

51. C. Switch to oral co-amoxiclav. A key component of good antibiotic management (stewardship) is daily review of all antimicrobial prescriptions in secondary care. At 48 hours after starting antibiotic treatment there are five prescribing decision options:

- Stop antibiotics if there is no evidence of infection.
- Switch antibiotics from IV to oral administration.
- Change antibiotics—ideally to a narrower spectrum if microbiological samples support this (or broader if no improvement or deterioration).
- Continue and review again at 72 hours.

- Set up outpatient parenteral antimicrobial therapy where a longer course of IV treatment is required.

In IV antibiotic therapy, oral switch should be considered if the patient is improving clinically and haemodynamically stable; they have a temperature <38°C for 48 hours; they show a trend to normalisation of CRP and white cell count (WCC); they can tolerate and absorb oral medications; and they do not have immunosuppression or deep-seated infection (e.g. abscess, bacterial meningitis) requiring prolonged IV therapy. Intravenous-to-oral switch is good practice as it reduces treatment complications and duration of inpatient stay as well as drug and administration costs.

Our patient meets the criteria for IV-to-oral switch. Her urine cultures grew *E. coli* sensitive to co-amoxiclav (see **Penicillins, broad-spectrum**) and so it would be reasonable to switch to an oral preparation of this drug. She is not deteriorating, so does not need to switch to a broader-spectrum antibiotic. Although her infection is sensitive to the narrower-spectrum antibiotic **nitrofurantoin**, this is only effective for lower UTIs where it has been concentrated in the urine and so would be inappropriate for her clinical infection of pyelonephritis. For pyelonephritis, the treatment duration should usually be 10–14 days.

52. D. Increase lamotrigine dosage. Lamotrigine is metabolised by glucuronidation. Other drugs, including **oestrogens** such as ethinylestradiol, can induce more rapid lamotrigine glucuronidation. This reduces lamotrigine concentrations and may lead to a loss of seizure control. If contraception with a systemic oestrogen is considered appropriate (alternative contraception, e.g. with an intrauterine device, may be preferable), higher dosages of lamotrigine may be required. This may be supported by plasma lamotrigine concentration measurement.

53. B. Citalopram. Antidepressants are indicated for moderate and severe depression, and for mild depression that has not responded adequately to psychological interventions, as in this case. A **selective serotonin reuptake inhibitor** (SSRI), such as citalopram, is first choice in most patients. Amitriptyline (a **tricyclic antidepressant**) and mirtazapine (a **tetracyclic antidepressant**) are also effective antidepressants, but as they cause more side effects they are generally reserved for cases in which SSRIs are deemed unsuitable. Olanzapine is a **second-generation antipsychotic** which is not indicated for non-psychotic depression.

54. B. Lamotrigine. Options for treating episodes of bipolar depression include the **second-generation antipsychotics** olanzapine (with or without the **selective serotonin reuptake inhibitor (SSRI)** fluoxetine) and quetiapine, and the antiepileptic drug **lamotrigine**. Lamotrigine is unusual in that it does not increase the risk of mania, which may make it preferable in this case.

Gabapentin is an anticonvulsant that is also efficacious in neuropathic pain. It is not used in bipolar disorder. Lithium has long been used as a mood stabiliser in bipolar disorder, but its antidepressant effect is slow to develop. This makes it a less suitable choice in acute depressive episodes, but in people already on established lithium treatment it should be continued and the dosage optimised. Sertraline is an **SSRI**; evidence for its efficacy in bipolar depression is limited and it may increase the risk of mania. **Valproate** is an antiepileptic drug which is efficacious in bipolar disorder, but because of the risk of precipitating mania other options are preferable for acute depressive episodes.

55. E. Zopiclone. Zopiclone (see **Z-drugs**) is a relatively short-acting sedative that is useful for short-term treatment of insomnia. Its use in this scenario may be justifiable given the acute and disabling nature of the insomnia. It would be prudent to discuss that zopiclone should not be taken for a prolonged period, as there is potential for dependence to develop. Diazepam and midazolam are **benzodiazepines**. Diazepam has a long half-life; sleepiness can persist for many hours after taking the drug, and so it would not be appropriate given his impending job interview. The duration of action of midazolam is too short to be useful for insomnia. Propofol (see **Anaesthetics, general**) is administered IV, and only in high-dependency settings (e.g. operating theatres or critical care units).

56. A. Amitriptyline. Amitriptyline, a **tricyclic antidepressant**, is a first-line option for treating neuropathic pain, most suitable in nocturnal pain that is interfering with sleep. Gabapentin and pregabalin (see **Gabapentinoids**) are alternatives, particularly where tricyclics are contraindicated, for example because of cardiovascular disease or epilepsy. **Carbamazepine** is used in trigeminal neuralgia, but other drugs are better studied in other neuropathic pain syndromes. The **opioids** tramadol and morphine may be considered if first-line treatments are insufficient. **NSAIDs**, such as ibuprofen, are not effective in the management of neuropathic pain.

57. E. Synaptic vesicles. Levetiracetam is an antiepileptic drug effective in focal, generalised, and myoclonic seizures. Its mechanism of action is not fully understood, but at a molecular level it appears to target a membrane glycoprotein called synaptic vesicle protein 2A (SV2A). Through this, it probably interferes with synaptic vesicle function, and therefore the release of neurotransmitters during depolarisation. Mechanisms of antiepileptic activity exhibited by other drugs include voltage-sensitive sodium channel inhibition (**carbamazepine**, **lamotrigine**, phenytoin), voltage-sensitive calcium channel inhibition (**gabapentinoids**) and modulation of the γ-aminobutyric acid$_A$ (GABA$_A$) receptor (**benzodiazepines**). Some antiepileptic drugs have multiple actions (e.g. **valproate**).

58. D. Rash. Although benign rashes are a common adverse effect of treatment with the antiepileptic agent **lamotrigine**, they may rarely be the first symptom of a hypersensitivity reaction. As these hypersensitivity reactions (Stevens–Johnson syndrome, toxic epidermal necrolysis, or drug reaction with eosinophilia and systemic symptoms) are serious and potentially life threatening, urgent medical review should be sought. The period of highest risk is the first 8 weeks of treatment, and rashes are more common with high initial doses. Rashes that occur later in therapy (after 2–3 months) are less likely to represent a hypersensitivity reaction to lamotrigine.

59. B. Haloperidol. Haloperidol is a **first-generation (typical) antipsychotic**. One of the many adverse effects of this drug class is prolongation of the QT interval.

First-generation antipsychotics should therefore be avoided in this case, as should other drugs that prolong the QT interval, including **amiodarone**, **quinine**, **macrolide antibiotics,** and **selective serotonin reuptake inhibitors**. Combining QT-prolonging drugs may have an additive effect, increasing the risk.

Lorazepam (a **benzodiazepine**) would be a reasonable alternative to haloperidol for rapid tranquilisation in this case.

60. E. Tramadol. You need to be particularly careful when prescribing for people with epilepsy, for two main reasons. First, antiepileptic drugs (including **lamotrigine**, **carbamazepine,** and **valproate**) have many potential drug interactions that may result in drug toxicity (either of the antiepileptic drug or the other interacting drug) or loss of seizure control. Second, there are several drugs that can lower the seizure threshold, including **antipsychotics** and **opioids**, particularly tramadol. The other opioids may also affect seizure threshold, but this is much less significant. In the context of severe pain, their benefits are likely to outweigh their risks. Naproxen (an **NSAID**) and **paracetamol** are not known to affect seizure threshold or interact with carbamazepine.

61. B. Ischaemic heart disease. Serotonin 5-HT$_1$-receptor agonists, such as sumatriptan, are an effective treatment for migraine symptoms. However, as they act through vasoconstriction, they can cause angina and, rarely, myocardial infarction. They are therefore contraindicated in people with established cardiovascular disease.

62. C. Meropenem. Drug interactions are a common problem with many antiepileptic agents, including **valproate**, **carbamazepine**, **lamotrigine**, and phenytoin. Valproate has a particularly serious interaction with **carbapenem** antibiotics, characterised by a rapid (within days) and profound (near-complete) reduction in serum valproate concentration. This may lead to a loss of seizure control. Concurrent administration should be avoided if possible. If treatment with a carbapenem is essential, the serum valproate concentration should be monitored closely.

63. E. Weight, lipid profile, and haemoglobin A$_{1c}$ (HbA$_{1c}$). Olanzapine is a **second-generation antipsychotic** drug. Metabolic effects, such as weight gain, diabetes mellitus, and lipid changes, are among the most common adverse effects of second-generation antipsychotics. Monitoring weight, lipid profile, and HbA$_{1c}$ at baseline, 12 weeks into therapy, then annually, is therefore advised. Weight is monitored more intensively at the start of treatment (e.g. weekly for the first 6 weeks). Fluoxetine is a **selective serotonin reuptake inhibitor** which does not have specific safety monitoring requirements.

64. E. Tablets can take up to 24 hours to reach full effect. A cause for abnormal menstrual bleeding should always be sought, so that serious and/or treatable underlying conditions such as cancer or fibroids are identified. However, it is reasonable to offer symptomatic treatment in parallel. A levonorgestrel intrauterine device (IUD) is usually the preferred treatment for menorrhagia, but she was unable to tolerate IUD insertion. Additionally, fibroids could be contributing to anatomical abnormalities that may make insertion difficult, so tranexamic acid is a reasonable alternative choice. It should be explained that tranexamic acid tablets take up to 24 hours to have an effect. Generally, tranexamic acid is well tolerated. It does not reduce the effectiveness of hormonal contraception. However, there is a small increased risk of deep vein thrombosis in combination with oral hormonal contraceptives, which should be discussed if relevant. Tranexamic acid acts by *stopping* the breakdown of clots, rather than helping their break down (which is how **fibrinolytics** like alteplase work). Tablets should be taken for the 4 days or so when her periods are at their heaviest. She does not need to take it in the interval between her periods.

65. B. Aromatase inhibition. Anastrozole is a **sex hormone antagonist used in breast cancer**. It acts by inhibiting aromatase, which prevents the peripheral conversion of androstenedione to oestradione. This reduces the amount of oestradione that can be converted to oestradiol (the active form of oestrogen). Reducing oestradiol decreases the amount able to bind oestrogen-receptor positive breast cancers, reducing tumour growth. Tamoxifen, which is an alternative option, acts as a selective oestrogen receptor modulator.

5α-**reductase inhibitors**, e.g. finasteride, are used in the treatment of benign prostatic enlargement. **Antifungals** such as fluconazole inhibit ergosterol synthesis. **Oestrogens and progestogens** suppress luteinising hormone (LH)/follicle-stimulating hormone (FSH) secretion.

66. C. Antagonism at the muscarinic M_3 receptor. Oxybutynin (see **Antimuscarinics, genitourinary uses**) blocks muscarinic acetylcholine receptors, including the M_3 receptor that predominates in the bladder. This inhibits the procontractile effect of parasympathetic stimulation, causing relaxation of the bladder smooth muscle and increasing bladder capacity. This makes it a useful option for treatment for urge incontinence and overactive bladder symptoms.

α_1-**blockers** (e.g. doxazosin) and 5α-**reductase inhibitors** (e.g. finasteride) are used in benign prostatic enlargement; they have no role in the treatment of overactive bladder. β_2-**agonists** are used to induce smooth muscle relaxation in the airways. They are not used for overactive bladder; however, mirabegron (a β_3-agonist) is an option. The nicotinic acetylcholine receptor is involved in neuromuscular transmission in skeletal muscle. Antagonists of this receptor are used in anaesthetic practice to induce muscle relaxation.

67. A. Doxazosin. Sildenafil is a **phosphodiesterase (type 5) inhibitor** that causes (among other things) vascular smooth muscle relaxation and vasodilation. Doxazosin is an α-**blocker**, which also has a vasodilator effect. Concomitant use may cause hypotension and collapse. A gap of 4 hours should be left between taking sildenafil and α-blockers.

68. E. Ramipril. ACE inhibitors (e.g. ramipril) commonly cause an increase in the serum potassium concentration. This can usually be tolerated provided it does not exceed 6.0 mmol/L. Other drugs with a significant potassium-elevating effect include **angiotensin-receptor blockers**, **aldosterone-receptor antagonists**, oral and IV **potassium** supplements, and potassium-sparing diuretics. **β-blocker** and **aspirin** can also increase the potassium concentration, but this effect is not usually significant. **Statins** and **clopidogrel** do not cause hyperkalaemia.

69. C. Solifenacin. Solifenacin (see **Antimuscarinics, genitourinary uses**) is used to treat urinary urgency and urge incontinence. Side effects of antimuscarinics include dry mouth, blurred vision, constipation, and confusion. Older people, especially those with dementia, are particularly vulnerable to these side effects. The reasons for susceptibility to confusion are complex but include alteration in drug distribution and metabolism as well as increased sensitivity to their neurological effects. Where possible, alternative therapies should be used.

The other drugs listed are unlikely to have been started in this case. Finasteride is a **5α-reductase inhibitor** and tamsulosin is an **α-blocker**; they are both used in benign prostatic enlargement, but not in overactive bladder. They are not known to cause confusion. Furosemide is a **loop diuretic** used in states of fluid overload such as heart failure and does not directly cause confusion (although over-diuresis leading to dehydration might). **Trimethoprim** is an antibiotic that acts by interfering with bacterial folate synthesis. It is commonly used to treat UTIs but not overactive bladder. It causes confusion very rarely.

70. B. Postural hypotension. Tamsulosin (an **α-blocker**) blocks α_1-adrenoceptors in the smooth muscle of the prostate gland, increasing urinary flow and relieving obstructive symptoms. As α_1-adrenoceptors are also found in the smooth muscle of blood vessels, α-blockers can cause hypotension, particularly postural hypotension. People taking other antihypertensive medications should be especially vigilant to these effects and may need to omit their usual treatment when starting an α-blocker. Bronchospasm and erectile dysfunction are adverse effects of **β-blockers** (not α-blockers). Tamsulosin does not cause gynaecomastia or prostate cancer.

71. B. Diltiazem. Sildenafil is a **phosphodiesterase (type 5) inhibitor**. It is metabolised by a member of the cytochrome P450 (CYP) enzyme family called CYP3A4. Diltiazem is a **calcium channel blocker** that inhibits CYP3A4 activity. If the drugs are taken together, the metabolism of sildenafil will be reduced and its concentration will rise. This increases the chance of dose-related adverse effects, such as headache. A reduced dose of sildenafil is recommended in people taking CYP inhibitors, other examples of which include **amiodarone** and **macrolide antibiotics**.

Diltiazem can also interact with digoxin, since they both reduce conduction at the AV node. This interaction may be exploited therapeutically, as in this case, to slow the ventricular rate in AF. There are no other clinically significant interactions between the drugs listed.

72. C. Indapamide. Gout is caused by deposition of uric acid in joints. The first metatarsophalangeal joint (of the big toe) is most commonly affected. The likely precipitant in this instance is indapamide, a **thiazide-like diuretic**, which reduces uric acid excretion by the kidneys. Other drug causes of gout include *low-dose*

aspirin, some anticancer drugs (by increasing uric acid production with tumour breakdown) and alcohol.

Allopurinol prevents gout by reducing uric acid production through xanthine oxidase inhibition. It should not be started or stopped in acute gout, where sudden fluctuations in uric acid levels can worsen attacks. **Calcium channel blockers** (e.g. amlodipine), **ACE inhibitors** (e.g. ramipril) and **statins** (e.g. simvastatin) do not cause or worsen gout.

73. D. β_2-adrenoceptors. β_2-adrenoceptors are activated by salmeterol, a long-acting β_2-**agonist** bronchodilator.

Doxazocin is an α-**blocker**, which antagonises α_1-adrenoceptors. Ipratropium and hyoscine butylbromide block muscarinic receptors (see **Antimuscarinics, bronchodilators** and **Antimuscarinics, cardiovascular, and GI uses**, respectively). Amlodipine is a **calcium channel blocker**. Fluticasone is an **inhaled corticosteroid** which activates glucocorticoid receptors to influence gene transcription.

74. E. Tiotropium. Tiotropium (see **Antimuscarinics, bronchodilators**) inhibits parasympathetic stimulation of salivation, causing a dry mouth. None of the other drugs listed cause a dry mouth, although inhaled fluticasone (an **inhaled corticosteroid**) can cause oral thrush, the risk of which is reduced by rinsing and gargling after inhalation.

75. E. Tiotropium. Tiotropium (see **Antimuscarinics, bronchodilators**) is a long-acting antimuscarinic (LAMA) administered by inhalation. Its side effects include urinary retention in people susceptible to this. It should therefore be avoided or used cautiously in people with a history of urinary retention or risk factors such as benign prostatic enlargement.

Salbutamol and salmeterol are, respectively, short- and long-acting β_2-**agonists**. Seretide and Symbicort are compound β_2-agonist–corticosteroid inhalers (see **Corticosteroids, inhaled**).

76. C. Naproxen. The most appropriate treatment for acute gout is an antiinflammatory. **NSAIDs**, e.g. naproxen, are the usual first-line choice in the absence of contraindications. In this case, however, they are strongly contraindicated by the history of aspirin-induced bronchospasm. Colchicine is an alternative option. It should be avoided in renal and hepatic impairment, and it has some important drug interactions (e.g. with the antibiotic fusidic acid). Where NSAIDs and colchicine are contraindicated or not tolerated, a short course of a **systemic corticosteroid** (e.g. oral prednisolone) is a useful option. Codeine, a weak **opioid**, may provide some pain relief, but it does not have any anti-inflammatory action.

77. A. Acetylcysteine. Acetylcysteine is a specific antidote for **paracetamol** poisoning. It is highly effective if started within 8–10 hours of the overdose. The decision about whether to administer acetylcysteine is guided by the nature of the overdose and the serum paracetamol concentration. If it was a single overdose taken at a known time, you should measure the paracetamol concentration 4 or more hours after the time of ingestion, then compare this with a paracetamol poisoning treatment graph (see the BNF for the graph recommended for UK practice). If the concentration is above the treatment line, acetylcysteine is indicated. If the overdose was staggered (i.e. the time between the first and last doses was more than 1 hour) or its timing is uncertain, you cannot interpret the paracetamol concentration. Your decision is then based on the amount of paracetamol ingested. If this exceeds 75 mg/kg, treatment with acetylcysteine is likely to be indicated.

Activated charcoal is used to reduce absorption of toxins, but in general, it is only effective if given within 1 hour of the overdose. Cyclizine is an antiemetic (see **Antiemetics, histamine H$_1$-receptor antagonists**). It may be an appropriate symptomatic treatment for nausea, but it is not as important as acetylcysteine at this stage. Omeprazole is a **proton pump inhibitor**, which is not indicated in this case. **Naloxone** is a specific antidote for **opioid** toxicity; it is not indicated.

78. D. Naloxone. The low Glasgow Coma Scale (GCS) score, pinpoint pupils and respiratory rate point toward **opioid** toxicity. **Naloxone** is useful here both diagnostically (it provides an indication of the extent to which his drowsiness is due to opioid toxicity) and therapeutically (it reverses the opioid effect—albeit only temporarily). The other most obvious culprit drug for causing low GCS is diazepam, a **benzodiazepine**. However, the antidote for benzodiazepines, flumazenil, should only be given in circumstances where it is certain that pure benzodiazepine toxicity has occurred, such as iatrogenic overdose. This is because flumazenil has significant adverse effects, including lowering the seizure threshold. If the benzodiazepine was taken as part of a mixed overdose with pro-convulsive drugs, this may precipitate seizures. Activated charcoal is useful for acute oral overdoses, but not for toxicity caused by reduced drug elimination. There is no history of **paracetamol** overdose and it is not eliminated by the kidneys, so there is no immediate indication for **acetylcysteine**. Sodium bicarbonate is used in the treatment of **tricyclic antidepressant** toxicity (e.g. amitriptyline). His antidepressant, fluoxetine, is a **selective serotonin reuptake inhibitor**.

79. C. Folinic acid. Methotrexate inhibits the enzyme dihydrofolate reductase, which converts dietary folic acid to tetrahydrofolate (FH4). FH4 is required for DNA and protein synthesis. Folinic acid is readily converted to FH4 (without the need for dihydrofolate reductase) and is therefore useful in methotrexate toxicity. Folic acid (see **Vitamins**) cannot be used, as in the absence of dihydrofolate reductase activity it cannot be converted to FH4 and is therefore not metabolically useful.

Activated charcoal is only useful where poisons have been recently ingested (e.g. within 1 hour). Toxicity in this case has occurred over weeks. Haemodialysis is not useful in removing methotrexate from the circulation, although may be necessary when managing the associated renal failure. Granulocyte colony-stimulating factor (G-CSF) has been used in the treatment of neutropenia as a result of methotrexate toxicity, but is not routinely part of initial management.

Methotrexate toxicity may be very serious and its management is complex. Advice should be sought from a poisons centre.

80. D. Temporarily stop acetylcysteine and give chlorphenamine. When administered intravenously at high doses (such as in **paracetamol** poisoning), **acetylcysteine** can cause an anaphylactoid reaction. Like anaphylaxis, anaphylactoid reactions are mediated by histamine and involve symptoms such as urticaria, angioedema, and bronchospasm. However, in contrast to anaphylaxis, they do not involve IgE antibodies. This means that the reactions tend to build up more gradually, such that they can usually be identified and treated before they become too severe.

At this stage, the management would be to stop the acetylcysteine and administer an IV **antihistamine** (H$_1$-receptor antagonist), such as chlorphenamine. Once the reaction has subsided, it is usually safe to restart the infusion at a lower rate. **Adrenaline**, administered by IM injection, is the key treatment for anaphylaxis, but it is not required for anaphylactoid reactions unless they are very severe or the diagnosis is in doubt. Ranitidine is an **H$_2$-receptor antagonist** used to suppress gastric acid production. It has little, if any, role in the treatment of anaphylactic and anaphylactoid reactions.

Prescribing questions

81.

Drug	GLYCERYL TRINITRATE
Dose	400–800 micrograms
Route	SL
Frequency	For chest pain, repeated at 5-minute intervals if required, to max three doses

Angina occurs when, as a result of narrowed atheromatous coronary arteries, insufficient blood is supplied to the myocardium to meet its oxygen demand. Short-acting **nitrates**, such as glyceryl trinitrate, are taken during an attack of angina to relieve chest pain. Glyceryl trinitrate (GTN) is prescribed sublingually as tablets or spray for immediate relief of chest pain; a spray is usually the most convenient formulation, because tablets have a short shelf-life (they must be discarded 8 weeks after opening the bottle). The BNF recommends a dosage of 400–800 micrograms under the tongue (SL), repeated up to three times at 5-minute intervals. Note that when prescribing this dose, 'micrograms' must be written in full.

82.

Drug	METFORMIN
Dose	500 mg

Route	Oral
Frequency	Once daily for 1 week, then twice daily. Doses to be taken with meals.

Metformin is the first-line choice for type 2 diabetes because it lowers blood glucose without causing weight gain or hypoglycaemia; it is associated with decreased risk of cardiovascular mortality; and it is cheap. To maximise tolerability, it is best to start metformin at a low dose and increase it gradually over several weeks. The model prescription illustrates the first two dosage increments; this may later be increased to a usual maximum of 1 g twice daily. Taking doses with meals (breakfast and evening meals in twice daily dosing) also contributes to maximising tolerability.

    Sodium–glucose co-transporter 2 inhibitors (e.g. empagliflozin), **dipeptidylpeptidase-4 (DPP-4) inhibitors** (e.g. sitagliptin) and **sulphonylureas** (e.g. gliclazide) are alternatives if metformin is not tolerated and may be added to metformin if monotherapy is insufficient. **Insulin** is reserved for situations in which combination therapy with oral agents is insufficient.

83.

Drug	LACTULOSE
Dose	30 mL
Route	Oral
Frequency	8-hrly

One of the main substances involved in the pathogenesis of hepatic encephalopathy is ammonia. Lactulose is an osmotic **laxative** that reduces absorption of ammonia by increasing the transit rate of colonic contents and by acidifying the stool, which inhibits the proliferation of ammonia-producing bacteria. This makes it an important treatment for people with, or at risk of, hepatic encephalopathy, regardless of whether they are constipated. For this indication, lactulose is typically started at a dose of 30 mL orally 8-hrly, titrated to achieve soft stools and two to three bowel movements per day.

84.

Drug	DALTEPARIN
Dose	5000 units
Route	SC
Frequency	Daily

People admitted to hospital should be assessed for the risk of developing venous thromboembolism (VTE). Pharmacological prophylaxis should be offered if thrombotic risk is high, and bleeding risk is low. Thrombotic risk factors in this case include her age, history of deep venous thrombosis (DVT) and likely immobility during her acute illness. The usual choice is a **low molecular weight heparin** (LMWH) prescribed at a 'prophylactic dose', such as dalteparin 5000 units SC daily or enoxaparin 40 mg SC daily. In practice, the correct choice will be dictated by local protocols.

85.

Drug	ACICLOVIR
Dose	750 mg
Route	IV infusion
Frequency	8-hrly
Duration	Review with results of cerebrospinal fluid analysis
Indication	Suspected herpes simplex encephalitis

Aciclovir is an **antiviral** which acts by inhibiting herpes-specific DNA polymerase. It is the antiviral of choice in suspected cases of herpes simplex encephalitis. Note the dose and route of administration vary widely by indication: for encephalitis (a severe infection), 10 mg/kg (750 mg for this patient) IV 8-hrly is recommended for at least 14 days. This should be started urgently. The diluted solution will be administered by infusion over 1 hour. In practice, it is not usually necessary to specify the infusion instructions in the prescription, as these will be detailed in a local IV drugs prescribing policy. It is, however, essential always to specify the indication and duration or review date in any inpatient prescription for an antimicrobial drug. In this case, the logical time-point for review is when results from cerebrospinal fluid analysis are available.

86.

Fluid (including any additives)	Volume	Rate/duration
Sodium chloride 0.9%	500 mL	10 min

This patient is sick and requires urgent review by a senior clinician. While arranging this, it would be appropriate to start fluid resuscitation. IV fluid solutions containing sodium at a concentration similar to that found in extracellular fluid (ECF), such as sodium chloride 0.9% and compound sodium lactate, are retained in the extracellular compartment. This means that, after distribution, a materially useful proportion (about 20%) of the fluid remains in the circulation, making these solutions a viable option for fluid resuscitation. In adults, it is recommended that 500 mL is infused rapidly (e.g. over 10 minutes). The effects of this on haemodynamics and markers of organ perfusion should then be assessed.

Fluids containing a supra-physiological concentration of **potassium** (e.g. sodium chloride 0.9% with potassium chloride 0.15% (20 mmol/L)) are never used for fluid resuscitation due to the risk of inducing hyperkalaemia. However, compound sodium lactate, which contains a physiological concentration of potassium (5 mmol/L), may be used. **Glucose** solutions should not be used for fluid resuscitation because (in the absence of sodium) they distribute throughout total body water, leaving only about 7% in the circulation. **Colloids** are designed to be preferentially retained in the plasma, but there is little evidence that they improve clinical outcomes. Moreover, they are considerably more expensive; not reliably stocked on general wards; and their constituents (e.g. gelatin) may have adverse effects.

87.

Fluid (including any additives)	Volume	Rate/duration
Sodium chloride 0.9%	500 mL	8 hours

For stable adults, the normal daily fluid and electrolyte requirements (often referred to as 'maintenance requirements') are, roughly:
- Water 25–30 mL/kg/day
- Sodium 1 mmol/kg/day
- Potassium 1 mmol/kg/day

These requirements can be met using a combination of **glucose** 5% (which effectively just provides water), **sodium chloride** 0.9% (which provides water and sodium) and **potassium** chloride (which is included as an 'additive' in the other fluids). As he has already received 2000 mL glucose 5% with potassium chloride 0.3% (K^+ 40 mmol/L), his potassium requirement has been met, along with part of his water requirement. However, he still needs approximately 80 mmol Na^+. A reasonable way to achieve this is to prescribe 500 mL sodium chloride 0.9% (Na^+ 154 mmol/L), providing Na^+ 77 mmol and increasing his total water provision to 2500 mL. **Compound sodium lactate** would be a reasonable alternative.

88.

Fluid (including any additives)	Volume	Rate/duration
Sodium chloride 0.9% with potassium chloride 0.3% (40 mmol/L)	1000 mL	4 hours

Hypokalaemia is a potentially dangerous electrolyte abnormality because of its association with arrhythmias. A serum potassium concentration <2.5 mmol/L is generally deemed to be 'severe', and this warrants IV treatment. On a general ward, this is administered through a peripheral cannula using a **potassium**-containing fluid, as illustrated in the example prescription. When treating hypokalaemia, potassium should be administered as part of a combined solution with **sodium chloride**. Solutions containing **glucose** should be avoided, because this may stimulate insulin production, which in turn stimulates cellular uptake of potassium. When infused peripherally, the maximum concentration of potassium chloride is 0.3% (40 mmol/L). It should be infused no faster than 10 mmol/hr, as higher rates can precipitate arrhythmias.

89.

Drug	LORAZEPAM
Dose	4 mg
Route	Slow IV injection
Frequency	Once only (repeated once at 10 min if seizure persists)

Broadly, status epilepticus may be defined as a state of unrelenting seizure activity. It is a life-threatening condition that requires urgent treatment. First-line pharmacological treatment is with a **benzodiazepine**, which in a hospital setting should be administered intravenously. The ideal choice is lorazepam because of its long duration of effect. In adults, this is usually given in an initial dose of 4 mg IV, injected slowly over about 2 minutes. This may be repeated once if the seizure does not terminate. Diazepam is a reasonable alternative if lorazepam is unavailable. If the seizure cannot be controlled with a benzodiazepine, an antiepileptic drug should be given. Options include **levetiracetam**, **valproate**, and phenytoin. If this is unsuccessful, the patient should be anaesthetised and managed in the intensive care unit.

90.

Drug	BECLOMETASONE metered dose inhaler with spacer
Dose	100 micrograms
Route	Inhaled
Frequency	12-hrly

Inhaled corticosteroids suppress inflammation in the airways, reducing the risk of asthma attacks. Topical administration by inhaler reduces systemic side effects. For children with asthma that is not controlled with a short-acting bronchodilator, guidelines recommend offering an inhaled corticosteroid as first-line maintenance therapy. Many products are available, and individual guidelines vary in their precise recommendations on drug choice and dosage; the model answer illustrates one option. Equivalent doses of budesonide or fluticasone would also be reasonable. You should state the device type in the prescription, or specify the brand. Brand-name prescribing is essential for combination inhalers (though combination treatment is not indicated at this stage).

Calculation questions

Note that there is often more than one way to solve a calculation. We present our method as an example only. You may have reached the correct answer by an alternative, equally acceptable method.

91. 12 mL/hr. The maximum infusion rate is 200 micrograms/minute, but we require a value in mL/hr. This requires us to convert the microgram dosage into mg, by dividing by 1000.

200 micrograms/min = 0.2 mg/min

The infusion solution has a glyceryl trinitrate concentration of 50 mg/50 mL, or 1 mg/mL, so the dosage in mass can simply be substituted for the volume in mL:

0.2 mg/min = 0.2 mL/min

Next we need to convert the unit of time from minutes to hours, by multiplying by 60:

0.2 mL/min × 60 min/hr = 12 mL/hr

For further discussion of glyceryl trinitrate, see **Nitrates**.

92. 20 mL. The maximum dose is 3 mg/kg or 200 mg, whichever is lower:

3 mg/kg × 75 kg = 225 mg

So, the maximum dose is 200 mg, because that is lower than the calculated dose. We now need to work out what volume of 1% solution contains 200 mg of lidocaine. This will be easier if we first convert the percentage concentration to a value in mg/mL. Recall that a percentage concentration (a form of ratio concentration) refers to the parts of solute (lidocaine) in 100 parts of solvent (water). As the solvent is water, its mass in grams can be substituted for its volume in mL, so:

1% = 1 g of lidocaine in 100 g water

   = 1000 mg in 100 mL   (because 1 g = 1000 mg, and for water, 1 g = 1 mL)

1000 mg ÷ 100 mL = 10 mg/L

To work out what volume of solution contains a certain mass of drug, we divide the mass of drug by the concentration of the solution:

Volume of solution required

   = mass of drug required ÷ concentration of drug in solution

   = 200 mg ÷ 10 mg/mL

   = 20 mL

For further discussion of lidocaine, see **Anaesthetics, local**.

93. 59.5 g. Two preliminary steps are required. One is to calculate the amount of glucose contained in 1 mL of the intravenous fluid preparation. For this calculation, the sodium chloride and potassium chloride content can be disregarded. The important information is that it contains glucose at a concentration of 5%. Recall that a percentage concentration (a form of ratio concentration) refers to the parts of solute (glucose) in 100 parts of solvent (water). As the solvent is water, its mass in grams can be substituted for its volume in mL, so:

Glucose 5% = glucose 5 g in water 100 mL   (because for water, 1 g = 1 mL)

   5 g glucose ÷ 100 mL water = 0.05 g/mL

The other preliminary step is to calculate the volume of the intravenous fluid that has been infused:

85 mL/hr × 14 hr = 1190 mL

Now we have the information we need to calculate the amount of glucose infused, by multiplying glucose concentration by the volume that has been given:

0.05 g/mL × 1190 mL = 59.5 g

94. 2880 mL/hr. The volume of the required fluid bolus is 20 mL/kg:

20 mL/kg × 24 kg = 480 mL

Next we need to calculate the rate of infusion:

480 mL ÷ 10 min = 48 mL/min

But we have been asked for the rate in mL/hr, so need to multiply this by 60:

48 mL/min × 60 min/hr = 2880 mL/hr

Note that most infusion pumps cannot accommodate infusion rates this high, so in practice, this would need to be administered manually (e.g. with a pressure bag, or syringe and three-way tap).

   For further discussion of the use of IV fluid in states of impaired tissue perfusion, see **Sodium chloride**.

95. Two spoonfuls. Two preliminary steps are required. One is to calculate amount of ferrous fumarate (see **Iron**) contained in 1 mL of the oral solution:

140 mg ÷ 5 mL = 28 mg/mL

The other is to calculate the amount of *elemental iron* per 1 mg of ferrous fumarate:

65 mg of iron ÷ 200 mg of ferrous fumarate

   = 0.325 mg of iron per mg of ferrous fumarate

Now we can calculate the amount of elemental iron per 1 mL of oral solution:

28 mg/mL × 0.325 mg/mg

   = 9.1 mg/mL

She requires 200 mg/day of elemental iron in two divided doses, so each dose will be 100 mg. To provide 100 mg iron, she will need:

100 mg[iron] ÷ 9.1 mg[iron]/mL = 10.98 mL, or approximately two spoonfuls

96. 400 mg. Adjusted body weight is calculated using the formula provided. Note the order of operations: first any calculations in brackets, then multiplication, then addition.

Adjusted body weight

= **[ideal body weight] + 0.4 × ([actual body weight] − [ideal body weight])**

= **68 kg + 0.4 × (94 kg − 68 kg)**

= **68 kg + 10.4 kg**

= **78.4 kg**

The dose required is 5 mg/kg, calculated from adjusted body weight. For practicality, we have been asked to round this to the nearest 40 mg.

5 mg/kg × 78.4 kg = 392 mg ≈ 400 mg

For further discussion about gentamicin, see **Aminoglycosides**.

97. Two bottles. You can approach this calculation either by working out the total mass of amoxicillin required for the course first, then converting it to the equivalent volume of suspension, or by calculating the volume of suspension required per dose first, then working out the total volume required for the course. Taking the former approach, the total mass of amoxicillin required is:

250 mg/dose × 3 doses/day × 5 days = 3750 mg

To convert this to an equivalent volume of amoxicillin suspension, we need to know its concentration:

125 mg ÷ 5 mL = 25 mg/mL

Now we can calculate the volume of suspension required, by dividing the mass required by the concentration of the solution:

3750 mg ÷ 25 mg/mL = 150 mL

And the number of 100-mL bottles:

150 mL ÷ 100 mL/bottle = 1.5 bottles

As this needs to be rounded up to a whole number of bottles, two bottles will be required for this course of treatment.

For further discussion about amoxicillin, see **Penicillins, broad-spectrum**.

98. 4.8 mL. The required dose is 400 micrograms per kg, or 5 mg, whichever is lower:

400 micrograms/kg × 12 kg = 4800 micrograms = 4.8 mg

So the dose will be 4.8 mg, because that is the lower number. Now work out what volume of adrenaline 1:1000 solution this equates to. This will be easier if we first convert the ratio concentration to a value in mg/mL. Recall that a 1:1000 ratio concentration means that there is 1 part solute (adrenaline) in 1000 parts solvent (water). As the solvent is water, its mass in grams can be substituted for its volume in mL, so:

1 : 1000 = 1 g of adrenaline in 1000 mL (because for water, 1 g 5 1 mL)

    = **1000 mg of adrenaline in 1000 mL** (converting mass of drug from g to mg)

    = **1 mg of adrenaline in 1 mL** (dividing mass and volume by 1000)

As this is a 1 mg/mL solution, the volume required to provide 4.8 mg is 4.8 mL.

The administration of adrenaline by nebuliser for croup is not licensed, but well established in practice. See **Adrenaline (epinephrine)** for further discussion.

99. Eight tablets. The total daily dose is calculated from body weight:

120 mg/kg/day × 62 kg = 7560 mg/day

Next, we divide this by the number of doses to be given per day:

7560 mg/day ÷ 2 doses/day = 3780 mg/dose

Now we divide this by the strength of the tablets:

3780 mg/dose ÷ 480 mg/tablet = 7.875 tablets/dose

As only whole or half tablets can be given, this rounds to eight tablets per dose.
See **Trimethoprim** for further discussion about co-trimoxazole.

100. 870 mmol. The amount of chloride contained in 1 L of sodium chloride 0.9% with potassium chloride 0.15% is calculated by summing the mmol/L content from each source:

154 mmol/L (from sodium chloride) + 20 mmol/L (from potassium chloride) = 174 mmol/L

Now we can calculate the amount of chloride in 5000 mL (5 L) of this solution:

5 L × 174 mmol/L = 870 mmol

See Sodium chloride and Potassium chloride for further discussion about their use in intravenous fluid therapy.

Index

Page numbers followed by "*b*" indicate boxes.